D1203318

Cases on Health Outcomes and Clinical Data Mining:
Studies and Frameworks

Patricia Cerrito
University of Louisville, USA

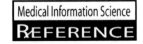

MEDICAL INFORMATION SCIENCE REFERENCE

Hershey · New York

Director of Editorial Content:	Kristin Klinger
Director of Book Publications:	Julia Mosemann
Acquisitions Editor:	Lindsay Johnston
Development Editor:	Christine Bufton
Publishing Assistant:	Sean Woznicki
Typesetter:	Deanna Zombro
Production Editor:	Jamie Snavely
Cover Design:	Lisa Tosheff
Printed at:	Yurchak Printing Inc.

Published in the United States of America by
Medical Information Science Reference (an imprint of IGI Global)
701 E. Chocolate Avenue
Hershey PA 17033
Tel: 717-533-8845
Fax: 717-533-8661
E-mail: cust@igi-global.com
Web site: http://www.igi-global.com/reference

Copyright © 2010 by IGI Global. All rights reserved. No part of this publication may be reproduced, stored or distributed in any form or by any means, electronic or mechanical, including photocopying, without written permission from the publisher.

Product or company names used in this set are for identification purposes only. Inclusion of the names of the products or companies does not indicate a claim of ownership by IGI Global of the trademark or registered trademark.

Library of Congress Cataloging-in-Publication Data

Cases on health outcomes and clinical data mining : studies and frameworks /
Patricia Cerrito, editor.
     p. ; cm.
  Includes bibliographical references and index.
  Summary: "Because so much data is now becoming readily available to
investigate health outcomes, it is important to examine just how statistical
models are used to do this. This book studies health outcomes research using
data mining techniques"--Provided by publisher.
  ISBN 978-1-61520-723-7 (h/c)
  1. Outcome assessment (Medical care) 2. Data mining. I. Cerrito, Patricia
B.
  [DNLM: 1. Outcome Assessment (Health Care) 2. Data Mining--methods. 3.
Models, Statistical. W 84.41 C338 2010]
  R853.O87C37 2010
  362.1--dc22
                        2009053483

British Cataloguing in Publication Data
A Cataloguing in Publication record for this book is available from the British Library.

All work contributed to this book is new, previously-unpublished material. The views expressed in this book are those of the authors, but not necessarily of the publisher.

Table of Contents

Section 2
Case Studies in Healthcare Delivery

Section 3
Modeling EEG Images for Analysis

Detailed Table of Contents

In this case, we provide some basic information concerning the statistical methods used throughout this text. These methods include visualization by kernel density estimation, regression and predictive models, time series, and text analysis. This case is not intended to provide extensive information concerning these techniques; references are provided for the interested reader who wants to follow up on the methodology. Some of the methodology is fairly well known while the predictive modeling and text analysis are relatively recent. One of the primary visualization techniques used is that of kernel density estimation. Since the patient base is relatively heterogeneous, we cannot assume that any health outcome is normally distributed. Kernel density estimation can find the entire population distribution so that we no longer have to rely upon averages and can relate the results more to individuals.

Section 1
Case Studies in Health Outcomes Research

The purpose of this study is to use data mining methods to investigate the physician decisions specifically in the treatment of osteomyelitis. Two primary data sets have been used in this study; the National Inpatient Sample (NIS) and the Thomson MedStat MarketScan data. We used online sources to obtain background information about the disease and its treatment in the literature. An innovative method was used to capture the information from the web and to cluster or filter that information to find the most relevant information, using SAS Text Miner. Other important innovations in investigating the data include finding the switches of medication and comparing the date of the switch with the date of procedures. We could study these medications switched at deeper levels, but this is not necessary in our study, especially with limited access to data. We also create a model to forecast the cost of hospitalization for patients with osteomyelitis.

In this case, the main objective is to examine information about patients with coronary artery disease who had invasive procedures (such as balloon angioplasty or stents), or coronary artery bypass surgery. We investigate the use of the drug- eluting stent as a treatment for coronary artery disease. The first section of this chapter is a brief background about coronary artery disease and different procedures that may be used as its treatment. Next, time series analysis as a statistical tool is discussed, and in the third section, the results of the time series analyses that are performed on the database are demonstrated. In this section, the effect of the drug-eluting stent as a new treatment on the demand of other procedures is discussed. The fourth section is about computing the risk of each procedure based on the claims database used. The last section includes the result, conclusion, and suggestions.

Chapter 4

Asthma is a common chronic disease in the United States, with increasing prevalence. Many patients do not realize therapeutic goals because of poor disease management. The purpose of this study is to examine the costs of the commonly used drugs used to treat asthma. We examined the contribution of individual, government and private agencies for medication payment. We next compared the prescription cost to the cost of emergency room visits. The data are taken from the Medical Expenditure Panel Survey. SAS Enterprise Guide was used for preprocessing and data visualization. It was found that prednisone is the cheapest drug and the drug, albuterol, is the most common, even if it is more expensive. The contribution of the government is higher than the amount paid by individuals and other agencies. We examined data from the National Inpatient Sample to investigate trends in asthma as well.

Chapter 5

In this case, we analyze breast cancer cases from the Thomson Medstat Market Scan® data using SAS and Enterprise Guide 4. First, we find breast cancer cases using ICD9 codes. We are interested in the age distribution, in the total charges of the entire treatment sequence and in the length of stay at the hospital during treatment. Then, we study two major surgery treatments: Mastectomy and Lumpectomy. For each one of them, we analyze the total charges and the length of stay. Then, we compare these two treatments in terms of total charges, length of stay and the association of the choice of treatment with age. Finally, we analyze other treatment options. The objective is to understand the methods used to obtain some useful information about breast cancer and also to explore how to use SAS and SAS Enterprise Guide 4 to examine specific healthcare problems.

Chapter 6

Guoxin Tang, University of Louisville, USA

Lung cancer is the leading cause of cancer death in the United States and the world, with more than 1.3 million deaths worldwide per year. However, because of a lack of effective tools to diagnose lung cancer, more than half of all cases are diagnosed at an advanced stage, when surgical resection is unlikely to be feasible. The purpose of this study is to examine the relationship between patient outcomes and conditions of the patients undergoing different treatments for lung cancer and to develop models to estimate the population burden, the cost of cancer, and to help physicians and patients determine appropriate treatment in clinical decision-making. We use a national database, and also claim data to investigate treatments for lung cancer.

Chapter 7

Jennifer Ferrell Pleiman, University of Louisville, USA

This research will use data fusion methodology to develop a process for sequential episode grouping data in medicine. By using data fusion, data from different sources will be combined to review the use of physical therapy in orthopedic surgical procedures. The data that were used to develop sequential episode grouping consisted of insurance claims data from the Thomson Medstat MarketScan database. The data will be reviewed as a continuous time lapse for surgery date; that is, the utilization of physical therapy for a defined time period both before and after surgery will be used and studied. The methodology of this research will follow a series of preprocessing cleaning and sequential episode grouping, culminating in text mining and clustering the results to review. Through this research, it was found that the use of physical therapy for orthopedic issues is not common and was utilized in under 1% of the data sampled.

Chapter 8

Xiao Wang, University of Louisville, USA

The purpose of this study is to examine the relationship between the diagnosis and the cost of patient care for those with diabetes in Medicare. In this analysis, the author used data sets about outpatient claim, inpatient claim as well as beneficiary demography information for the year 2004, all of which were taken from the Chronic Condition Data Warehouse provided by the Centers for Medicare and Medicaid. The author analyzed the cases for diabetic inpatients and outpatients by different methods. For outpatient analysis, exploratory data analysis and linear models were used .The results show that the total charges for diagnoses are reduced considerably for payment. The distribution of the total charges follows a

Gamma distribution. The output of the generalized linear model demonstrates that only 15 out of the top 20 primary treatments for charges are statistically significant to the expenditures on outpatients.

This case examines the issue of compliance by patients at the University of Louisville School of Dentistry (ULSD). The focus is defining compliance and constructing a measurement scale. Confidence interval estimation and bootstrapping were explored to assist with the allocation of patients to compliance levels. Patients who were within the 95% confidence interval of the median for visit intervals at least 80% of the time were defined as fully compliant, with decreasing levels of compliance as the percentage decreases. Research on compliance has developed over the past few years, but a lot of work still needs to be done. A new measure of compliance could assist in understanding the patients' needs and concerns other than the obvious financial, fear and psychological reasons as well as shedding some light on the way dentists operate and how that affects compliance. A new way of defining and measuring compliance is proposed in this research study.

This case study describes the use of SAS technology in streamlining cross-sectional and retrospective case-control studies in the exploration of the co-morbidity of depression and gastrointestinal disorders. Various studies in Europe and America have documented associations between irritable bowel syndrome and psychological conditions such as depression and anxiety disorders; however, these were observational studies. Because it is impossible to randomize symptoms, it is difficult to isolate patients with these co-morbidities for randomized trials. Therefore, studies will continue to use observational data. In this study, all steps are conducted electronically in a rapid development environment provided by SAS technology. In addition, it examines the potential rate of health-care utilization particularly for GI disorders among individuals with depressive symptoms and anxiety disorders. We find that the proportion of patients with gastrointestinal problems and psychological disorders is typically higher than the proportion of patients with only gastrointestinal problems.

Hydrocephalus is a disorder where cerebrospinal fluid (CSF) is unable to drain efficiently from the brain. This paper presents a set of exploratory analyses comparing attributes of inpatients under one-year old diagnosed with hydrocephalus provided by the Agency for Healthcare Research and Quality (AHRQ) as part of the National Inpatient Sample (NIS). The general methods include calculation of summary statistics, kernel density estimation, logistic regression, linear regression, and the production of figures and charts using the statistical data modeling software, SAS. It was determined that younger infants show higher mortality rates; additionally, males are more likely to present hydrocephalus and cost slightly more on average than females despite the distribution curves for length of stay appearing virtually identical between genders. Diagnoses and procedures expected for non-hydrocephalic infants showed a negative correlation in the logistic model. The study overall validates much of the literature and expands it with a cost analysis approach.

Section 2
Case Studies in Healthcare Delivery

Chapter 12

Patricia B. Cerrito, University of Louisville, USA
Aparna Sreepada, University of Louisville, USA

The study presents the analysis of the results of a health survey that focuses on the health risk behaviors and attitudes in adolescents that result in teenage obesity. Predictive models are built and charts are plotted to map variations in childhood physical health with respect to their weight behavior and to compare the impact of each weight control plan. The analysis provides many useful observations and suggestions that can be helpful in developing child health policies. We also investigate another aspect of child health by examining the severity of immediate risk from disease versus the immediate risk from childhood vaccination by comparing mortality rates from the disease to the mortality rates from the vaccination. Results show that for some individuals, the risk from the vaccine can be higher than the risk from the disease. Therefore, individual risk should be taken into consideration rather than uniform risk across the population.

Chapter 13

Joseph Twagilimana, University of Louisville, USA

The outcome of interest in this study is the length of stay (LOS) at a Hospital Emergency Department (ED). The Length of stay depends on several independent clinical factors such as treatments, patient demographic characteristics, hospital, as well as physicians and nurses. The present study attempts to identify these variables by analyzing clinical data provided by electronic medical records (EMR) from an emergency department. Three analysis methodologies were identified as appropriate for this task. First, data mining techniques were applied, and then generalized linear models and Time series followed. In spite of the fact that Data Mining and Statistics share the same objective, which is to extract useful information from data, they perform independently of each other. In this case, we show how the two methodologies can be integrated with potential benefits. We applied decision trees to select important variables and used these variables as input in the other models.

Chapter 14

David Nfodjo, University of Louisville, USA

The primary role of the Emergency Department (ED) is to treat the seriously injured and seriously sick patients. However, because of federal regulations requiring the ED to treat all who enter, EDs have become the providers of a large number of unscheduled, non-urgent care patients. The role of the ED has changed considerably in recent years to treat those without insurance, and without primary care physicians. The main purpose of this study is to investigate the use of the hospital ED for non-urgent care in relationship to socio-economic status and payer type. This study will identify the Socio-economic factors related to the utilization of the emergency department for health care. The study will identify for the purpose of shifting patients that use the Ed as primary care to a nearby clinic. The clinic is within a mile of the ED. It is a Nurse-managed health center that provides free care.

The purpose of this project is to develop time series models to investigate prescribing practices and patient usage of medications with respect to the severity of the patient condition. The cost of medications is rising from year to year; some medications are prescribed more often compared to others even if they have similar properties. It would be of interest to pharmaceutical companies to know the reason for this. In this case, we predict the cost of medications, private insurance payments, Medicaid payments, Medicare payments, the quantity of medications, total payment and to study why the cost is rising in one medication compared to others. We investigate how much patients are spending on average for their prescriptions of medications, taking the inflation rate into account as a time-dependent regressor. Both forecasts, the one that incorporates the inflation rates and the one that does not are compared.

Government reimbursement programs, such as Medicare and Medicaid, generally pay hospitals less than the cost of caring for the people enrolled in these programs. For many patient conditions, Medicare and Medicaid pay hospitals a fixed amount based upon average cost for a procedure or treatment with local conditions taken into consideration. In addition, while the hospital provides the services, it has little control over the cost of delivery of that service, which is determined more by physician orders. The physician is under no real obligation to control those costs as the physician bills separately for services that are independent of orders charged. However, some patients who are severely ill will cost considerably more than average. This has caused providers to lose money. In this study, we investigate the reimbursement policies and the assumptions that have been made to create these reimbursement policies.

Section 3
Modeling EEG Images for Analysis

The brain is the most complicated and least studied area of Neuro Sceince. In recent times, it has been one of the fastest growing areas of study in the Medical Sciences. This is mostly due to computers and computational techniques that have emerged in the last 10-15 years. Cognitive Neuropsychology aims to understand how the structure and function of the brain relates to psychological processes. It places emphasis on studying the cognitive effects of brain injury or neurological illness with a view to inferring models of normal cognitive functioning. We investigate the relationship between sleep apnea and learning disorders. Sleep apnea is a neural disorder, where individuals find it difficult to sleep because they stop breathing. We want to see if patients with learning disabilities should be treated for sleep apnea.

Foreword

A pressure of competitiveness is growing in the healthcare sector while quality demands are rising. These trends confront medical institutions more than ever with the necessities of critically reviewing their own efficiency and quality under both medical and economical aspects. At the same time, growing capture of medical data and integration of distributed and heterogeneous databases create a completely new environment for medical quality and cost management. These advances have come to the foreground with the vast amounts of biomedical and genomic data in an electronic form, the Internet ability to transfer the data efficiently, and the wide application of computer use in all aspects of medical, biological, and health care research and practice. In medical and health care areas, due to regulations, a large amount of data is becoming available, and practitioners are expected to use these data in their everyday work. But such a large amount of data cannot be processed by humans in a short time to support timely and accurate medical decisions. Medical datasets have reached enormous capacities. Just as an illustration, note that almost a billion persons living in North America and Europe have at least some of their medical information collected in electronic form, at least transiently. These data may contain valuable information that awaits extraction, and a new knowledge may be encapsulated in various patterns and regularities that were hidden in the data. Such knowledge may prove to be priceless in future medical decision making.

This book presents several case studies of medical data mining developed by faculty and graduates of the University of Louisville's PhD program in Applied and Industrial Mathematics. Each contributor provides valued insights in the utilization of data mining technology supporting various aspects of a data mining process (e.g. data collection, reduction, cleansing and data integration). The book is organized in three main sections covering physician decision making, healthcare delivery, and medical data modeling. The studies include data analyses of the treatment of osteomyelitis, cardiovascular bypass versus angioplasty, the treatment of asthma, and both lung and breast cancer. Generally, the cases in this book use datasets that are publicly available for the purpose of research including the National Inpatient Sample and the Medical Expenditure Panel Survey, while data mining techniques used include market basket analysis, predictive modeling, time series analysis, survival data mining, kernel density estimation, and text mining.

This book describes applications of data mining in a very accessible form: both as a text to give ideas to the next generation of data mining practitioners, and to inform lifelong learners about potentials of data mining technology in the medical field. No chapter in this book will give you the full and final explanation about how to solve problems with data mining technology; every chapter will give you insights into how unpredictable and messy is a data mining process. Medical data mining must not be regarded as an independent effort, but it should rather be integrated into the broader environment that is aligned with decision-making processes in the medical field. The collection of papers illustrates the importance of maintaining close contact between data mining practitioners and the medical community in order to keep a permanent dialogue in order to identify new opportunities for applications of existing data mining technologies.

Mehmed Kantardzic
Louisville, February 10, 2009

Mehmed Kantardzic *received B.S., M.S., and Ph.D. degrees in computer science from University of Sarajevo, Bosnia. Currently, he is a Professor at the Computer Engineering and Computer Science Department, University of Louisville. He is also Director of CECS Graduate Programs, Director of Data Mining Lab, and Co-Director of Data Mining Graduate Certificate Program. His research interests are: data mining & knowledge discovery, machine learning, soft computing, click fraud detection, text mining & link analysis, sequence mining, and distributed intelligent systems. His recent research projects are supported by NSF, KSTC, US Treasury Department, and NASA. Dr. Kantardzic published more than 200 articles in refereed journals and conference proceedings including two books on data mining and applications. His book on data mining, published by John Wiley, is accepted as a textbook at universities all over the world. Dr. Kantardzic is a member of IEEE, IEE, ISCA, WSEAS, and SPIA. He is on editorial board or guest editor for several international journals, NSF and NSERC panel member and reviewer, program or conference chair for several international conferences and ICMLA Steering Committee member.*

Preface

This book gives several case studies developed by faculty and graduates of the University of Louisville's PhD program in Applied and Industrial Mathematics. The program is generally focused on applications in industry, and many of the program members focus on the study of health outcomes research using data mining techniques. Because so much data are now becoming readily available to investigate health outcomes, it is important to examine just how statistical models are used to do this. In particular, many of the datasets are large, and it is no longer possible to restrict attention to regression models and p-values.

Clinical databases tend to be very large. They are so large that the standard measure of a model's effectiveness, the p-value, will become statistically significant with an effect size that is nearly zero. Therefore, other measures need to be used to gauge a model's effectiveness. Currently, the only measure used in medical studies is the p-value. In linear regression or the general linear model, it would not be unusual to have a model that is statistically significant but with an r^2 value of 2% or less, suggesting that most of the variability in the outcome variable remains unaccounted for. It is a sure sign that there are too many patient observations in a model when most of the p-values are equal to '<0.00001'. The simplest solution, of course, is to reduce the size of the sample to one that is meaningful in regression. However, sampling does not utilize all of the potential information that is available in the data set and a reduction in the size of the sample requires a reduction in the number of variables used in the model so as to avoid the problem of over-fitting. Unfortunately, few studies that have been published in the medical literature using large samples take any of these problems into consideration.

An advantage of using data mining techniques is that we can investigate outcomes at the patient level rather than at the group level. Typically in regression, we look to patient type to determine those at high risk. Patients above a certain age represent one type. Patients who smoke represent another type. However, with data mining, we can examine and predict specific outcomes for a patient of a specific age who smokes 10 cigarettes a week, who drinks one glass of wine on weekends, and who is physically in good shape.

The purpose of using data mining is to explore the data so that the information gathered can be used to make decisions. In healthcare, the purpose is to make decisions with regard to patient treatment. Decision making does not necessarily require that a specific hypothesis test is generated and proven (or disproven). Exploration without a preconceived idea as to what will be discovered is also a valid means of data investigation.

A measure of the relationship of treatment decisions to patient outcomes that we can consider stems from the fact that physicians vary in how they treat similar patients. That variability itself can be used to examine the relationship between physician treatment decisions and patient outcomes. Once we determine which outcome is "best" from the patient's viewpoint, we can determine which treatment decisions are more likely to lead to that decision. This is particularly true for patients with chronic illness where there is a sequence of treatment outcomes followed by multiple patient outcomes. For example, a patient with diabetes can start with medication tablets, and then progress to insulin injections. Such patients can potentially end up with organ failure: failure of the heart, kidney, and so on. We can examine treatments that prolong the time to such organ failure. In this way, data mining can find optimal treatments as a decision making process.

Health outcomes research depends upon datasets that are routinely collected in the course of patient treatment, but are observational in nature and are very large. Traditional statistical methods were developed for randomized trials that are typically small in terms of the number of subjects where the main focus is on just one outcome variable. Only a few independent, input variables were needed because of the property of randomness. With large, observational datasets, there are some very important issues that cannot be disregarded. In particular, there is always the potential of confounding factors that must be considered.

There are many examples in the medical literature of observational studies that did ignore confounding factors. For example, the study of cervical cancer initially focused on the birth control pill, ignoring the reasons that women chose to use the pill. More recently, the association between the HPV infection and cervical cancer has been established. Because of a general perception that bacteria cannot exist in the acid content of the stomach, there was a general perception that peptic ulcers were caused by stress. The treatment offered was psychological, and H.pylori was not even considered as a possibility. More recently, hormone replacement therapy was considered as a way to reduce heart disease in women until a randomized trial debunked the treatment. It became popular because many women with heart disease were initially denied the therapy because of a perception that the therapy could increase heart problems. Observational studies that ignore confounders and rely on the standard regression models can often result in completely wrong conclusions.

Large data sets are required to examine rare occurrences. There needs to be a sufficient number of rare occurrences in the database to be comparable. For example, if a condition occurs 0.1% of the time, there would be approximately one such occurrence for every 1000 patients, 10 occurrences for 10,000 patients, and so on. A minimum of 100,000 patients in the dataset would be required to find 100 occurrences. However, all 100,000 patients cannot be used in a model to predict these occurrences. The model would be nearly 99% accurate, but would predict nearly every patient as a non-occurrence. In the absence of large samples and long-term follow up, surrogate endpoints are still used. For example, instead of looking at the mortality rate or rate of heart attacks to test a statin medication, the surrogate endpoint of cholesterol level is used. Instead of testing a new vaccine to see if there is a reduction in the infection rate, blood levels are measured.

Instead of using traditional statistical techniques, the studies in this book use exploratory data analysis and data mining tools. These tools were designed to find patterns and trends in observational data. In large datasets, data mining can examine enough variables to investigate potential confounders. One of the major potential confounders is the collection of co-morbidities that many patients have. Interactions between medications and conditions needs to be examined within the model, and such interactions are costly in terms of degrees of freedom in traditional regression models. They require large samples for analysis.

Chapter 1 gives a brief introduction to the data mining techniques that are used throughout the cases. The methods are used to drill down and discover important information in the datasets that are investigated in this casebook. These techniques include market basket analysis, predictive modeling, time series analysis, survival data mining, and text mining. In particular, it discusses an important, but little used technique known as kernel density estimation. This is a means of estimating the entire population distribution. While it is typical to assume that the population has a normal distribution with a bell-shaped density curve, that assumption is not valid if the population is heterogeneous, or is skewed. Using observational data concerning patient treatment, the population is always heterogeneous and skewed. Therefore, the standard assumptions used for defining linear and regression models are not valid. Other techniques must be used instead.

Generally, the cases in this book use datasets that are publicly available for the purpose of research. These include the National Inpatient Sample (NIS) and the Medical Expenditure Panel Survey (MEPS) available via the National Center for Health Statistics. The National Inpatient Sample contains a stratified sample of all inpatient events from 1000 different hospitals scattered over 37 states. It is published every year, two years behind the admission dates. The Medical Expenditure Panel Survey collects information about all contacts with the healthcare profession for a cohort of 30,000 individuals scattered over approximately 11,000 households. A different cohort has been collected each year since 1996. Each individual has data collected for two years. It contains actual cost and payment information; most other publicly available datasets contain information about charges only. Therefore, the MEPS is used to make estimates on healthcare expenditures by the population generally.

In addition, data from Thomson Medstat were used for some of the cases. Thomson Medstat collects all claims data from 100 insurance providers for approximately 40 million individuals. These individuals are followed longitudinally. These data were used in several of the cases as well. The remaining data were from local sources and used to investigate more specific questions of healthcare delivery. Thomson has a program to make its data available for student dissertation research, and we greatly appreciate the support.

The first section of the casebook contains various studies of outcomes research to investigate physician decision making. These case studies include an examination into the treatment of osteomyelitis, cardiovascular by-pass surgery versus angioplasty, the treatment of asthma, and the treatment of both lung cancer and breast cancer. In addition, there is a chapter related to the use of physical therapy as an attempt to avoid surgery for orthopedic problems and a study related to patient compliance with treatment in relationship to diagnosis. In particular, it discusses the importance of data visualization techniques as a means of data discovery and decision making using these large healthcare datasets.

One of the major findings from this section is that amputation is in fact the primary treatment for osteomyelitis for patients with diabetes, as discussed in detail in Chapter 2. Physicians are reluctant to prescribe antibiotics and often use inappropriate antibiotics for too short durations, resulting in recurrence of the infection. Amputation is assumed to eradicate the infection even though the amputations can often become sequential. This study demonstrates very clearly how treatment perception can be used for prescribing in the absence of information from the study of these outcomes datasets.

Chapter 3 examines the results in cardiovascular surgery where the major choice is CABG (cardiovascular bypass graft) or angioplasty. The introduction of the eluting stent in 2002 changed the dynamics of that choice. It appears that the eluting stent yields results that are very comparable to bypass surgery. The data here were examined using survival data mining. It shows the importance of defining an episode of care from claims datasets, and to be able to distinguish between different episodes of treatment.

The next chapter, 4, examines treatment choices for the chronic condition of asthma. This chapter investigates the various medications that are available for treatment, and how they are prescribed by physicians. It also examines the treatment of patients in the hospital for patients who have asthma. This study used both the NIS and MEPS to investigate both medication and inpatient treatment of asthma.

The next two chapters look at two different types of cancer, breast cancer and lung cancer. The purpose is to examine different treatment choices. In the first case, the purpose is to investigate the choice between a lumpectomy and mastectomy, and the patient conditions that might be related to these choices. In the second, we are also looking at treatment choices and the various regimens of chemotherapy.

A similar question motivates Chapter 7, which looks at the tendency to require physical therapy with the intent of preventing the need for surgery for orthopedic complaints. This chapter also examines the preprocessing necessary to investigate healthcare data. This study, too, relies upon the definition of an episode, and also on the definition of the zero time point. In this example, the zero point starts at physical therapy and the survival model ends with surgery. Patients are censored if they do not undergo the surgery.

Chapter 8 examines the relationship of patient procedures to inpatient care. It demonstrates that the compliance of patients in testing blood glucose reduces the cost of treatment. The importance of this monitoring cannot be understated. Similarly, chapter 9 looks at patient compliance and the patient condition in dental care. It shows that patients with the worst dental problems have the least compliance with treatment. Do they have such problems because of a lack of compliance, or are the most compliant the ones who have the best dental outcomes?

The final three chapters in section one examine the treatment of gastrointestinal problems and their relationship to mental disorders, the condition of hydrocephalus in infants, and common problems in childhood and adolescence. In particular, this chapter examines the issue of adolescent obesity and also some issues with vaccines in childhood and adolescents.

The second section of this book is related to case studies in healthcare delivery. Two of the studies examine healthcare delivery in the hospital emergency department. The first examines the scheduling of personnel; the second examines the patients who present at the emergency department. The objective of the first study concerning the emergency department is to use time series techniques to predict the need for personnel throughout the day. The second study looked at the detailed demographic information of patients presenting to the emergency department to determine the relationship between the demographics and the type of visit, non-urgent, urgent, or emergency conditions. The goal was to determine which patients should be referred to a no-cost clinic that treats patients with chronic conditions at no charge. It introduces another type of analysis, that of spatial data and spatial analysis using geographic information systems (GIS).

A third case study in the section examines time trends in physician prescribing of antibiotics and a fourth looks at the current process of reimbursing hospital providers by negotiated amount for a specific DRG code. One additional paper in this section relates to the information contained within the voluntary reporting of adverse events as supported by the Centers for Disease Control, or CDC. It looks at some standard issues in the treatment of pediatric patients, including the issue of obesity and exercise. Many of the studies in this section rely upon the use of time series methods to investigate health and treatment trends.

The third section in the book looks at the use of data mining techniques to model the relationship between brain activity and cognitive functioning. It is possible that some children are treated for learning disabilities when they should be treated instead for sleep apnea. This can have considerable impact on the type and amount of medication that is typically prescribed for problems such as ADHD. The techniques shown in this final chapter can also be used in microbiology research related to gene networks and interactions.

All of these examples can give the reader some excellent concepts of how data mining techniques can be used to investigate these datasets to enhance decision making. These large databases are invaluable in investigating general trends, and also to provide individual results.

Patricia Cerrito
Editor

Acknowledgment

We appreciate the efforts of the students involved in and graduated from the University of Louisville. It is their hard work and effort that made this book possible.

We also appreciate the support from Thom Medstat (now Thomson Reuters), who so willingly provided their MarketScan data for graduate dissertations. We appreciate the help of the IGI Global staff in getting the book to publication.

Patricia Cerrito
Editor

Chapter 1
Introduction to Data Mining Methodology to Investigate Health Outcomes

Patricia Cerrito
University of Louisville, USA

ABSTRACT

In this case, we provide some basic information concerning the statistical methods used throughout this text. These methods include visualization by kernel density estimation, regression and predictive models, time series, and text analysis. This case is not intended to provide extensive information concerning these techniques; references are provided for the interested reader who wants to follow up on the methodology. Some of the methodology is fairly well known while the predictive modeling and text analysis are relatively recent. One of the primary visualization techniques used is that of kernel density estimation. Since the patient base is relatively heterogeneous, we cannot assume that any health outcome is normally distributed. Kernel density estimation can find the entire population distribution so that we no longer have to rely upon averages and can relate the results more to individuals.

INTRODUCTION

The "gold standard" for investigating medical treatments is the randomized, controlled, double-blind study. Volunteers are recruited and randomized into a control or treatment group; the physician is blinded as to which patients receive the treatment and which receive a placebo. The patients are also blinded and unaware of whether they receive the actual treatment or not. Because such studies are

expensive, they can only be performed on a small number of potential treatments. They are done using a minimum number of subjects, usually on the patients at highest risk. Randomized studies are usually relatively short term and often use surrogate endpoints because it would take too long to examine real endpoints.

Because of informed consent requirements, such randomized, blinded studies are impossible to examine the effectiveness of a surgical procedure. Also, patients are usually excluded if they have multiple conditions that require more than one medication.

DOI: 10.4018/978-1-61520-723-7.ch001

Copyright © 2010, IGI Global. Copying or distributing in print or electronic forms without written permission of IGI Global is prohibited.

Until recently, young women with the potential to become pregnant were excluded from such trials for fear of damaging the woman's baby; children were excluded as well. Therefore, there are many studies that cannot be performed using a randomized design. We cannot, for example, look to the randomization of patients into levels of cigarette use, alcohol use, or level of sexual activity.

In this book, we present a number of examples of using data mining techniques and healthcare databases to examine healthcare decision making. Because any dataset collected in the routine of treating patients, including billing data, is quite extensive, the more traditional statistical methods cannot be used to investigate the data. (Cerrito, 2009a) This chapter is not intended to be a complete discussion of data mining; for more information, we refer the reader to texts by Cerrito (2009b) and deVille (2006).

DATA MINING TECHNIQUES

There are many different methods that can be used to investigate the data. We will discuss them briefly here. For more information, we refer the reader to Cerrito. (Cerrito, 2009a) These techniques include data visualization, predictive modeling, market basket analysis, time series analysis, and text analysis. Data mining is a process as well as a collection of techniques. We will list some of the differences between data mining and traditional statistical techniques.

Data mining deals with heterogeneous data, sometimes with a complex internal structure such as multimedia; including images, video, and text. Because most data collected in healthcare related to the routine of patient treatment consists of heterogeneous populations, the techniques of data mining are ideal to use with the various healthcare datasets. Data mining starts with the assumption that the raw data set is not of sufficient quality to apply a statistical model directly without some appropriate preprocessing techniques such that

the preprocessing will have as much or even more influence on the quality of the final results compared to the selected statistical technique. Data mining uses flexible predictive techniques that often are based on algorithmic foundations, but may have weak formal statistical justification. The data mining process often uses hidden variables as tools to perform a step-by-step compression of raw input data. Data mining attempts to find not only general, global models based on a data set, but also to find basic patterns in the data. Data mining is more concentrated on the aspects of data management and optimization of a search through the data while statistics is more oriented toward formalisms for final model representation, and score function formalization in the data space to perform inference. Data mining has been more focused on estimation, and the process generally ignores inferential models.

Data mining and statistics have generally developed in different domains. Statisticians are primarily interested in inference; data miners in exploratory data analysis. Nevertheless, there are some instances where data mining and statistics have blended. Many statisticians remain dubious about the data mining process. (Lee, 1995) Others are concerned with the lack of a theoretical framework similar to the one for inferential statistics, especially since data mining tends to be algorithmic-based. (Giudiei & Passerone, 2002; Hand & Bolton, 2004; Sargan, 2001)

Statistics and data mining differ in the use of machine learning methods, the volume of data, and the role of computational complexity. Our need for analysis is exceeding our abilities to handle the complexity. (Hosking, Pednault, & Sudan, 1997; Keim, Mansmann, Schneidewind, & Ziegler, 2006) Preprocessing is far more important with large datasets, especially as we approach the petabyte level, although healthcare data have yet to approach that level of size, with gigabytes considered to be extensively large. (Mannila, 1996) However, there are indications that data mining is focused on the data mining process itself with little emphasis on the knowledge actually extracted. (Pazzani, 2000) We need to know whether the extracted pattern is real or spurious, meaningful or meaningless. Will the extracted knowledge motivate positive action? Will it motivate decision making? Can the extracted information be interpreted?

While some of the methodologies are similar in both data mining and statistical analysis, the desired outcomes can differ substantially. For example, market segmentation is a problem of clustering; however, in the data mining approach, the clustering is acceptable if the result is increased sales or better prediction. (Bruin, Cocx, Kosters, Laros, & Kok, 2006; Jiang & Tuxhilin, 2006) In the statistical approach, the clustering is good if there is homogeneity within clusters and heterogeneity across clusters. (Jiang & Tuxhilin, 2006) On the other hand, an association rule or market basket analysis is a technique of data mining used almost exclusively in marketing applications. (Wang & Zhou, 2005; R. C.-W. Wong & Fu, 2005) The primary concern of this type of analysis is sales, and more recently to distinguish between customers with higher levels of sales. (Brus, Swinnen, Vanhoof, & Wets, 2004) However, in other, non-marketing applications, the optimal goal might be to change behavior rather than to just model customer behavior. (P. B. Cerrito & J. C. Cerrito, 2006; Giudier & Passerone, 2002) Therefore, the potential of market basket analysis still needs to be exploited statistically.

Another difference in approach occurs with binary or ordinal outcomes. Typically in a logistic regression analysis from a statistical perspective, the sample size is too small to allow us to over-sample rare occurrences. (Foster & Stine, 2004) This over-sampling is necessary because logistic regression performs poorly if the group sizes are not similar. In the process of over-sampling, probabilities should reflect the actual population proportions. Yet, especially in medical studies, logistic regression is used frequently to predict

rare occurrences without over-sampling or adjusting prior probabilities. Often, high rates of accuracy in the model are not examined in terms of differing false positive and false negative rates, resulting in a very inflated outcome. (Barlow et al., 2006) Sometimes, attempts are made to find matching cohorts; however, they are only matched on parameters defined by the investigator; the rare occurrence remains rare. (Claus, 2001; Ried, Kierk, Ambrosini, Berry, & Musk, 2006) The prior probabilities remain unchanged. While there are concerns about the use of statistical models in medicine, the issue of sampling rare occurrences is not considered important. (A. N. Freedman et al., 2005) High risk versus low risk is often the binary outcome under consideration. In statistical models, linear and logistic models are used to distinguish between population groups. Often risk, particularly patient risk, is assumed uniform across the population base. (Gaylor, 2005; Louis Anthony Cox, 2005; Thompson & Tebbins, 2006) For example, we consider the risk of polio as uniform when the disease now occurs from a vaccine, or potentially from the risk of bioterrorism. (Tebbins et al., 2006) We assume that each individual is equally likely to be exposed. The risk is still assumed uniform across the population. (Siegrist, Keller, & Kiers, 2005) Pooled risk, too, assumes that risk is uniform throughout the pool. (Tsanakas & Desli, 2005) The use of more input variables allows for individual assessment so that in data mining, risk is defined by individuals in the population base.

While statistical software simplifies the development of predictive models, there is danger in the inapplicability of models that must be clearly understood. (CHi-Ming et al., 2005) In the data mining approach, the number of rare occurrences is sufficiently large so that over-sampling still results in a sufficiently large sample. (Xiangchun, Kim, Back, Rhee, & Kim, 2005) Therefore, we can change the focus from the prediction of risk to the prediction of diagnosis. Data mining procedures can also rank observations to determine those most likely to predict accurately. (Sokol, Garcia, West, Rodriguez, & Johnson, 2001)

One of the major problems with either data mining or statistical analysis is the requirement of preprocessing data. (Popescul, Lawrence, Ungar, & Pennock, 2003; Sokol et al., 2001) Often, different pieces of the databases are located at different sources that are not necessarily compatible. This is particularly true in healthcare. Information publicly available, but located at different web locations, is also problematic to use for analysis because it is difficult to collect. Even in relatively cleaned claims data, inpatient claims are often separated from outpatient and physician visits, requiring them to be joined. Different coding requirements must also be reconciled.

There are indications that 80-90% of available data are in text form. (Menon, Tong, Sathiya-keerthi, Brombacher, & Leong, 2004) For too long, such data have been largely ignored, or used to define simple frequency counts. Text mining can now be used to analyze smaller and smaller pieces of text, allowing it to be used to compress large, categorical variables. (Cerrito, Badia, & Cerrito, 2005; Yuhua Li, Bandar, O'Shea, & Crockett, 2006) Text mining can also be used to find a natural ordering in the data for the purpose of ranking clusters. (Moches, 2005)

Much of the data collected in databases in the present time is incomplete and noisy. This may be deliberate as, for example, when a customer refuses to provide an accurate date of birth or accidental, as due to input error. Also, there is always the danger that data may be old or redundant. Thus, it is essential to researchers to base their analysis on what is described as *"clean data"*. Cleaning data or preprocessing the data prior to mining is designed to eliminate the following anomalies:

1. Missing field values.
2. Outliers.
3. Obsolete and/or redundant data.
4. Data in clear contradiction of common sense or well established industry norms.
5. Data in inconsistent state or format.

It is estimated the 50-60% of researchers' time is spent in data preprocessing to create databases suitable for data mining. Thus, it is no surprise that data preparation is an integral phase of the data mining process as a whole.

It is also the case that data preprocessing requires an understanding of the data and of the statistical analysis that is necessary to manipulate the data in order to remove any anomalies. (Hernandez & Stolfo, 1998; K. Wong, Byoung-ju, Bui-Kyeong, Soo-Kyung, & Doheon, 2003; Zhu, Wu, & Chen, 2006) Another issue in preprocessing is the need to define the observational unit. For example, the dataset might focus on individual claims from one inpatient hospital stay. However, there would be separate claims for the hospital, the physicians, the medications prescribed on discharge, and any home health care required. Institutional and hospice care can also be included. In order to examine the entire cost of one visit, the observational unit must be changed from claim to inpatient process. Data mining routinely considers the preprocessing requirements of the data, making its methodology critical for our proposed project. In particular, we will want to transpose information so that observational units are patients, not claims.

Data Visualization

With large datasets, data visualization becomes an important tool to understand the data. There are many different methods of data visualization, including bar and pie graphs, line plots and scatter plots. In addition, there is a method of visualization called kernel density estimation. It provides a way of investigating the entire population distribution instead of focusing on just the mean and variance. Since most healthcare outcome variables tend to have a gamma distribution that is highly skewed, the mean may misrepresent the true distribution. When a known distribution does not work to estimate the population, we can just use an estimate of that distribution. (Silverman, 1986) The formula for computing a kernel density estimate at the point x is equal to

$$f(x) = \frac{1}{na_n} \sum_{j=1}^{n} K\left(\frac{x - X_j}{a_n}\right)$$

where n is the size of the sample and K is a known density function. The value, a_n, is called the bandwidth. It controls the level of smoothing of the estimate curve. As the value of a_n approaches zero, the curve, f(x), becomes very jagged. As the value of a_n approaches infinity, the curve becomes closer to a straight line.

There are different methods available that can be used to attempt to optimize the level of smoothing. However, the value of a_n may still need adjustments because it is an approximation. If it first appears too jagged, the value of a_n is increased; if it first appears too smooth, the value of a_n is decreased. Note that for most standard density functions K, where x is far in magnitude from any point X_j, the value of f(x) will be very small. Where many data points cluster together, the value of the density function will be high because the sum of $x - X_j$ will be large and the probability defined by the kernel function will be large. However, where there are only scattered points, the value will be small. K can be the standard normal density, the uniform density, or any other density function. Simulation studies have demonstrated that the value of K has very limited impact on the value of the density estimate. It is the value of the bandwidth, a_n, that has substantial impact on the smoothness of the density estimate. The true value of this bandwidth must be estimated, and there are several methods available to optimize this estimate.

Market Basket Analysis

Market basket analysis, also called association rules, was developed to examine customer purchasing habits. The technique can be used to examine physician prescribing practices to determine which medications and which procedures are related. Market basket analysis defines a series of rules A→B and provides a measure of the probability that event A leads to event B where A and B can be a series of medications, a series of treatments, or a combination of both. There are a number of measures of the usefulness of the rule, and rules are generally ranked by the measure of usefulness. For example, if we want to investigate the rule {Metformin, Rosaglitazone}→{Insulin}, then the probability of the antecedent (Metformin, Rosaglitazone) is called the support for the rule. The confidence is the conditional probability of the consequent (Insulin) given the antecedent (Metformin, Rosaglitazone). Because there are so many available treatments and medications, we use the methodology that was developed to examine so many different combinations.

One major problem with market basket analysis is that a large number of the rules may be trivial and well known. If you require rules to have a high minimum support level and a high confidence level, you may miss some useful results. Differential market basket analysis can be used to investigate differences across different healthcare providers.

One good way of examining the results of market basket analysis is through the data visualization technique of link graphs. A link graph is a series of nodes and links. The nodes represent treatment items; the links represent the connections between the items. The strength of the connection is shown through the color and the width of the link; the importance of the treatment item is shown by color and size as well. Another way to investigate these links is through a combination of text mining and association rules. Text mining allows for a reduction in the problem so that fewer rules are generated and the interpretation becomes much easier.

Predictive Modeling

Regression is one type of predictive modeling, which also includes decision trees and artificial neural networks. The purpose of predictive modeling is to estimate an outcome variable, Y, given a series of input variables, X_1, X_2, …, X_n. The standard regression model is defined by

$$Y=\alpha+\beta_1 X_1+\beta_2 X_2+\ldots+\beta_n X_n$$

where the regression equation is optimized to minimize the error term. In healthcare, most of the continuous patient outcomes have a gamma-type distribution with a very large tail. Consider, for example, the relationship of age to health. The relationship between a person's age and various indicators of health is most likely not linear in nature: During early adulthood, the average health status of someone 30 years old compared to the average health status of someone 40 years old is not all that different. However, the difference in health status of a 60 year old compared to a 70 year old person is very likely much greater.

For this reason, the standard regression models are not applicable as they generally assume that the population distribution is normal. Therefore, the generalized linear model is much more applicable when investigating healthcare data. With the generalized model, we assume that

$$Y=g(\alpha+\beta_1 X_1+\beta_2 X_2+\ldots+\beta_n X_n)$$

where the inverse of g() is called a link function. Various functions are available to define the link function. In particular, the gamma function can be modeled using this approach.

Generally, discrete patient outcomes are rare occurrences and are modeled using logistic regression. For example, mortality is one such outcome but generally occurs in less than 10% of the patient population (unless we restrict our attention to patients with life-threatening conditions). Unless a stratified model is used so that the rare occurrence consists of 50% of the sampled observations, the resulting logistic regression will be highly accurate, but will have almost no practical predictive ability. That is because the logistic regression will predict virtually the entire population into the nonoccurrence group.

A decision tree creates a tree-shaped structure that represents sets of decisions. It consists of a series of leaves, and each leaf splits the data into two parts. These decisions generate rules for the classification of the dataset. Specific decision tree methods include Classification and Regression Trees (CART) and Chi Square Automatic Interaction Detection (CHAID). The neural network is considered a "black box" since the connections between the outcome variable and the input variables are hidden.

Predictive modeling generally allows for the use of prior probabilities and decision weights because some misclassification of outcomes is more costly compared to others. In addition, the predictive model can determine which observations can be more readily predicted compared to other observations.

Time Series Analysis

Time series techniques are generally used to examine trends over time. They can be used to examine trends such as medication use over time, or surgical procedures that can change as new techniques and devices are developed. Generally, we assume that the future can be predicted based upon the past and the present.

A time series model takes into consideration the following characteristics of the data:

- *Autocorrelation.* A positive deviation from the mean is likely to stay positive; a negative deviation is likely to stay negative.

- *Trend.* A positive or negative trend requires a first or second difference.
- *Seasonality.* The data have a seasonal trend.
- *Transformation.* To maintain the assumption of normality, a transformation is sometimes required.

A purely autoregressive (with autocorrelations) model indicates that the current value $Y(t)$ depends on a specific number of previous values. If the number of previous values is equal to p, then an autoregression of size p is equal to

$$Y(t) = \mu + \alpha_1(Y(t-1) - \mu) + \alpha_2(Y(t-2) - \mu) + \ldots + \alpha_p(Y(t-p) - \mu) + \varepsilon(t)$$

Estimation of the number of lags in the model is based on the autocorrelations. The moving average component expresses the current value $Y(t)$ in terms of future shocks (or errors):

$$Y(t) = \mu + \varepsilon(t) - \theta_1\varepsilon(t-1) - \ldots - \theta_q\varepsilon(t-q)$$

In the existence of a trend, a first or second difference is used. That is, a new model $W(t)$ is defined so that

$$W(t) = Y(t) - Y(t-1)$$

and the model is then defined for the difference $W(t)$. Once this is estimated, $Y(t)$ is estimated as equal to

$$Y(t) = W(t) + Y(t-1)$$

The number of differences is defined by the parameter d. The three components of autocorrelation, seasonality, and trend make up the ARIMA model (AR=autoregressive, I=integrated, MA=moving average). It is identified as of order (p,d,q). It estimates both the autocorrelation and the trend.

Seasonality is added to the model by using an ARIMA$(p,d,q)x(P,D,Q)$ model, where

P is the number of seasonal autoregressive terms

D is the number of seasonal differences

Q is the number of seasonal moving average terms

In the seasonal part of the model, all of these factors operate across multiples of lag s (the number of periods in a season). If the seasonality changes yearly, then the value of s is 12.

If the seasonal pattern is both strong and stable over time (for example, high in the summer and low in the winter or vice versa), then your model should probably use a seasonal difference (regardless of whether the first, nonseasonal part uses a difference) to prevent the seasonal pattern from fading in long-term forecasts.

Sometimes a log transformation is included as part of the model. Seasonal ARIMA models are inherently additive models, so to capture a multiplicative seasonal pattern, use the log transformation with the data prior to fitting the ARIMA model. If the residuals show a marked increase in variance over time, the log transformation should be used.

Unfortunately, many investigators still attempt to use time series data in a linear model. This is totally incorrect, and will lead to incorrect results. The most egregious error is needed when the time units are split into smaller intervals to inflate the degrees of freedom in a linear model, thereby guaranteeing statistical significance.

Survival Analysis

Survival analysis is used when the variable under study is the time to an event. In healthcare, the event can be cancer recurrence, death, or healed. Survival data mining occurs when there can be multiple events that can occur in sequence. For example, cancer recurrence can occur before death, as can disease progression. Survival data mining is an important process when investigating different patient outcomes as they relate to patients with chronic diseases.

Survival data will usually follow some type of exponential distribution. However, since it is not always possible to observe all subjects until the event of interest (for example, mortality) occurs, there will be censored observations at the end of the study, meaning subjects for whom the event has not yet occurred at the end of the data collection period. One parameter of interest when examining survival data is the hazard rate. For discrete time, the hazard rate is the probability that a subject will experience an event at time t while that individual is at risk for having an event. In other words, the hazard rate is really just the unobserved rate at which events occur.

There are two primary techniques for survival analysis. The first is log rank statistics, assuming a nonparametric model. It is also called a Kaplan-Meier estimate of survival. It is somewhat limited in that survival cannot be investigated in relationship to patient parameters. The second is the more flexible Cox Regression, which must make the assumption that the hazard rate is constant for each time interval. In other words, it must assume that the risk of mortality between the ages of 30 and 40 will be the same as between the ages of 70 and 80.

The survival function, S(t), is defined as S(t)=P(T>t) where t is some time point and T is a random variable that denotes the time of the event. The hazard rate is defined as

$$\lambda(t)dt = \frac{S'(t)dt}{S(t)}$$

As traditional survival analysis cannot be used, we turn toward survival data mining. The technique has been developed primarily to examine the concept of customer churn, again where

multiple end points exist. (Linoff, 2004; Potts, 2000) However, medical use of survival is still generally limited to one defined event, although some researchers are experimenting with the use of predictive modeling rather than survival analysis. (Berzuini & Larizza, 1996; Eleuteri et al., 2003; John & Chen, 2006; Pinna et al., 2000; Seker et al., 2002; Shaw & Marshall, 2006; Xie, Chaussalet, & Millard, 2006) Nevertheless, in a progressive disease, the event markers of that progression should be considered. However, to first construct survival curves to visualize the recurrence outcome of the procedure, we use the variables for time 1 and time 2. We also limit the starting procedure, or stratify by starting procedure to compute comparisons. We can also use this code to determine the proportion of patients with only one procedure during the period of study.

Once we have identified the episodes, we want to use a model for recurrent events data, or survival data mining. The intensity model is given by

$$\lambda_z(t)dt = E\{dN(t) \mid F_{t_-}\} = \lambda_0 e^{\beta'Z(t)}dt$$

where F_t represents all the information of the processes N and Z up to time t, $\lambda_0(t)$ is an arbitrary baseline intensity function, and β is the vector of regression coefficients. The instantaneous intensity is the hazard rate. This model has two components: 1) the covariates assume multiplicative effects on the instantaneous rate of the counting process and 2) the influence of prior events on future recurrences is mediated through the time-dependent covariates. The hazard rate function is given by

$$d\mu_z(t) = E\{dN(t) \mid Z(t)\} = e^{\beta'Z}\mu_0(t)$$

where $\mu_0(t)$ is an unknown continuous function and β is the vector of regression parameters. We compute the estimates of the regression coefficients by solving the partial likelihood function. A subject with K events contributes K+1 observations to the input data set. The kth observation of the subject identifies the time interval from the $(k-1)^{th}$ event or time 0 (if k=1) to the kth event, k=1,2,…,K. The $(K=1)^{th}$ observation represents the time interval from the Kth event to time of censorship.

Text Analysis

Text analysis uses techniques of natural language processing to quantify words, sentences, and paragraphs. It can also be used to examine relationships between nominal and categorical variables. In this book, text analysis will be used to investigate coded information. Healthcare datasets generally identify patient diagnosis and procedure information through the use of codes. There are three major types of codes: ICD9, CPT, and DRG codes. ICD9 codes were developed by the World Health Organization and are used in hospitals. CPT codes are used by physicians. DRG codes were developed by Medicare largely for billing purposes. There are hundreds and possibly thousands of codes. Each patient can have multiple codes assigned with one assigned as a primary condition or a primary procedure.

In this casebook, text analysis is used to define classes of patient severity so that outcomes can be investigated in terms of the general condition of each patient. Text analysis uses linkage between patient diagnoses to classify them.

The basics of text analysis are as follows:

1. Transpose the data so that the observational unit is the identifier and all nominal values are defined in the observational unit.
2. Tokenize the nominal data so that each nominal value is defined as one token.
3. Concatenate the nominal tokens into a text string such that there is one text string per identifier. Each text string is a collection of tokens; each token represents a noun.
4. Use text mining to cluster the text strings so that each identifier belongs to one cluster.

5. Use other statistical methods to define a natural ranking in the clusters.
6. Use the clusters defined by text mining in other statistical analyses.

The first step in analyzing text data is to define a term by document matrix. Each document forms a row of the matrix; each term forms a column. The resulting matrix will be extremely large, but very sparse, with most of the cells containing zeros. The matrix can be compressed using the technique of singular value decomposition with the matrix restricted to a maximum of N dimensions. For defining patient severity, each patient represents a document and each code represents a term. Each cell contains a count of the number of times a code appears for a patient. Since there are only a handful of diagnoses connected to any one patient, most of the cells will contain the value, '0'. Therefore, the matrix will be very large, but most of the cells will be empty.

Singular value decomposition is based upon an assignment of weights to each term in the dataset. Terms that are common and appear frequently, such as 'of', 'and', 'the' are given low or zero weight while terms that appear in only a handful of documents are given a high weight (entropy). Other weighting schemes take into consideration target or outcome variables (information gain, chi-square). When working with patient condition codes, the less common diagnoses are given higher weights compared to more common diagnoses such as hypertension. Generally, we use the standard entropy weighting method, so that the most common ICD9 codes (hypertension, disorder of lipid metabolism or high cholesterol) will be given low weights while less common (uncontrolled Type I diabetes with complications) will be given higher weights.

Clustering was performed using the expectation maximization algorithm. It is a relatively new, iterative clustering technique that works well with nominal data in comparison to the K-means and hierarchical methods that are more standard.

The clusters are identified by the terms that most clearly represent the text strings contained within the cluster. It does not mean that every patient has the representative combination of terms. It does mean that the linkages within the terms are the ones that have the highest identified weights.

DISCUSSION

Each case in this book will use several of the data mining techniques listed in this chapter. The cases will clearly demonstrate how data mining can very effectively find meaningful information in the data. This information can either examine standard practice, or it can define optimal practice; hopefully, but not always, standard practice will coincide with optimal practice. In the future, data mining will become standard practice in health outcomes research because of the important findings that are resulting from the use of data mining techniques.

REFERENCES

Barlow, W. E., White, E., Ballard-Barbash, R., Vacek, P. M., Titus-Ernstoff, L., & Carney, P. A. (2006). Prospective breast cancer risk prediction model for women undergoing screening mammography. *Journal of the National Cancer Institute*, *98*(17), 1204–1214.

Berzuini, C., & Larizza, C. (1996). A unified approach for modeling longitudinal and failure time data, with application in medical monitoring. *IEEE Transactions on Pattern Analysis and Machine Intelligence*, *16*(2), 109–123. doi:10.1109/34.481537

Bruin, J. S. d., Cocx, T. K., Kosters, W. A., Laros, J. F., & Kok, J. N. (2006). *Data mining approaches to criminal career analysis*. Paper presented at the Proceedings of the Sixth International Conference on Data Mining, Hong Kong.

Brus, T., Swinnen, G., Vanhoof, K., & Wets, G. (2004). Building an association rules framework to improve produce assortment decisions. *Data Mining and Knowledge Discovery*, *8*, 7–23. doi:10.1023/B:DAMI.0000005256.79013.69

Cerrito, P., Badia, A., & Cerrito, J. C. (2005). *Data Mining Medication Prescriptions for a Representative National Sample*. Paper presented at the Pharmasug 2005, Phoenix, Arizona.

Cerrito, P. B. (2009a). *Data Mining Healthcare and Clinical Databases*. Cary, NC: SAS Press, Inc.

Cerrito, P. B. (2009b). *Text Mining Techniques for Healthcare Provider Quality Determination: Methods for Rank Comparisons*. Hershey, PA: IGI Publishing.

Cerrito, P. B., & Cerrito, J. C. (2006). *Data and text mining the electronic medical record to improve care and to lower costs*. Paper presented at the SUGI31, San Francisco.

CHi-Ming, C., Hsu-Sung, K., Shu-Hui, C., Hong-Jen, C., Der-Ming, L., Tabar, L., et al. (2005). Computer-aided disease prediction system: development of application software with SAS component language. *Journal of Evaluation in Clinical Practice*, *11*(2), 139–159. doi:10.1111/j.1365-2753.2005.00514.x

Claus, E. B. (2001). Risk models used to counsel women for breast and ovarian cancer: a guide for clinicians. *Familial Cancer*, *1*, 197–206. doi:10.1023/A:1021135807900

Eleuteri, A., Tagliaferri, R., Milano, L., Sansone, G., Agostino, D. D., Placido, S. D., et al. (2003). *Survival analysis and neural networks*. Paper presented at the 2003 Conference on Neural Networks, Portland, OR.

Foster, D. P., & Stine, R. A. (2004). Variable selection in data miing: building a predictive model for bankruptcy. *Journal of the American Statistical Association*, *99*(466), 303–313. doi:10.1198/016214504000000287

Freedman, A. N., Seminara, D., Mitchell, H., & Hartge, P., colditz, G. A., Ballard-Barbash, R., et al. (2005). Cancer risk prediction models: a workshop on developmnet, evaluation, and application. *Journal of the National Cancer Institute, 97*(10), 715–723.

Gaylor, D. W. (2005). Risk/benefit assessments of human diseases: optimum dose for intervention. *Risk Analysis, 25*(1), 161–168. doi:10.1111/j.0272-4332.2005.00575.x

Giudiei, P., & Passerone, G. (2002). Data mining of association structures to model consumer behaviour. *Computational Statistics & Data Analysis, 38*, 533–541. doi:10.1016/S0167-9473(01)00077-9

Giudier, P., & Passerone, G. (2002). Data mining of association structures to model consumer behavior. *Computational Statistics & Data Analysis, 38*(4), 533–541. doi:10.1016/S0167-9473(01)00077-9

Hand, D. J., & Bolton, R. J. (2004). Pattern discovery and detection: a unified statistical methodology. *Journal of Applied Statistics, 8*, 885–924. doi:10.1080/0266476042000270518

Hernandez, M. A., & Stolfo, S. J. (1998). Real-world data is dirty: data cleansing and the merge/purge problem. *Data Mining and Knowledge Discovery, 2*, 9–17. doi:10.1023/A:1009761603038

Hosking, J. R., Pednault, E. P., & Sudan, M. (1997). Statistical perspective on data mining. *Future Generation Computer Systems, 13*(2-3), 117–134. doi:10.1016/S0167-739X(97)00016-2

Jiang, T., & Tuxhilin, A. (2006). *Improving personalization solutions through optimal segmentation of customer bases.* Paper presented at the Proceedings of the Sixth International Conference on Data Mining, Hong Kong.

John, T. T., & Chen, P. (2006). Lognormal selection with applications to lifetime data. *IEEE Transactions on Reliability, 55*(1), 135–148. doi:10.1109/TR.2005.858098

Keim, D. A., Mansmann, F., Schneidewind, J., & Ziegler, H. (2006). Challenges in visual data analysis. *Information Visualization, 2006*, 9–16.

Lee, S. (1995). *Predicting atmospheric ozone using neural networks as compared to some statistical methods.* Paper presented at the Northcon 95. IEEE Technical Applications Conference and Workshops Northcon95, Portland, OR.

Linoff, G. S. (2004). Survival Data Mining for Customer Insight. Retrieved 2007. from www.intelligententerprise.com/showArticle.jhtml?articleID=26100528

Louis Anthony Cox, J. (2005). Some limitations of a proposed linear model for antimicrobial risk management. *Risk Analysis, 25*(6), 1327–1332. doi:10.1111/j.1539-6924.2005.00703.x

Mannila, H. (1996). *Data mining: machine learning, statistics and databases.* Paper presented at the Eighth International Conference on Scientific and Statistical Database Systems, 1996, Stockholm.

Menon, R., Tong, L. H., Sathiyakeerthi, S., Brombacher, A., & Leong, C. (2004). The needs and benefits of applying textual data mining within the product development process. *Quality and Reliability Engineering International, 20*, 1–15. doi:10.1002/qre.536

Moches, T. A. (2005). *Text data mining applied to clustering with cost effective tools.* Paper presented at the IEEE International Conference on Systems, Mand, and Cybernetics, Waikoloa, HI.

Pazzani, M. J. (2000). Knowledge discovery from data? *IEEE Intelligent Systems*, (March/April): 10–13. doi:10.1109/5254.850821

Pinna, G., Maestri, R., Capomolla, S., Febo, O., Mortara, A., & Riccardi, P. (2000). Determinant role of short-term heart rate variability in the prediction of mortality in patients with chronic heart failure. *IEEE Computers in Cardiology, 27*, 735–738.

Popescul, A., Lawrence, S., Ungar, L. H., & Pennock, D. M. (2003). *Statistical relational learning for document mining.* Paper presented at the Proceedings of the Third IEEE International Conference on Data Mining, Melbourne, FL.

Potts, W. (2000). Survival Data Mining. Retrieved 2007, from http://www.data-miners.com/resources/Will%20Survival.pdf

Ried, R., Kierk, N. d., Ambrosini, G., Berry, G., & Musk, A. (2006). The risk of lung cancer with increasing time since ceasing exposure to asbestos and quitting smoking. *Occupational and Environmental Medicine, 63*(8), 509–512. doi:10.1136/oem.2005.025379

Sargan, J. D. (2001). Model building and data mining. *Econometric Reviews, 20*(2), 159–170. doi:10.1081/ETC-100103820

Seker, H., Odetayo, M., Petrovic, D., Naguib, R., Bartoli, C., Alasio, L., et al. (2002). *An artificial neural network based feature evaluation index for the assessment of clinical factors in breast cancer survival analysis.* Paper presented at the IEEE Canadian Conference on Electrical & Computer Engineering, Winnipeg, Manitoba.

Shaw, B., & Marshall, A. H. (2006). Modeling the health care costs of geriatric inpatients. *IEEE Transactions on Information Technology in Biomedicine, 10*(3), 526–532. doi:10.1109/TITB.2005.863821

Siegrist, M., Keller, C., & Kiers, H. A. (2005). A new look at the psychometric paradigm of perception of hazards. *Risk Analysis, 25*(1), 211–222. doi:10.1111/j.0272-4332.2005.00580.x

Silverman, B. W. (1986). *Density Estimation for Statistics and Data Analysis (Monographs on Statistics and Applied Probability.* Boca Raton, FL: Chapman & Hall/CRC. Sokol, L., Garcia, B., West, M., Rodriguez, J., & Johnson, K. (2001). *Precursory steps to mining HCFA health care claims.* Paper presented at the 34th Hawaii International Conference on System Sciences, Hawaii.

Tebbins, R. J. D., Pallansch, M. A., Kew, O. M., Caceres, V. M., Jafari, H., & Cochi, S. L. (2006). Risks of Paralytic disease due to wild or vaccine-derived poliovirus after eradication. *Risk Analysis, 26*(6), 1471–1505. doi:10.1111/j.1539-6924.2006.00827.x

Thompson, K. M., & Tebbins, R. J. D. (2006). Retrospective cost-effectiveness analyses for polio vaccination in the United States. *Risk Analysis, 26*(6), 1423–1449. doi:10.1111/j.1539-6924.2006.00831.x

Tsanakas, A., & Desli, E. (2005). Measurement and pricing of risk in insurance markets. *Risk Analysis, 23*(6), 1653–1668. doi:10.1111/j.1539-6924.2005.00684.x

Wang, K., & Zhou, X. (2005). Mining customer value: from association rules to direct marketing. *Data Mining and Knowledge Discovery, 11,* 57–79. doi:10.1007/s10618-005-1355-x

Wong, K., Byoung-ju, C., Bui-Kyeong, H., Soo-Kyung, K., & Doheon, L. (2003). A taxonomy of dirty data. *Data Mining and Knowledge Discovery, 7,* 81–99. doi:10.1023/A:1021564703268

Wong, R. C.-W., & Fu, A. W.-C. (2005). Data mining for inventory item selection with cross-selling considerations. *Data Mining and Knowledge Discovery, 11,* 81–112. doi:10.1007/s10618-005-1359-6

Xiangchun, K. X., Back, Y., Rhee, D. W., & Kim, S.-H. (2005). *Analysis of breast cancer using data mining & statistical techniques.* Paper presented at the Proceedings of the Sixth International Conference on Software Engineering, Artificial Intelligence, Networking, and Parallel/Distributed Computing, Las Vegas, NV.

Xie, H., Chaussalet, T. J., & Millard, P. H. (2006). A model-based approach to the analysis of patterns of length of stay in institutional long-term care. *IEEE Transactions on Information Technology in Biomedicine, 10*(3), 512–518. doi:10.1109/TITB.2005.863820

Yuhua Li, D. M., Bandar, Z. A., O'Shea, J. D., & Crockett, K. (2006). Sentence similarity based on semantic nets and corpur statistics. *IEEE Transactions on Knowledge and Data Engineering*, *18*(6), 1138–1148.

Zhu, X., Wu, X., & Chen, Q. (2006). Bridging local and global data cleansing: identifying class noise in large, distributed data datasets. *Data Mining and Knowledge Discovery*, *12*(2-3), 275. doi:10.1007/s10618-005-0012-8

ADDITIONAL READING

Cerrito, P. B. (2009a). *Data Mining Healthcare and Clinical Databases*. Cary, NC: SAS Press, Inc.

Cerrito, P. B. (2009b). *Text Mining Techniques for Healthcare Provider Quality Determination: Methods for Rank Comparisons*. Hershey, PA: IGI Publishing.

Cerrito, PB. A Casebook on Pediatric Diseases, Bentham Science Publishing: Oak Park, Illinois.

Section 1
Case Studies in Health Outcomes Research

Chapter 2
Data Mining to Examine the Treatment of Osteomyelitis

Hamid Zahedi
University of Louisville, USA

ABSTRACT

The purpose of this study is to use data mining methods to investigate the physician decisions specifically in the treatment of osteomyelitis. Two primary data sets have been used in this study; the National Inpatient Sample (NIS) and the Thomson MedStat MarketScan data. We used online sources to obtain background information about the disease and its treatment in the literature. An innovative method was used to capture the information from the web and to cluster or filter that information to find the most relevant information, using SAS Text Miner. Other important innovations in investigating the data include finding the switches of medication and comparing the date of the switch with the date of procedures. We could study these medications switched at deeper levels, but this is not necessary in our study, especially with limited access to data. We also create a model to forecast the cost of hospitalization for patients with osteomyelitis.

BACKGROUND

Preprocessing is an essential aspect of outcomes research. Dealing with multiple data sources is essential. We demonstrate the needed preprocessing. Our data contain multiple observations for each patient. We convert this dataset from a one-to-many to a one-to-one observation for each patient; we developed the necessary SAS coding required to

perform the preprocessing steps. In other words, we need to have a one-to-many relationship between patients and their procedures (instead of many-to-many). We also show how disparate datasets such as inpatients, outpatients and RX datasets can be merged to examine the relationship of antibiotics to disease treatment. (Cerrito, 2010)

Using MedStat MarketScan data, we show that physicians do not use proper antibiotics if antibiotics are used at all, resulting in unnecessary amputations and amputations performed sequentially on patients

DOI: 10.4018/978-1-61520-723-7.ch002

Copyright © 2010, IGI Global. Copying or distributing in print or electronic forms without written permission of IGI Global is prohibited.

with osteomyelitis. Other conclusions discovered include the result that physicians assume amputation is the primary treatment for Osteomyelitis. Injection of antibiotics was performed on only a small portion of patients with Osteomyelitis. In many cases, infection has recurred and amputation was performed more than once.

MRSA

Methicillin-Resistant Staphylococcus Aureus (MRSA) is a type of bacteria that is resistant to most antibiotics known as beta-lactams that include Methicillin, Amoxicillin, and Penicillin. *Staphylococcus Aureus* (Steph) bacteria commonly live on the skin. They can cause infection when they enter inside the body from a cut, or through a catheter or breathing tube. This infection occurs in people with weak immune systems, the patients with long stays in hospitals or care facilities, and people receiving certain, invasive treatments such as dialysis. People with diabetes are at a great risk of infection since they usually have a weaker immune system compared to others, and they also have a greater chance to be exposed to the bacteria. In some cases, MRSA infection has occurred in people not considered at high risk; these infections are known as community-associated MRSA (CA-MRSA). They occur in healthy people who have no history of hospitalization in the past. Many such infections have occurred among athletes who share equipment or personal items, and children in daycare facilities. (MedlinePlus, n.d.) More recently, infections have occurred as a result of tattoos.(MRSA, n.d.) Another study showed homosexuals are at greater risk of infection than others. (Binan Dep, et.al., 2008)

One of the main ways of transmission to other patients is through human hands, especially worker's hand. Hands may be contaminated with MRSA by infected contact or colonized patients. If healthcare providers do not wash hands after contact with a patient, the bacteria can be spread when that provider touches other patients.

Osteomyelitis

Osteomyelitis is an acute or chronic bone infection, usually caused by bacteria. The infection that causes osteomyelitis often is in another part of the body and spreads to the bone via the blood. Affected bone may have been predisposed to infection because of recent trauma. The objective of treatment is to eliminate the infection and prevent it from getting worse. Antibiotics are given to destroy the bacteria that cause the infection.

If left untreated, the infection can become chronic and cause a loss of blood supply to the affected bone. When this happens, it can lead to the eventual death of the bone tissue.

For infections that are not eradicated, surgery may be needed to remove dead bone tissue (Amputation). Antibiotic choice and duration can help reduce the chance of amputation.

Osteomyelitis can affect both adults and children. The bacteria or fungus that can cause osteomyelitis, however, differ among age groups. In adults, osteomyelitis often affects the vertebrae and the pelvis. In children, osteomyelitis usually affects the adjacent ends of long bones. Long bones are large, dense bones that provide strength, structure, and mobility. They include the femur and tibia in the legs, and the humerus and radius in the arms.

Osteomyelitis does not occur more commonly in a particular race or gender. However, some people are more at risk for developing the disease, including: (Cleveland Clinic, n.d.)

- People with diabetes
- Patients receiving hemodialysis
- People with weakened immune systems
- People with sickle cell disease
- Intravenous drug abusers
- The elderly

The symptoms of osteomyelitis can include:

- Pain and/or tenderness in the infected area
- Swelling and warmth in the infected area
- Fever
- Nausea, secondarily from being ill with infection
- General discomfort, uneasiness, or ill feeling
- Drainage of pus through the skin

Additional symptoms that may be associated with this disease include:

- Excessive sweating
- Chills
- Lower back pain
- Swelling of the ankles, feet, and legs
- Changes in gait (walking pattern that is painful, yielding a limp)

ICD9 Codes

ICD9 codes are provided in The *International Statistical Classification of Diseases and Related Health Problems* (most commonly known by the abbreviation ICD) to classify diseases and a wide variety of signs, symptoms, abnormal findings, complaints, social circumstances and external causes of injury or disease. Every health condition can be assigned to a unique category and given a code, up to six characters long. Such categories can include a set of similar diseases that can be converted to a diagnosis.

The ICD9 codes used in this project translate to: (ICD9, n.d.)

Procedures:

84.1 Amputation of lower limb
84.3 Revision of amputation stump
99.21 Injection of antibiotic
00.14 Injection or infusion of Oxazolidinone class of antibiotics

Diagnoses:

730 Osteomyelitis, periostitis, and other infections involving bone
895 Traumatic amputation of toe(s) (complete) (partial)
905.9 Late effect of traumatic amputation
997.6 Amputation stump complication
E878.5 Amputation of limb(s)
V49.6 Upper limb amputation status
V49.7 Lower limb amputation status

DRG Codes

The original objective of diagnosis related groupings (DRGs) was to develop a patient classification system that related types of patients treated to the resources they consumed. Since the introduction of DRGs in the early 1980's, the healthcare industry has evolved and developed an increased demand for a patient classification system that can serve its original objective at a higher level of sophistication and precision. To meet those evolving needs, the objective of the DRG system had to expand in scope. Today, there are several different DRG systems that have been developed in the US.

The DRG codes used in this project translate to:

DRG 113: Amputation for circulatory system disorders except upper limb & toe
DRG 114: Upper limb & toe amputation for circulatory system disorders
DRG 213: Amputation for musculoskeletal system & connective tissue disorders
DRG 238: Osteomyelitis
DRG 285: Amputation of lower limb for endocrine, nitrite & metabolic disorders

The complete table of DRG codes was provided with our data. It is also available online at http://health.utah.gov/opha/IBIShelp/codes/DRGCode.htm.

Antibiotics

Zyvox (Linezolid): (Zyvox, 2007)

To reduce the development of drug-resistant bacteria and to maintain the effectiveness of

Zyvox formulations and other antibacterial drugs, Zyvox should be used only to treat or prevent infections that are proven or strongly suspected to be caused by bacteria. The generic label for Zyvox is linezolid. Zyvox is a synthetic antibacterial agent of the oxazolidinone class. The empirical formula is $C16H20FN3O4$. The Zyvox I.V. Injection is supplied as a ready-to-use sterile isotonic solution for intravenous infusion. Each mL contains 2 mg of linezolid. Inactive ingredients are sodium citrate, citric acid, and dextrose in an aqueous vehicle for intravenous administration. The sodium (Na+) content is 0.38 mg/mL (5 mEq per 300-mL bag; 3.3 mEq per 200-mL bag; and 1.7 mEq per 100-mL bag).

Vancomycin: (Vancomycin, 2006)

Sterile Vancomycin Hydrochloride, USP, intravenous, is a chromatographically (chromatography is a technique used to separate the components of a chemical mixture by moving the mixture along a stationary material, such as paper or gelatin) purified tricyclic glycopeptide antibiotic derived from Amycolatopsis orientalis (formerly Nocardia orientalis) and has the molecular formula $C_{66}H_{75}C_{12}N_9O_{24} \cdot HCl$. Vancomycin is poorly absorbed after oral administration; it is given intravenously for the therapy of systemic infections. Intramuscular injection is painful.

Oral Vancomycin is used to treat colitis (inflammation of the intestine caused by certain bacteria) that may occur after antibiotic treatment. Vancomycin is in a class of medications called glycopeptide antibiotics. It works by killing bacteria in the intestines. Vancomycin will not kill bacteria or treat infections in any other part of the body when taken by mouth. Antibiotics will not work for colds, flu, or other viral infections. Vancomycin comes as a capsule to take by mouth. It is usually taken 3-4 times a day for 7-10 days.

Data Mining

Data Mining is an analytic process designed to explore data (usually large amounts of data, typically business, market or healthcare related) in search of consistent patterns and/or systematic relationships between variables, and then to validate the findings by applying the detected patterns to new subsets of data. The ultimate goal of data mining is prediction. Predictive data mining is the most common type of data mining and one that has the most direct applications. The process of data mining consists of three stages: (1) the initial exploration, (2) model building or pattern identification with validation/verification, and (3) deployment (i.e., the application of the model to new data in order to generate predictions). Of course, domain knowledge is necessary before starting these stages. (Statsoft, 2004)

SETTING THE STAGE

The purpose of this study is to consider a cohort of patients undergoing treatment for Osteomyelitis by examining large databases of clinical information and investigating the treatment options for Osteomyelitis. The two main treatments of Osteomyelitis are amputation and long-term antibiotics. We want to determine whether there are limb-preserving treatment choices.

Objective 1 is to consider whether the physicians attempt to eradicate the infection with antibiotics before considering amputation. It is hypothesized that amputation is performed on the patients before considering the antibiotic usage with the recommended duration and dosage.

Table 1. The list of antibiotics included in the survey

No.	Generic Name	Brand Names	Other names
1	Co-trimoxazole	Bactrim®, Septra®	Sulfamethoxazole and Trimethoprim, SMX-TMP, TMP-SMX
2	Clindamycin	Cleocin®, Clinda-Derm®,	Clindagel®, Clindets® Pledgets
3	Doxycycline	Vibramycin®, Doryx®,	Monodox®, Vibra-Tabs®
4	Piperacillin/ Tazobactam	Zosyn®	
5	Various	Vancomycin	Vancocin®
6	Linezolid	Zyvox®	
7	Ciprofloxacin	Cipro®	
8	Levofloxacin	Levaquin®	
9	Rifampin	Rifadin®	Rimactane®

Objective 2 is to investigate whether recommended drugs with recommended lengths of treatment are used. It is hypothesized that there is a difference between actual treatment and recommended treatment. We want to see if patients are getting antibiotic drugs that are not recommended in the literature.

Objective 3 is to consider antibiotic choice and duration used to treat the patient before amputation. Does amputation become sequential because of a failure to eradicate the infection? It is hypothesized that there are many records of infection recurrence in patients with infection. There is a sequence of amputations for most patients due to the failure of treatment.

We will use multiple databases to examine these objectives, starting with the National Inpatient Sample and then using the Thomson MedStat MarketScan data containing all patient claims for 40 million people followed for the years 2000-2001. (The National Inpatient Sample, nd.; Thomson MedStat MarketScan Data, nd).

We first wanted to examine treatment options by surveying healthcare providers. We requested a list of Physicians and Pharmacists from the Kentucky Board of Medical Licensure and the Kentucky Board of Pharmacists, respectively. The surveys were sent out to all Infectious Disease specialists in Kentucky, and we systematically sampled other specialists, including Endocrinology Diabetes & Metabolism, Family Practice, Orthopedic Surgery and General Surgery. Pharmacists were selected randomly from the list of Kentucky Pharmacists. A total of 121 surveys were sent with a 10% response rate. However, the returned surveys were relatively similar in responses. We asked Physicians and Pharmacists to evaluate the antibiotics in their clinical experience as it relates to the treatment of MRSA-infected diabetic foot ulcers. Antibiotics included in the survey are shown in Table 1.

Physicians were asked if they ever used these antibiotics to treat MRSA, and if yes, what time period was used for the treatment of MRSA for Osteomyelitis (bone infection), Deep Tissue Wounds, and Surface Wounds. The survey was reviewed by John Cerrito, Pharm.D., prior to distribution. A copy of the survey is included in the appendix.

We also investigated the medical literature and other Internet sources to see how the drug manufacturers and clinical studies recommended antibiotics for the treatment of MRSA, starting with Medline. (MedlinePlus, n.d.) We used the keywords MRSA + one choice of antibiotic. SAS Enterprise Miner was used to accumulate the study information from other Internet sources such as search.yahoo.com.

Figure 1. Time period in weeks used for the treatment of MRSA for Osteomyelitis

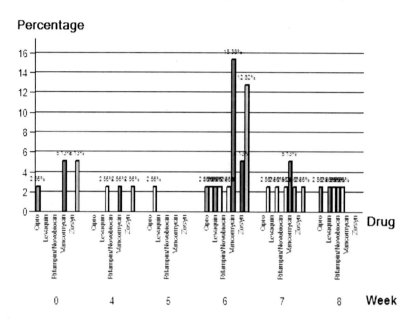

Figure 2. Physicians and Pharmacist who have not used these Antibiotics for Osteomyelitis

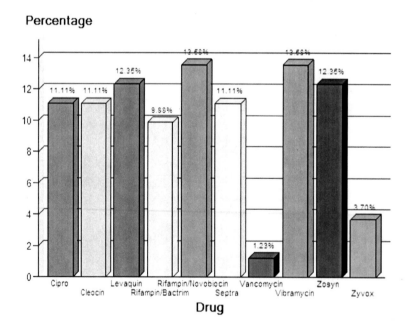

We asked Physicians and Pharmacists to evaluate the antibiotics in their clinical experience as it relates to the treatment of MRSA-infected diabetic foot ulcers. Physicians were asked if they ever used these antibiotics to treat MRSA, and if yes, what time period was used for the treatment of MRSA for Osteomyelitis (bone infection), Deep Tissue Wounds, and Surface Wounds.

Figure 3. Time period in days used for the treatment of MRSA for Deep Tissue Wounds

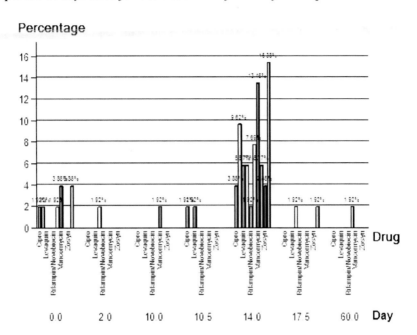

The surveys were transferred to three spreadsheets. The first one contained information related to the drugs used for the treatment of Osteomyelitis, the 2nd listed treatment for deep tissue wounds, and the last one listed the treatment of Surface Wounds. We filtered the data to separate the results for specialists who used the antibiotics to treat MRSA.

Survey Results

Figure 1 shows the length of treatment of Osteomyelitis using different antibiotics. Vancomycin has the highest percentage followed by Zyvox. They are both used for about six weeks to treat MRSA. In this graph, 0 is used to show the physicians who use the named antibiotics, but who did not specify the length of treatment. We also see the highest percentage for Vancomycin and Zyvox in this part of the figure.

Figure 2 shows the statistics of physicians who have not used these antibiotics to treat MRSA. We see that Vancomycin and Zyvox have the lowest percentages since they are the most commonly used antibiotics to treat MRSA for osteomyelitis.

Figure 3 shows the length of treatment of Deep Tissue Wounds using different antibiotics. Zyvox has the highest percentage, with Vancomycin next. They are both used for about 14 days to treat MRSA. In this graph, 0 is used to show the physicians who use the named antibiotics, but who did not specify the length of treatment.

Figure 4 shows the statistics of physicians who have used these antibiotics to treat MRSA. We see that Vancomycin and Zyvox have the lowest percentage since they are the most commonly used antibiotics for MRSA for Deep Tissue Wounds.

Figure 5 shows the length of treatment of Surface Wounds using different antibiotics. Zyvox has the highest percentage followed by Vancomycin, Septra and Levaquin. They are all used for about 10 days to treat MRSA. Cleocin also has the highest percentage for 7 days of treatment. We see other antibiotics are used for different lengths of treatment for Surface Wounds. In this graph, 0 is used to show the physicians who use the named antibiotics but who did not specify

Figure 4. Physicians and Pharmacists who have not used these Antibiotics for Deep Tissue Wounds

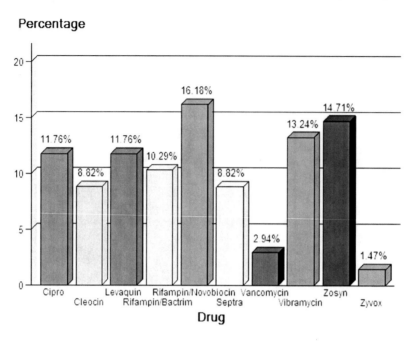

Figure 5. Time period in days used for the treatment of MRSA for Surface Wounds

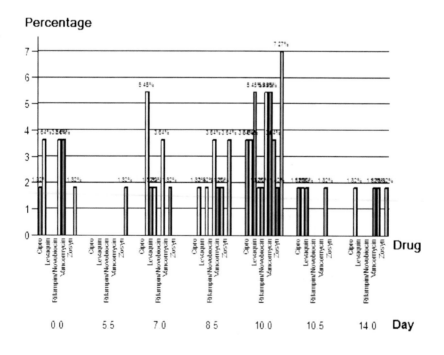

the length of treatment. We also see the highest percentage for Vancomycin, Septra and Cleocin in this part of the figure.

Physicians use different antibiotics for MRSA, and some of these antibiotics are ineffective; they are not recommended in any source to treat MRSA.

Table 2. Clustering the SAS data set in Text Miner (MRSA + Zyvox)

Cluster #	Descriptive Terms	Frequency	Percentage	RMS Std.
1	Zyvox, + cause, + result, + infection, mrsa, back, previsou, + version, + treat, + receive	30	0.117	0.119
2	+ do, + see, + good, + create, + have, + do, + make, + will, + find, + not	68	0.266	0.148
3	+ preference, with, + sign, + add, + save, + tool, + help, + bookmark, guest, mail	139	0.543	0.096
4	+ subscription, + find, + will, all, +service, more, + not, +site, +have, +home	19	0.074	0.146

After comparing the data set from our research, there is a noticeable difference between recommended and actual treatment. We can also see that physicians assume the same length of treatment for all antibiotics even if it is not validated in the literature. Actual treatment will result in a higher rate of amputation because of recurrence of the infection. The current studies of Zyvox and osteomyelitis indicate that treatment should be for 12-15 weeks, not the 6 weeks indicated by physicians in the survey. (Senneville, et.al., 2006, Aneziokoro, et.al., 2005)

Text Analysis on the Web

We also investigated the medical literature and other Internet sources to see how the drug manufacturers and clinical studies recommended antibiotics for the treatment of MRSA, starting with Medline. We used the keywords MRSA + one choice of antibiotic, and repeated this step for all antibiotics in the list. We had no results from our search in Medline except for MRSA + Vancomycin and MRSA + Zyvox (Linezolid). The other antibiotics were not recommended nor approved in the medical literature. Then we searched using some popular search websites such as yahoo.com. The macro, %tmfilter, from Enterprise Miner, was used to accumulate the study information from these other Internet sources. The code below shows an example of the macro, %tmfilter, for searching for "MRSA and Septra":

```
%tmfilter(url=%NRSTR(http://search.ya
hoo.com/search?p=Mrsa+Septra&fr=FP-tab-
webt400&toggle=1&cop=&ei=UTF-8),
depth=2,
dir=c:\micro\dir1,
destdir=c:\micro\destdir1,
norestrict=1,
dataset=sasuser.sepra1, numbers=3200);
```

Text Miner Results

Using SAS Text Miner, we first clustered the website information. Table 2 shows an example of the clustered data set for MRSA + Zyvox. In this example, the first cluster (highlighted) is the only useful cluster. We filtered the cluster(s) to focus on the most relevant information.

We may not always get wanted results from filtering the clusters. Another way to filter our data set is to filter the Terms as shown in Table 3; the result of restricting the terms to MRSA + Zosyn.

We can use the results from filtering the terms and then re-cluster them. Table 4 is another example of re-clustering. It shows the result from clustering the data set from MRSA + Zyvox.

Enterprise Miner lets us study the relationship between the terms as concept links. We can view terms that are highly associated with the selected term in a hyperbolic tree display. The tree display shows the selected term in the center of the tree structure. The selected term is surrounded by the

Table 3. Term Filtered SAS data set in Text Miner (MRSA + Zosyn)

Term	Frequency	# Documents	Role
Mrsa	135	27	Prop
Mrsa	5	4	Adj
Zosyn	55	27	Prop
Zosyn	3	3	Noun
Zosyn ®	6	6	Prop

Table 4. Re-Clustering the SAS data set in Text Miner (MRSA + Zyvox)

Cluster #	Descriptive Terms	Frequency	Percentage	RMS Std.
1	Zyvox, + cause, + result, + infection, mrsa, back, previsou, + version, + treat, + receive	30	0.117	0.119

terms that correlate the strongest with it. Using the tree display, we can select a term associated with the first term to view its associated terms, and so on.

Figure 6 shows an example for the term "mrsa" in search files of "MRSA + Zyvox". Associated terms such as "zyvox", "linezolid", "resistant" and "infection" appear for "mrsa".

We expanded the term, "infection," to view its associated link terms (Figure 7). In this way, we can study the relationship between infection and other terms. These terms are associated with

"mrsa," but not as strongly as terms in Figure 1, since they are associated through the term "infection". This search was for MRSA + Zyvox, but we see vancomycin as one of the terms associated with infection in this search. Pneumonia is another term seen in Figure 7. Pneumonia is another disease that can be caused by MRSA.

Concept links can be used on other terms, too. Figure 8 shows links to the term, "vancomycin". Very similar terms are associated with vancomycin and zyvox. In fact, these two drugs are those most recommended and effective for MRSA.

Figure 6. Concept Links for MRSA in "MRSA + Zyvox" Search

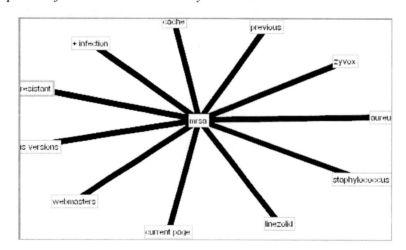

Figure 7. Secondary Concept Links to MRSA and Infection

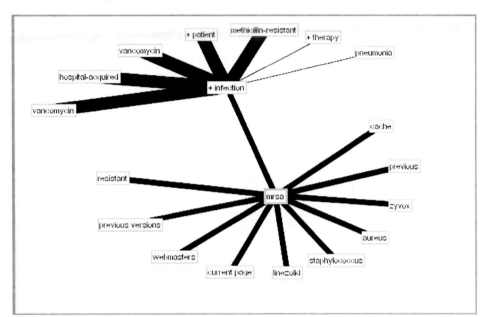

After clustering/filtering our data set, we will have the useful internet files available. We studied the information from the filtered web sites and observed that Vancomycin is the only commonly used antibiotic for the treatment of MRSA for

Osteomyelitis (bone infection) and deep wound with a specific time period of treatment. Zyvox is also recommended for MRSA; other antibiotics were suggested to use to treat MRSA, mostly for skin wounds from community-acquired MRSA as

Figure 8. Concept Links for MRSA in "MRSA + Vancomycin" Search

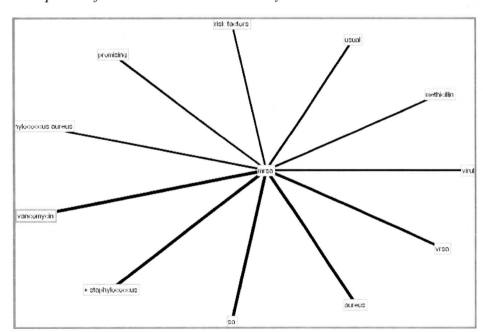

opposed to an infection acquired in the hospital. However, in some other (personal) websites, physicians have different opinions. They are treating (or trying to treat) MRSA with other antibiotics such as Septra, Cleocin, etc. We also have the same results from the survey.

Physicians use different antibiotics for MRSA, and some of these antibiotics are ineffective; they are not recommended in any source to treat MRSA. (Mauldin, After comparing the data set from our research, there is a noticeable difference between recommended and actual treatment. We can also see that physicians assume the same length of treatment for all antibiotics even if the antibiotic has not been approved. Actual treatments used will result in a higher rate of amputation because of recurrence of the infection.

CASE DESCRIPTION

National Inpatient Sample (NIS Data)

We first used NIS data. The NIS (National Inpatient Sample) is part of the Healthcare Cost and Utilization Project (HCUP), sponsored by the Agency for Healthcare Research and Quality (AHRQ), formerly the Agency for Health Care Policy and Research. (NIS, n.d.) The NIS is a database of hospital inpatient stays. Researchers and policymakers use the NIS to identify, track, and analyze national trends in health care utilization, access, charges, quality, and outcomes.

The NIS is the largest all-payer inpatient care database that is publicly available in the United States, containing data from 5 to 8 million hospital stays from about 1,000 hospitals sampled to approximate a 20-percent stratified sample of U.S. community hospitals. The NIS is available for a 17-year time period, from 1988 to 2004, allowing analyses of trends over time.

The NIS is the only national hospital database with charge information on all patients, regardless of payer, including persons covered by Medicare,

Medicaid, private insurance, and the uninsured. The NIS's large sample size enables analyses of rare conditions, such as congenital anomalies; uncommon treatments, such as organ transplantation and special patient populations, such as the uninsured.

Inpatient stay records in the NIS include clinical and resource use information typically available from discharge abstracts. Hospital and discharge weights are provided for producing national estimates. The NIS can be linked to hospital-level data from the American Hospital Association's Annual Survey of Hospitals and county-level data from the Bureau of Health Professions' Area Resource File, except in those states that do not allow the release of hospital identifiers.

The data files had to be expanded and converted to SAS format. The SAS code was provided with the NIS data. PROC FORMAT was used for this procedure. All discharges from sampled hospitals are included in the NIS database.

There are over 110 variables in this dataset. The variables are in the form of characters or numbers. Variables such as AGE (Age in years at admission), AMONTH (Admission month), DRG (DRG in effect on discharge date), TOTCHG (Total charges) are in number format and variables such as DX1 (Principal diagnosis), DX2 to DX15 (Diagnosis2 to 15), PR1 (Principal procedure), PR2 to PR15 (Procedures 2 to 15) are in character format. Most studies consider the Principle diagnosis and Principle procedure only; however, there is other important information in columns of diagnosis 2 to 15 that also contain diagnosis codes, and also procedures 2 to 15, representing procedures that have been performed on patients. Other datasets have similar codes that may differ in total number. Working with only one nominal variable with thousands of levels is already complicated; considering all fifteen variables is an even more difficult problem. In this project, we try to filter this large, healthcare database to a cohort of patients undergoing treatment for Osteomyelitis. We consider these codes as characters and introduce a method using SAS Text Miner that gives us a summary of these fields.

We used these datasets from NIS to investigate a summary of the treatment of osteomyelitis. We had five years of data, 2000 to 2004. Each year of data included about 8 million records. We filtered the patients who have Osteomyelitis (bone infection) or amputation using the DRG codes 113, 114, 213, 238 and 285. The Diagnosis-Related Groups (DRG) coding is used in health care data to group different diagnoses. The codes translate to

DRG 113: Amputation for circ system disorders except upper limb & toe

DRG 114: Upper limb & toe amputation for circ system disorders

DRG 213: Amputation for musculoskeletal system & conn tissue disorders

DRG 238: Osteomyelitis

DRG 285: Amputation of lower limb for endocrine, nitrite & metabol disorders

After preprocessing the data, we had 117,577 patient records involving Osteomyelitis with or without amputation.

Diagnosis codes are given in a variety of digits/characters. The codes have a 3-digit stem (diagnosis codes) and 2-digits for specifics. Procedure codes have a 2-digit stem. For example, the code "84" represents "Procedures on musculoskeletal system", 84.1 represents "Amputation of lower limb" and 84.11 is for "Amputation of toe". The decimal point is omitted in the data columns in the dataset. There are also some codes starting with the letter "V" or "E". It is not possible to treat these codes as numbers and they have to be considered as strings of characters. Working with these types of datasets requires a large amount of time for preprocessing.

The best way to work with all fifteen variables is to bring all of them into one column as a string of codes, using the CATX function, which concatenates character strings, removes leading and trailing blanks, and inserts separators. (SAS,

2008) The expression below shows an example of using this function to create a text string for the procedure codes.

```
CATX (' ', finalhcup.PR1, finalhcup.PR2,
..., finalhcup.PR15)
```

This expression makes a string of codes from Column PR1 to PR15 with a space between them. We also do the same for the fifteen diagnosis variables. As a result, we have two new columns carrying strings of procedures and diagnoses. This substring contains all information of PR1 to PR15, so we use it to find the match codes for osteomyelitis.

We were interested in Osteomyelitis only, so we needed to keep the records that have an Osteomyelitis code (730) in any of the fifteen columns of diagnosis. We filtered the created text strings with a defined diagnosis substring containing 730, using the code:

```
data sasuser.Osteomyelitis;
set sasuser.Query_For_finalhcup;
if (rxmatch('730',STR_DX) > 0) then os-
teom=1;
else osteom=0;
run;
```

We created a new column that indicates whether a patient is diagnosed with Osteomyelitis or not. We may count the number of patients with Osteomyelitis by filtering the data on the defined column as 1. In the filtered dataset, we have 44,035 records containing at least one diagnosis for Osteomyelitis. To consider the patients with amputation of lower limb (841), we should use the similar code for the string of procedures and create a column to indicate whether patients had amputation or not, using the code below:

```
data sasuser.amputation;
set sasuser.Query_For_Osteomyelitis;
if (rxmatch('841',STR_PR) > 0) then
```

```
amp=1;
else amp=0;
run;
```

Then we count the number of records that have a one to represent amputation. There were a total of 22,662 patients with amputation of lower limb (841). To investigate other diagnoses and/ or other procedures, we need to repeat the above procedure to get the result.

We examined all occurrences of osteomyelitis in the National Inpatient Sample by filtering DRG 238, consisting of 20,177 inpatient visits without amputation from 2000-2004, the last year available. We identify patient severity based upon secondary diagnosis, and determine how severity relates to a patient's length of stay in the treatment of osteomyelitis. We also examined the identified procedures that are used to treat the infection. We use data mining techniques and exploratory analysis to examine the treatment differences.

Of the 20,177 cases, 12,304 are identified as located in the lower leg and/or foot. The primary procedure for the treatment of osteomyelitis is venous catheterization for 5368 patients, antibi-

otic infusion for 417 patients, joint aspiration for 460 patients, drainage of skin and subcutaneous tissue for 860 patients, and blood transfusion for 384 patients. One patient only had a primary procedure of 00.14, or an infusion of Zyvox for the treatment of the infection; three others had it as a secondary procedure out of the 20,177. A total of 888 had previous leg or foot amputations; 57 had previous upper extremity amputations, suggesting recurrence requiring more aggressive treatment.

Text Miner Results

An alternative approach is to use SAS Text Miner. We use the dataset, including the concatenated columns defined using the CATX function in Enterprise Miner. Then, we use SAS Text Miner on the defined text string; since we work with numbers (ICD9 codes), we need to change the default setting on Text Miner and switch Numbers from No to Yes. We also need to change "Different Parts of Speech" from Yes to No, so we can put the codes with or without the letters "V" and "E" in an equivalent group. Figure 9 shows the changes to the default settings for Text Miner.

Figure 9. Changing the default setting for text mining

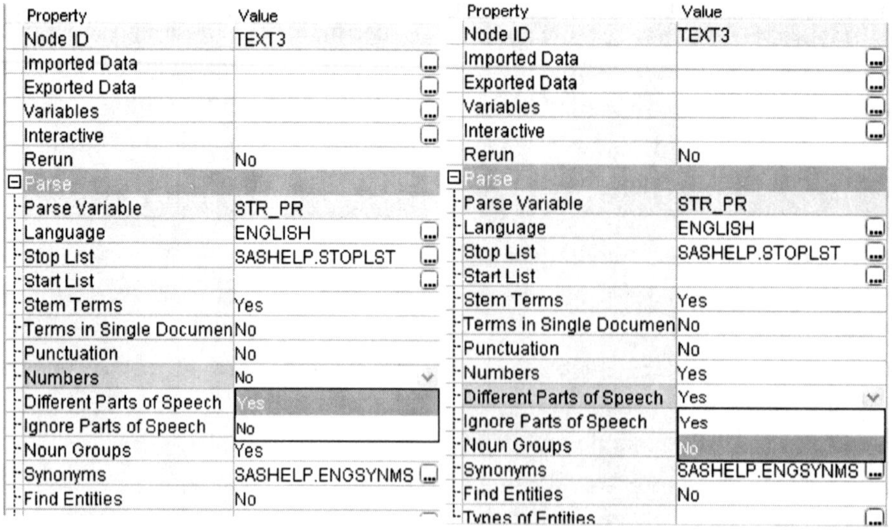

Property	Value			Property	Value	
Node ID	TEXT3			Node ID	TEXT3	
Imported Data		...		Imported Data		...
Exported Data		...		Exported Data		...
Variables		...		Variables		...
Interactive		...		Interactive		...
Rerun	No			Rerun	No	
⊟ Parse				⊟ Parse		
Parse Variable	STR_PR			Parse Variable	STR_PR	
Language	ENGLISH	...		Language	ENGLISH	...
Stop List	SASHELP.STOPLST	...		Stop List	SASHELP.STOPLST	...
Start List		...		Start List		...
Stem Terms	Yes			Stem Terms	Yes	
Terms in Single Documen	No			Terms in Single Documen	No	
Punctuation	No			Punctuation	No	
Numbers	No	⌄		Numbers	Yes	
Different Parts of Speech	Yes			Different Parts of Speech	Yes	⌄
Ignore Parts of Speech	No			Ignore Parts of Speech	Yes	
Noun Groups	Yes			Noun Groups	No	
Synonyms	SASHELP.ENGSYNMS	...		Synonyms	SASHELP.ENGSYNMS	...
Find Entities	No			Find Entities	No	
				Types of Entities		...

The terms window in the output gives the frequency and number of documents for each code. We were interested in Osteomyelitis only, so we needed to keep the records that have an Osteomyelitis code (730) in any of the fifteen columns of diagnosis. Thus, we filtered in Text Miner where the defined diagnosis substring contained 730. We did this by right clicking on the document window and using the option of "Filter Where Documents" as shown in Figure 10.

We then choose the strings of diagnosis codes containing 730 to filter the selected rows from the documents as shown in Figure 11.

After filtering, we had 44,035 patients with Osteomyelitis in this dataset. Osteomyelitis (730) might have been recorded in any of fifteen columns of diagnosis codes.

Now we have the dataset that contains patients with Osteomyelitis and we need to investigate the procedures that have been done on these patients, especially amputation in the lower limb (841). In this case, the codes we have to consider are 841, 8410, 8411, 8412 ... 8419. The fourth digit indicates the location of the amputation in the lower limb.

We sort the results by Terms to find these codes. We have the number of patients for each of these codes, but there are some patients who have more than one of these procedures, so if we add all the numbers of these rows, we might count some patients twice or more. To avoid this, we treat these terms as equivalent by selecting them and then right clicking on terms and choosing "Treat as Equivalent Terms" as shown in Figure 12. We choose 8410 to represents this group.

Out of 44,035 patients with Osteomyelitis, 22,649 patients (over 51%) had an Amputation of the lower limb (84.1).

To see what procedures have been done on these patients, we sort by the number of documents in the Terms window. We have the group of 84.1 (amputation of lower limb) with 22,649 patients and 38.93 (Venous catheterization) with 11,341 patients in the first two places followed by 9904 (Transfusion of packed cells) with 4,302 patients, 8622 (Excisional debridement of wound, infection, or burn) with 3,907 patients, 3995 (Hemodialysis) with 2,787 patients and 843 (Revision of amputation stump) with 2408 patients. The sorted results are shown in Table 5.

Figure 10. Document window; select "filter where documents" for filtering

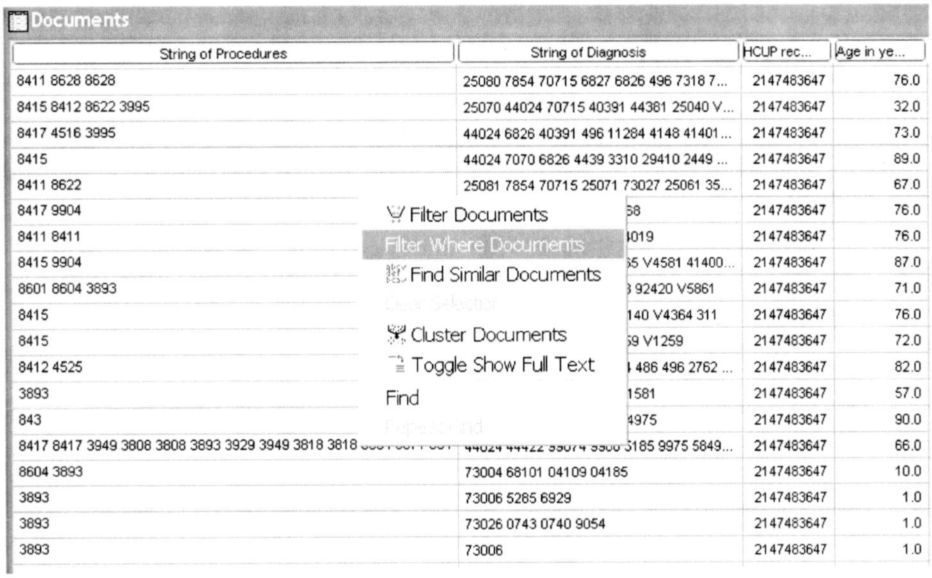

String of Procedures	String of Diagnosis	HCUP rec...	Age in ye...
8411 8628 8628	25080 7854 70715 6827 6826 496 7318 7...	2147483647	76.0
8415 8412 8622 3995	25070 44024 70715 40391 44381 25040 V...	2147483647	32.0
8417 4516 3995	44024 6826 40391 496 11284 4148 41401...	2147483647	73.0
8415	44024 7070 6826 4439 3310 29410 2449 ...	2147483647	89.0
8411 8622	25081 7854 70715 25071 73027 25061 35...	2147483647	67.0
8417 9904	58	2147483647	76.0
8411 8411	019	2147483647	76.0
8415 9904	5 V4581 41400...	2147483647	87.0
8601 8604 3893	92420 V5861	2147483647	71.0
8415	140 V4364 311	2147483647	76.0
8415	9 V1259	2147483647	72.0
8412 4525	486 496 2762 ...	2147483647	82.0
3893	1581	2147483647	57.0
843	4975	2147483647	90.0
8417 8417 3949 3808 3808 3893 3929 3949 3818 3818	44024 44422 35074 3500 5185 9975 5849...	2147483647	66.0
8604 3893	73004 68101 04109 04185	2147483647	10.0
3893	73006 5285 6929	2147483647	1.0
3893	73026 0743 0740 9054	2147483647	1.0
3893	73006	2147483647	1.0

Filter Documents
Filter Where Documents
Find Similar Documents
Cluster Documents
Toggle Show Full Text
Find

Figure 11. Filtering for osteomyelitis (ICD9 code 730)

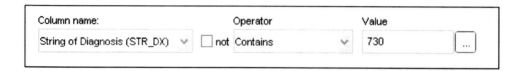

Figure 12. Treating as equivalent terms and choosing a representation for them

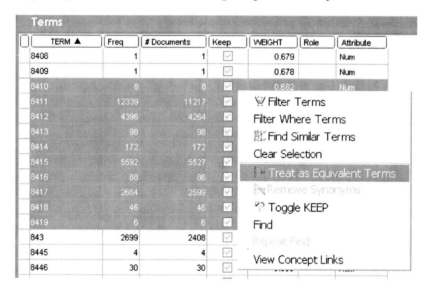

Table 5. Sorted table of terms by number of documents

Term	Translation	Frequency	# of Patients
8410	Lower limb amputation, not otherwise specified	25409	11649
3893	Venous catheterization, not elsewhere classified	11832	11341
9904	Transfusion of packed cells	4442	4302
8622	Excisional debridement of wound, infection, or burn	4756	3907
3995	Hemodialysis	3146	2787
843	Revision of amputation stump	2699	2408
8604	Other incision with drainage of skin and subcutaneous tissue	2198	2057
9921	Injection of antibiotic	1869	1836
8848	Arteriography of femoral and other lower extremity arteries	1887	1787
8628	Nonexcisional debridement of wound, infection or burn	1232	1116
8842	Aortography	1039	1030
9214	Bone scan	1039	1026

We also investigated the previous amputations as identified in the diagnosis codes; we took the resulting dataset from Text Miner and did the text mining again, but this time on the strings of diagnoses to find the number of patients with previous amputations.

From the total of 44,035 patients, 4,673 patients had previous amputation. We used ICD9 codes of 895, 905.9, and 997.6, E878.5, V49.6 and V49.7 to find previous amputations.

These ICD9 codes translate to:

895 Traumatic amputation of toe(s) (complete) (partial)
905.9 Late effect of traumatic amputation

997.6 Amputation stump complication
E878.5 Amputation of limb(s)
V49.6 Upper limb amputation status
V49.7 Lower limb amputation status

Table 6 shows the terms for the above ICD9 codes.

We also considered previous amputations for the patient with current amputation, so we filtered the procedure codes with ICD9 Codes of 84.1 and 84.3 as shown in Figure 13.

84.1 Amputation of lower limb
84.3 Revision of amputation stump

Table 6. Previous amputations of patients with osteomyelitis

Term	Translation	Frequency	Number of Documents
V4970	Lower limb amputation status (unspecified level)	5745	4673
V4966	Upper limb amputation status (above elbow)	3	3
V4960	Upper limb amputation status (unspecified level)	3	3
99760	Amputation stump complication (type unspecified)	16	16
E8785	Surgical operation and other surgical procedures as the cause of abnormal reaction of patient, or of later complication, without mention of misadventure at the time of operation (amputation of limbs)	539	505
V4973	Lower limb amputation status (foot)	197	197
V4965	Upper limb amputation status (below elbow)	5	5
V4961	Upper limb amputation status (thumb)	5	5
V4970	Lower limb amputation status (unspecified level)	22	22
V4974	Lower limb amputation status (ankle)	5	5
99769	Amputation stump complication	691	691
V4977	Lower limb amputation status (hip)	6	6
99762	Amputation stump complication (chronic infection)	1742	1742
9059	Late effect of traumatic amputation	6	6
V4972	Lower limb amputation status (other toe(s))	837	837
99761	Neuroma of amputation stump	9	9
V4975	Lower limb amputation status (below knee)	896	896
V4971	Lower limb amputation status (great toe)	338	338
V4976	Lower limb amputation status (above knee)	368	368
8951	Traumatic amputation of toe(s) (complete) (partial) (complicated)	3	3
V4962	Upper limb amputation status (finger(s))	49	49
V4963	Upper limb amputation status (hand)	3	3

Figure 13. Filtering for amputation (ICD9 codes 841 or 843)

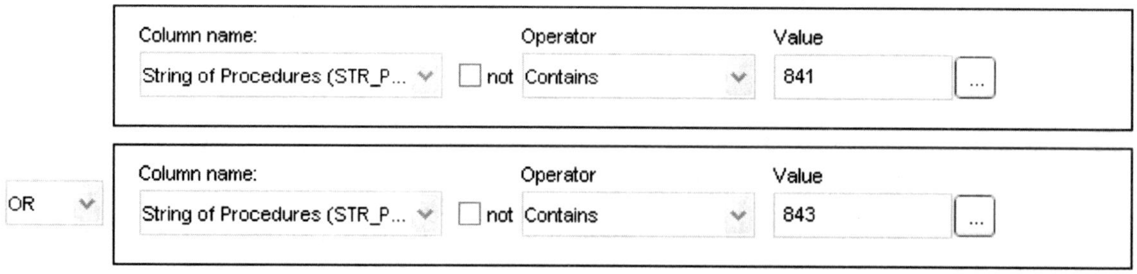

We have a total of 23,773 patients. There are 3,586 patients with previous amputation (ICD9 Codes of 895, 905.9, and 997.6, E878.5, V49.6 and V49.7). Table 7 shows the terms table of the results for these patients.

Previous amputation shows that amputation did not eliminate the problem completely, and the patients have to come back for another (current) amputation. In other words, amputation did not prevent the recurrence of infection.

There are some effective antibiotics to treat Osteomyelitis. Our results show that Amputation was assumed to be the primary treatment of Osteomyelitis. Of the 44,035 patients, 22,649 patients had an amputation of a lower limb and 1,836 patients had an injection of antibiotics (ICD9 code 99.21). Only 10 patients had an Injection or infusion of the Oxazolidinone class of antibiotics (Linezolid injection) with ICD9 code 00.14. Comparing the number of patients with amputation and the number of patients with antibiotic injections, we observed that in many cases, amputation is performed without trying the different antibiotics for treatment of Osteomyelitis before or after amputation.

Some antibiotics must be used in hospitals, and by having the supervision of experts, for example, Vancomycin and some antibiotics can be used orally at home. However, as the amputation was performed in the hospital, the antibiotic should be started then. Choosing the right antibiotics and the right length of treatment are very important parts of the treatment. Making the right choice of antibiotics will decrease the number of amputations in the treatment of Osteomyelitis.

We started with 117,577 records (patients). After filtering down to Osteomyelitis using the strings of diagnosis codes, we reduced the dataset to 44,035 records. By looking at procedure codes, we found 22,649 cases have had amputation, which is more than half (51%) of the patients with Osteomyelitis.

We can also sort the result in Text Miner by the number of documents and see that the first two procedures that were performed on patients with Osteomyelitis are 84.1 (Amputation of lower limb) with 22,649 patients and 38.93 (Venous catheterization) with 11,341 patients. We found only 3,133 patients with an injection of antibiotics and only 10 patients with Linezolid (Zyvox) injection.

Considering the result on this particular dataset, amputation was performed the most frequently compared to other procedures for patients with Osteomyelitis. Physicians assume amputation is the first (and best) treatment for Osteomyelitis. Injection of antibiotics was performed on only about 4% of the patients with Osteomyelitis. In many cases, infection has recurred and amputation was performed more than once.

MarketScan Database Overview

The MarketScan Databases capture person specific *clinical utilization, expenditures, and enrollment across inpatient, outpatient, prescription drug,*

Table 7. Previous amputations of patients with current amputation

Term	Translation	Frequency	Number of Documents
V4970	Lower limb amputation status (unspecified level)	4511	3586
V4971	Lower limb amputation status (great toe)	226	226
99762	Amputation stump complication (chronic infection)	1595	1595
e8785	Surgical operation and other surgical procedures as the cause of abnormal reaction of patient, or of later complication, without mention of misadventure at the time of operation (amputation of limbs)	506	474
V4972	Lower limb amputation status (other toe(s))	554	554
V4975	Lower limb amputation status (below knee)	599	599
99769	Amputation stump complication	646	646
V4970	Lower limb amputation status (unspecified level)	7	7
99761	Neuroma of amputation stump	8	8
9059	Late effect of traumatic amputation	6	6
V4966	Upper limb amputation status (above elbow)	1	1
V4973	Lower limb amputation status (foot)	130	130
V4976	Lower limb amputation status (above knee)	190	190
V4974	Lower limb amputation status (ankle)	2	2
V4965	Upper limb amputation status (below elbow)	2	2
V4962	Amputation stump complication (chronic infection)	19	19
99760	Amputation stump complication (type unspecified)	12	12
V4961	Upper limb amputation status (thumb)	3	3
V4963	Upper limb amputation status (hand)	2	2
8951	Traumatic amputation of toe(s) (complete) (partial) (complicated)	3	3

and carve-out services from approximately 45 large employers, health plans, and government and public organizations. The MarketScan Databases link paid claims and encounter data to detailed patient information across sites and types of providers over time. The annual medical databases include private sector health data from approximately 100 payers. Historically, more than 500 million claim records are available in the MarketScan Databases. These data represent the medical experience of insured employees and their dependents for active employees and early retirees, COBRA continues and Medicare-eligible retirees with employer-provided Medicare Supplemental plans. (Thomson, n.d.)

Diagnosis Codes in MarketScan data use the International Classification of Disease, 9th Division, Clinical Modifications (ICD-9-CM) classification system. Up to two diagnosis codes (DX1, DX2) are recorded on every Inpatient Service record. The principal diagnosis on the Inpatient Admissions Table is generally identified as the discharge diagnosis on a hospital claim. Up to 14 secondary diagnosis codes (DX2 through DX15) from individual Inpatient Service records are included on the corresponding Inpatient Admission record. Up to two diagnosis codes (DX1, DX2) are recorded on each Outpatient Service record.

Procedure Codes in MarketScan data are three to five digits in length depending on the classification system used. The CPT-4 (Current Procedural Terminology, 4th Edition) coding system is most prevalent. CPT-4 procedure codes appear on physician claims and many outpatient facility claims. CPT-4 codes are five-digit numeric codes. ICD-9-CM procedure codes are found on hospital claims. These codes are three to four digits in length and are all numeric. There is an implied decimal between the second and third digits.

HCPCS (HCFA Common Procedural Coding System) procedure codes are found less often than CPT and ICD procedure codes in the MarketScan data. These codes are five digits in length. The first character is alpha; all other characters are numeric. HCPCS codes beginning with "J" are included in the MarketScan databases and represent injectable drugs. One procedure code (PROC1) is stored on each Inpatient Service record. From the individual Inpatient Services comprising one Inpatient Admission record, one procedure code is identified and assigned as the principal procedure (PPROC). Up to 14 secondary procedure codes (PROC2 through PROC15) from individual Inpatient Service records are included on the corresponding Inpatient Admission record. One procedure code (PROC1) is included on each Outpatient Service record.

The variable, PROCTYP (Procedure Code Type), identifies the type of procedure code (HCPCS, CPT-4, etc.). We use this variable in conjunction with the PROC1 (Procedure Code 1) variables on the Inpatient Service and Outpatient Service records to designate the coding system of interest. The quality of diagnosis and procedure coding varies among the approximately 100 payers or administrators represented in the MarketScan Databases.

We can define a group of procedures and treat them as one episode to investigate the frequency of occurrence. In many studies, only the primary procedure and diagnosis are considered when there is more than one procedure and/or diagnosis column, since important information could be in those other columns. In our database used for the study, there are fifteen procedure and fifteen diagnosis columns that we use to find episodes of patient care. We also combine information from multiple datasets: inpatient, outpatient, and phar-

macy information. Another approach is to consider a sequence of treatments on patients and to study the effectiveness of treatment by looking at this sequence for each patient. Studying the physician decisions and the results of them is interesting to many health care organizations.

We want to find the frequency of a given input (code) for a variable, or more than one variable in health care data. Using the Thomson MedStat MarketScan data containing all patient claims for 40 million observations, the primary diagnosis code is given for each patient as well as fifteen possible secondary diagnoses. We use SAS Text Miner to demonstrate a simplified method to search these fifteen columns. We use ICD9 and CPT codes to find treatments for osteomyelitis. We also look for sequential treatments for recurrence of osteomyelitis.

The quality of diagnosis and procedure coding varies among the approximately 100 payers or administrators represented in the MarketScan Databases. We want to find the frequency of a given input (code) for a variable, or more than one variable in the health care data. Using the Thomson MedStat MarketScan data containing all patient claims for 40 million observations, the primary diagnosis code is given for each patient as well as fourteen possible secondary diagnoses.

We need to filter patients with osteomyelitis and we have to consider all fifteen diagnosis columns. Inpatient Services data have been given in two different data files, so we will filter each of them to find osteomyelitis and then append the data into one file.

The best way to work with all fifteen variables is to bring all of them into one column as a string of codes, using the CATX function, which concatenates character strings, removes leading and trailing blanks, and inserts separators. (SAS, n.d.) The expression below shows an example of using this function to create a text string for the diagnosis codes.

```
CATX (' ', ccaei001.DX1, ccaei001.DX2, …,
ccaei001.DX15)
```

This expression makes a string of codes from Column DX1 to DX15 with a space between them. We also do the same for the fifteen procedure variables. As a result, we have two new columns carrying strings of procedures and diagnoses. We can use this column to identify patients with a specific diagnosis or procedure.

We were interested in Osteomyelitis only, so we needed to keep the records that have an Osteomyelitis code (730) in any of the fifteen columns of diagnosis. This code can be recorded with extra detail. For example, code 730.0 means "Acute Osteomyelitis" and it is recorded in data as 7300, without the decimal point, or 7302 for "Unspecified Osteomyelitis". This is the main reason we do not consider the numerical value of these codes and treat them as characters. We filtered the created text strings, where a defined diagnosis substring contains 730.

We created a new column that indicates whether a patient is diagnosed with Osteomyelitis or not. We may count the number of patients with Osteomyelitis by filtering the data on the defined column as 1. In the filtered dataset, we have 18,721 records containing at least one diagnosis for Osteomyelitis.

We would like to study the patients with amputation and summarize the statistics of these patients; we need to use the procedure codes in our dataset; however, these procedures have been recorded with a different code format than is given in the PROCTYP variable. We have ICD-9-CM, CPT and HCPCS formats. We split these data in three parts in order to do the analysis using the appropriate formatting. About 90% of our filtered data is in CPT format. After filtering the data for Osteomyelitis, there are 18,721 observations in Inpatients and 233,001 observations in Outpatients.

We have repeated observations in our data for the same patients, so the number of records in the data does NOT represent the number of patients. We can use "Summary Statistics" in SAS Enterprise Guide to find the number of patients in each part of the data. We take patient ID (PATID) as the Analysis Variable and for the Classification Variable; we also use patient ID.

There are total of 78,957 patients in outpatients data filtered for osteomyelitis. We found 498 Amputations in the outpatient data. There are a total of 2,661 patients in inpatients filtered data. We found 773 amputations in the inpatients data. It appears to have the rate of about 30% for amputation in inpatients with osteomyelitis as patient procedures with counting repeated amputations for each patient. There are not many amputations performed on an outpatient basis, as is expected.

Now we have a dataset with repeated observations. We counted the non-repeated number of patients using the above methods; however, we need to follow the procedures performed on each patient with the procedure date. In other words, we need to have a one-to-many relationship between patients and their procedures (instead of many-to-many).

We combine the results from the above programs to have a data file including procedures and their dates together. This coding was repeated for outpatient data; as a result, we have a clean dataset with one observation for each patient containing all the procedures and procedure dates for them.

Now we use this dataset in Text Miner and consider the terms that show different types of amputation. We look at the number of patients versus amputations. For example, there are 608 amputations for 198 patients in Inpatients data, which is the average of about 3 per patient, and 495 amputations for 202 patients in Outpatients data, the average of about 2.5 amputations per patient receiving an amputation. It shows that there must be a sequence of amputations for some patients.

We would like to study the disease progress in patients by looking at the amputations. We use the program below on the dataset that results from the above program that contains one observation per patient with their procedures and the date of service. We look for the switch in codes when the amputation changes from one part to a (usually) higher part of the body. For example, the amputation of toe switched to amputation of foot. We also wanted to detect the amputations that have the same code, but were performed on different dates as the infection progresses. For example, amputation of toe is different from amputation of (another) toe on a different date. (Cerrito, PC and Cerrito, JC, 2008)

The variable, proc_num, in this program shows the number of amputations for each patient. In the result of the above code, we see that there are patients with up to 14 amputations. There are more than 22% of these patients with sequences of amputations (more than one amputation). Note that these are data for the years 2000 and 2001, only two years of data. There probably are more amputations for the same patients in years after 2001 for which we do not have access. This rate of sequential amputation is high for two years of data. We study the treatment of patients with osteomyelitis using different antibiotics by examination of the pharmacy data. We studied 8 different

antibiotics for osteomyelitis and focused on those antibiotics. The prescription data are available in ten different data files. We filtered our data for the eight antibiotics to study the treatment of osteomyelitis.

There are two variables specifying the drug used in the treatment; one is the NDC number (NDCNUM) and another one is the generic product ID (GENERID). The converter for NDC numbers is available at the FDA website. (FDA, n.d.) There are many NDC numbers for each drug due to their dosage and type, and there are a few Generic ID values. Therefore, it is faster to use generic IDs; however, we had no information about Generic IDs. We found the Generic IDs of each antibiotic using NDC numbers in two or three datasets (out of ten) and then filtered the rest using those Generic IDs. We appended all ten filtered datasets in the end.

We created a column "drug" containing the name of the antibiotic to make the analysis easier. We combined all datasets resulting from the above procedure to have one file containing all RX data for our study.

We use programming similar to what we used for procedures, but this time for antibiotic so as to follow the antibiotics prescribed for each

Figure 14. Joining two data files in enterprise guide

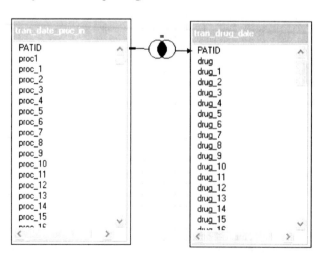

patient with the date. In other words, we need to have a one-to-many relationship between patients and their prescriptions (instead of many-to-many).

We have a dataset containing all patients who have been treated with one of eight listed antibiotics; however, we need to focus on osteomyelitis in our study, so we use the filtered dataset of osteomyelitis patients to join with these data, and as

Table 8. Result of text mining RX data filtered for patients with osteomyelitis

Antibiotics	No. of Prescriptions	No. of Patients
Septra	89	33
Cleocin	88	51
Vancomycin	37	8
Zyvox	27	8
Rifampin	24	6
Levaquin	9	4
Zosyn	7	3
Vibramycin	4	3

a result, we will have information about patients with osteomyelitis, including their procedures and prescriptions in the same dataset. In this section, we will focus on antibiotics, so we only keep the drug column of the joined table with patient IDs (Figure 14).

After summarizing the resulting data in Text Miner, we see that the total number of prescriptions is more than three times the number of patients, meaning that each patient had an average of three prescriptions. Table 8 below shows the number of prescriptions and the number of patients for each antibiotic.

Figure 15 shows the same information in graphical form. Note that the total number of prescriptions is nowhere close to the number of patients with osteomyelitis.

Now we filter for Zyvox and patients who had Zyvox as one of their prescriptions.

We see the results in Table 9. There are only eight patients treated with Zyvox, and they have been treated with other antibiotics such as Septra, Rifampin, Cleocin and Zosyn.

Figure 15. Graph of the result for all antibiotics

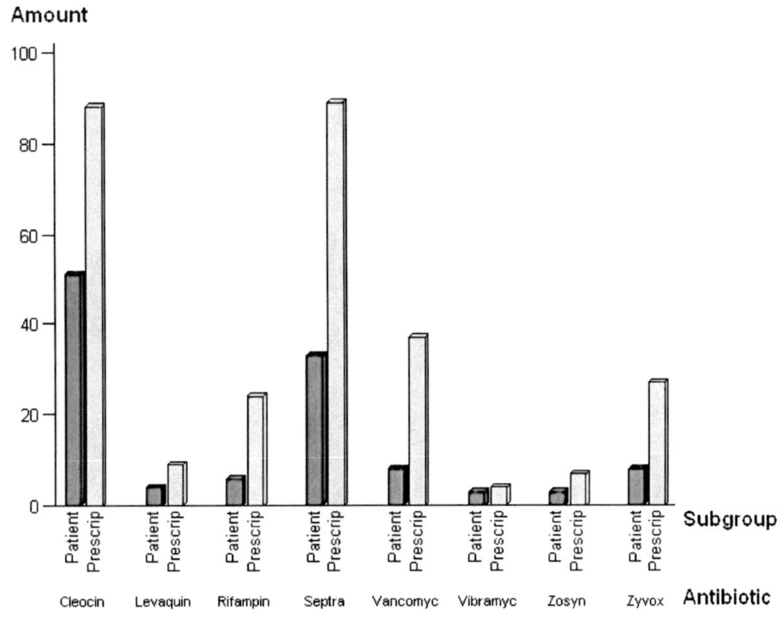

Table 9. Terms remaining after filtering the result of text mining for Zyvox

Antibiotics	No. of Prescriptions	No. of Patients
Zyvox	27	8
Septra	19	4
Rifampin	15	2
Cleocin	9	5
Zosyn	1	1

Table 10. Terms remaining after filtering the result of text mining for Vancomycin

Antibiotics	No. of Prescriptions	No. of Patients
Vancomycin	37	8
Septra	5	2
Zosyn	2	1
Rifampin	2	1
Cleocin	1	1
Vibramycin	1	1

The graph of the result is shown in Figure 16.

We can also study the patients treated with Vancomycin by filtering the data for vancomycin. The result is shown in Table 10 and Figure 17.

With the same method, we can find the patients who have not been treated with either Zyvox or Vancomycin as shown in Figure 18.

The result of above filtering is shown in Table 11 and Figure 19.

As we see, there are many patients treated with antibiotics other than Zyvox and Vancomycin, the opposite of what was recommended in the literature for resistant infection.

If we cluster the results of text mining, we get only two clusters, since there are not many terms in the data. One cluster has Zyvox and another one contains Vancomycin as was expected, since these two are the most effective antibiotics. Note that both clusters contain Septra. We assume Septra was used in the beginning of treatment, and due to its ineffectiveness, treatment switched to other antibiotics. The clusters are shown in Table 12.

One factor in the treatment of osteomyelitis is antibiotic choice from the beginning of the treatment. We may study the switch in prescriptions in our data using the same method we used in

Figure 16. Graph of result after filtering for Zyvox

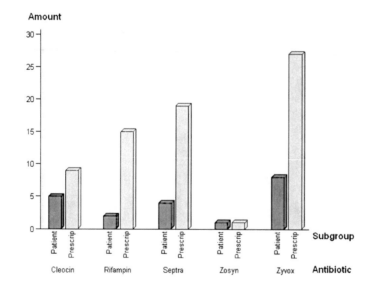

Figure 17. Graph of result after filtering for Vancomycin

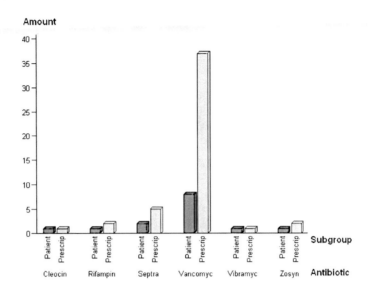

Figure 18. Filtering the text string of drugs for Zyvox and Vancomycin

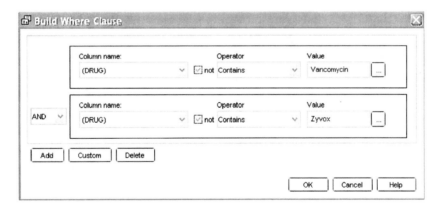

switching the procedures to find the number of different amputations.

There are up to 16 switches of antibiotics in the treatment of osteomyelitis. Note that if a patient is on Septra, for example, and switched to Levaquin, it counts as one switch; if the same patient switched back to Septra, we count it as another switch. We have the rate of about 27% of the total number of patients who had a switch in their prescriptions. This rate is 20% in Inpatient data and 35.5% in Outpatients. We also can find the switch for a specific medication such as zyvox

Table 11. Result of filtering the text string of drugs for Zyvox and Vancomycin

Antibiotics	No. of Prescription	No. of Patient
Cleocin	78	45
Septra	65	27
Levaquin	9	4
Rifampin	7	3
Zosyn	4	1
Vibramycin	3	2

Figure 19. Graph of result after filtering

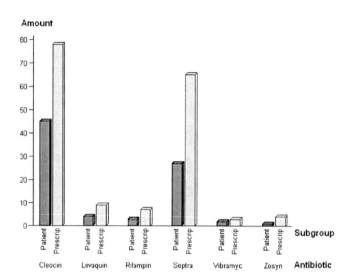

Table 12. Clustering the text mining result of RX data for patients with Osteomyelitis

Cluster Number	Descriptive Terms
1	Zyvox, levaquin, cleocin, septra, rifampin
2	Vancomycin, vibramycin, zosyn, septra

or vancomycin. This censoring will let us find the change of medication.

We can now apply survival analysis. We let time = 0 for the start date of January 1, 2000. We assume that future medication choice depends on the present medications and not the past medications. We use the code below;

```
PROC LIFETEST DATA=Medstat.medication
data ALPHA=0.05;
BY medchange;
STRATA drug_1;
TIME date_num * censor (1);
RUN;
```

We have the data from years 2000 and 2001. This does not show the long term treatment and we do not get very meaningful results from the

code above; however, this method can be used if more data are available. In this small population, most drugs have the 100% or near 100% censored, meaning they have not been switched to another medication. This does not mean the drugs were effective, but we do not have enough switches of medications. We filter for the patients with a second medication and then find the third medication, given that patients have already used two medications.

Since we filtered to patients with a second medication, our dataset is even smaller and again, it is very hard to get meaningful information from these data. Note that for a larger dataset, we could even study the fourth switch, and so on. We have to see if finding the next switch will be helpful or not.

We consider the date difference to be the minimum elapsed time between a procedure and switching medications. Table 13 shows the summary statistics of date difference (diff). The mean is 127 days and the median is 93 days.

We study the kernel density estimation in Figure 20. It shows that the peak of the distribution occurs in about 60 days with a tail up to 420 days.

Table 13. Summary statistics of date difference (diff)

Basic Statistical Measures			
Location		Variability	
Mean	127.4651	Standard Deviation	137.00910
Median	93.0000	Variance	18771
Mode	102.0000	Range	685.0000

Therefore, there is mostly a 0-60 day difference between a procedure and a new medication.

We can define a group of procedures and treat them as one episode to investigate the frequency of occurrence. Preprocessing is an essential aspect of outcomes research. Dealing with multiple data sources is essential. While amputation does not occur as often as debridement, we wanted to examine the sequence of treatments to see whether amputation follows a pattern of debridement.

The difference between the number of observations and the number of distinct patient IDs shows that most patients have a sequence of procedures during their treatment.

After sorting the data by procedures, the most frequent (20%) is "Dorsal and dorsolumbar fusion, posterior technique", the second is "Excisional debridement of wound, infection, or burn" (15%), third "Amputation of toe" (9%), and in fourth place, "Revision of amputation stump" (7%). In the outpatient data, the most frequent procedure is code 86.59 (Closure of skin and subcutaneous tissue of other sites) with 4,021 records out of 8,711 records. We found that about 8% of patients with osteomyelitis from inpatient data and about 0.3% from outpatient data had amputation.

Sequences of amputations are found in these data for patients with osteomyelitis. Note that we only have two years (2000 and 2001) of data and there might be more amputations performed on the same patients in the year 2002 or after. We do not have access to more recent data to verify

Figure 20. Kernel density and Histogram of date difference variable (diff)

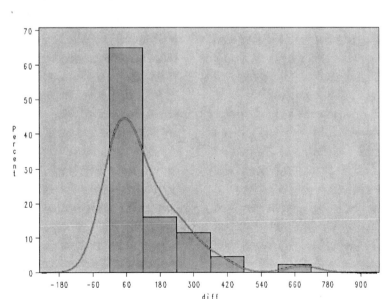

these anticipated amputations. By studying the antibiotics prescribed for these patients, we do not see the most effective antibiotics prescribed from the beginning of the treatment. There are many switches in antibiotics used to treat the patients with osteomyelitis. There are also many patients with osteomyelitis with no antibiotics prescribed.

Since there are not many patients with antibiotics, the number of switches is small. This limited dataset does not completely satisfy our study, and a larger dataset with a longer length of information is needed to study switches of medications. The method is provided here and can be used on other data. Switching or adding the medications shows that treatment was not very effective. Studying the switches of medication can determine the effectiveness or ineffectiveness of prescriptions.

CURRENT AND FUTURE CHALLENGES FACING THE ORGANIZATION

The purpose of this project was to investigate the treatment of patients with Osteomyelitis by examining large databases of clinical information and investigating the treatment options for Osteomyelitis. The two main treatments of Osteomyelitis are amputation and long-term antibiotics. We also studied the antibiotic choices for the patients with osteomyelitis. Antibiotic choice and length of treatment are critical for these patients.

We used four different sources to study in this project. First, we surveyed the physicians and analyzed the results; then, we gathered information from the web using Text Miner and compared it to survey results. We also used two large databases to examine our objectives starting with the National Inpatient Sample for the years of 2000 to 2004 and then using the Thomson MedStat MarketScan data containing all patient claims for 40 million people followed for the years 2000-2001.

Surveys showed us that physicians use different antibiotics for MRSA, and some of these antibiotics are ineffective; they are not recommended in any source to treat MRSA. After comparing the data set from our research, there is a noticeable difference between recommended and actual treatment. We can also see that physicians assume the same length of treatment for all antibiotics even if it is not validated in the literature. Actual treatment will result in a higher rate of amputation because of recurrence of the infection.

No antibiotic treatment is FDA approved for osteomyelitis with MRSA; Zyvox is approved for treatment of MRSA in the skin and soft tissues only. However, previous amputation does not prevent recurrence of osteomyelitis; more aggressive antibiotic treatment should be considered.

Considering the result on the NIS dataset, amputation was performed the most frequently compared to other procedures for patients with Osteomyelitis. Physicians assume amputation is the first (and best) treatment for Osteomyelitis. Injection of antibiotics was performed on only about 4% of the patients with Osteomyelitis. In many cases, infection has recurred and amputation was performed more than once.

Preprocessing is an essential aspect of outcomes research. Dealing with multiple data sources is essential. While amputation does not occur as often as debridement, we wanted to examine the sequence of treatments to see whether amputation follows a pattern of debridement.

The difference between the number of observations and number of distinct patient IDs in the Thomson MedStat MarketScan shows that most patients have a sequence of procedures during their treatment. There are sequences of amputations found in these data for patients with osteomyelitis. Note that we only have two years (2000 and 2001) of data and there might be more amputations performed on the same patients in the year 2002 or beyond. We do not have access to more recent data to verify it. Because we had such a short time period to work with, we could not investigate the patients as sequentially as desired. Future challenges will require additional and long term data to continue the investigation of sequential data.

Nevertheless, by studying the antibiotics prescribed for these patients, we do not see the most effective antibiotics prescribed from the beginning of the treatment. There are many switches in antibiotics used to treat the patients with osteomyelitis. There are also many patients with osteomyelitis with no antibiotics prescribed.

ACKNOWLEDGMENT

The author wishes to thank Thomson Medstat for providing the MarketScan Data for use with this project as part of the author's dissertation. The author also wishes to thank John C. Cerrito, PharmD, for his help in developing the survey and in interpreting the data results.

REFERENCES

Aneziokoro, C. O., Cannon, J. P., Pachucki, C. T., & Lentino, J. R.. The effectiveness and safety of oral linezolid for the primary and secondary treatment of osteomyelitis. *Journal of Chemotherapy (Florence, Italy)*, *17*(6), 643–650.

Binh An Diep, P. H. F. C., Graber, C. J., Szumowski, J. D., Miller, L. G., Han, L. L., Chen, J. H., et al. (n.d.). *Emergence of Multidrug-Resistant, Community-Associated, Methicillin-Resistant Staphylococcus aureus Clone USA300 in Men Who Have Sex with Men (Annals of Internal Medicine website)*. Retrieved February 19, 2008, from: http://www.annals.org/cgi/content/full/0000605-200802190-00204v1

Cerrito, P. (2010). *Clinical Data Mining for Physician Decision Making and Investigating Health Outcomes*. Hershey, PA: IGI Global Publishing.

Cerrito, P. C., & Cerrito, J. (2008). C. *Survival Data Mining: Treatment of Chronic Illness*. in *SAS Global Forum*, SAS Institute Inc. Retrieved 2009, from http://sasglobalforum.org

Cleveland Clinic. (n.d.). Retrieved from: http://www.clevelandclinic.org/health/health-info/docs/2700/2702.asp?index=9495

ICD9.chrisendres website (n.d.). *Free online searchable ICD-9-CM*. Retrieved 2009, from www.ICD9.chrisendres.com

Mauldin, P. D., Salgado, C. D., Durkalski, V. L., & Bosso, J. A. (2008). (n.d.). Nosocomial infections due to methicillin-resistant Staphylococcus aureus and vancomycin-resistant enterococcus: relationships with antibiotic use and cost drivers. *The Annals of Pharmacotherapy*, *42*(3), 317–326. doi:10.1345/aph.1K501

MedlinePlus. (n.d.). *MedlinePlus*. Retrieved 2009, from: www.medlineplus.gov

Medscape.com. (2006, July 10). *Methicillin-Resistant Staphylococcus aureus Skin Infections Among Tattoo Recipients — Ohio, Kentucky, and Vermont, 2004–2005*. Retrieved from http://www.medscape.com/viewarticle/537433

Medstatmarketscan.com. (n.d.). *Marketscan Research Database, Thomson MedStat; Ph.D. Dissertation Support Program*. Retrieved from http://www.medstatmarketscan.com/

NIS. (n.d.). *The National Inpatient Sample*. Retrieved 2009, from http://www.ahrq.gov.n.d

Pfizer (2007, March). *Zyvox*. (distributed by Pfizer). Retrieved 2009, from http://www.pfizer.com/files/products/uspi_zyvox.pdf

SAS.com. (n.d.). *SAS 9.1.3 Help and Documentation*. Retrieved 2009, from http://www.sas.com

Senneville, E., Legour, L., Valette, M., Yazdanpanah, Y., Beltrand, E., & Caillaux, M. (2006). Effectiveness and tolerability of prolonged linezolid treatment for chronic osteomyelitis: a retrospective study. *Clinical Therapeutics, 28*(8), 1155–1163. doi:10.1016/j.clinthera.2006.08.001

StatSoft. (1984-2004)., *Inc.* Retrieved 2009, from www.statsoft.com

USFDA. (n.d.). *US. Food and Drug Administration website*,www.fda.org;*used to concert NDC Numbers*. Retrieved 2009, from http://www.fda.gov/cder/ndc/database/Default.htm

Vancomycin (n.d.). *vancomycin Description.* Retrieved 2009, from http://www.drugs.com/pro/vancomycin.html

ADDITIONAL READING

Cerrito, P. B. (2009a). *Data Mining Healthcare and Clinical Databases.* Cary, NC: SAS Press, Inc.

Cerrito, P. B. (2009b). *Text Mining Techniques for Healthcare Provider Quality Determination: Methods for Rank Comparisons.* Hershey, PA: IGI Publishing.

Concia, E., Prandini, N., Massari, L., Ghisellini, F., Consoli, V., & Menichetti, F. (2006). Osteomyelitis: clinical update for practical guidelines. [Review]. *Nuclear Medicine Communications, 27*(8), 645–660. doi:10.1097/00006231-200608000-00007

Henke, P. K., Blackburn, S. A., Wainess, R. W., Cowan, J., Terando, A., Proctor, M., et al. (2005). Osteomyelitis of the foot and toe in adults is a surgical disease: conservative management worsens lower extremity salvage.[see comment]. *Annals of Surgery, 241*(6), 885-892; discussion 892-884.

Mader, J. T., Norden, C., Nelson, J. D., & Calandra, G. B. (1992). Evaluation of new anti-infective drugs for the treatment of osteomyelitis in adults. Infectious Diseases Society of America and the Food and Drug Administration. [Guideline Practice Guideline Research Support, U.S. Gov't, P.H.S.]. *Clinical Infectious Diseases, 15*(Suppl 1), S155–S161.

Wimalawansa, S. J., & Wimalawansa, S. J. (2008). Bisphosphonate-associated osteomyelitis of the jaw: guidelines for practicing clinicians. [Review]. *Endocrine Practice, 14*(9), 1150–1168.

Zahedi, H. (2009). Data Mining to Examine the Treatment of Osteomyelitis . In Cerrito, P. (Ed.), *Cases on Health Outcomes and Clinical Data Mining: Studies and Frameworks.* Hershey, PA: IGI Publishing.

Data Mining to Examine the Treatment of Osteomyelitis

APPENDIX. SURVEY TO PHYSICIANS

1. Please evaluate the following antibiotics in your clinical experience as it relates to the treatment of MRSA-infected diabetic foot ulcers:

Antibiotic	Use in Treatment of Surface Wounds for ____ days	Use in Treatment of Deep Tissue Wounds for ____ days	Use in Treatment of Osteomyelitis for ____ weeks	Never Use to treat MRSA
Septra (Sulfamethoxyasole/ Trimethoprim_				
Cleocin (Clindamycin)				
Vibramycin (Doxycycline)				
Zosyn (Piperacillin/ Tazobactam)				
Vancomycin (Various)				
Zyvox (Linezolid)				
Cipro (ciprofloxacin)				
Levaquin (levofloxacin)				
Rifampin/novobiocin				
Rifampin/bactrim				

2. I would supplement antibiotic treatment with hyperbaric oxygen for

____ Surface wounds, ____ Deep wounds, ____ Osteomyelitis

For Osteomyelitis, I would use hyperbaric oxygen for _____ weeks, for deep wounds for ____ weeks.

3. Do you consider the following factors when deciding upon the treatment of patients with infected foot ulcers caused by MRSA

	Important	Somewhat Important	Somewhat un-important	Not important
Ability of Patient to carry out therapy				
Amount of help the Patient may need				
Physical Lay Out of Home, if antibiotic is to administered at home				
Cost to Payer				
Cost to Patient				
Length of Therapy				
Convenience to Patient or Care givers				

4. What is your Specialty? _____

5. Age? __31-38 __39-44 __45-49 __50-55 __56-60 __Over 60

6. Gender? __Male ___Female
7. Additional Comments Concerning Treatment of MRSA:

_____

Chapter 3
Outcomes Research in Cardiovascular Procedures

Fariba Nowrouzi
Kentucky State University, USA

ABSTRACT

In this case, the main objective is to examine information about patients with coronary artery disease who had invasive procedures (such as balloon angioplasty or stents), or coronary artery bypass surgery. We investigate the use of the drug- eluting stent as a treatment for coronary artery disease. The first section of this chapter is a brief background about coronary artery disease and different procedures that may be used as its treatment. Next, time series analysis as a statistical tool is discussed, and in the third section, the results of the time series analyses that are performed on the database are demonstrated. In this section, the effect of the drug-eluting stent as a new treatment on the demand of other procedures is discussed. The fourth section is about computing the risk of each procedure based on the claims database used. The last section includes the result, conclusion, and suggestions.

BACKGROUND

According to the results of a number of studies (P. Cerrito & J. C. Cerrito, 2006; Igor Singer, ; Loren, n.d.), heart disease is known as the number one killer of women in the United States. More than 250,000 women die from heart disease each year. In addition, 10 percent of women aged 45 to 64, and 25 percent of women over 65 have some kind of heart disease. Studies confirm that heart disease is the number

one killer of Americans (Loren, n.d.). The cost of bypass surgery is very high. There is one hypothesis that a reasonable way to reduce the cost of treating heart disease while maintaining patient quality is to shift treatment from bypass to angioplasty with the drug-eluting stent. To investigate this hypothesis, a dataset provided by an insurance company has been used. It contained about 6,500,000 patient claims that were related to the years 2000-2005. This dataset was very multifaceted, and data processing was time consuming. In order to estimate the effect of the drug-eluting stent on bypass surgery as the two

DOI: 10.4018/978-1-61520-723-7.ch003

Copyright © 2010, IGI Global. Copying or distributing in print or electronic forms without written permission of IGI Global is prohibited.

alternative treatments, time series analyses was used. Different time series analyses are performed and compared to forecast the demand for each procedure and their costs. The risk of re-blocking an artery after each procedure (bypass surgery, drug-eluting stent, and bare stent) are estimated based on the probabilities of repetition of a procedure or having another procedure for the second or third time. Finally, for cost productivity and cost-effectiveness analysis of the drug-eluting stent as an advanced treatment, the Markov chain method was used.

Heart disease has the highest mortality rate of any chronic disease, particularly in the United States (Loren, n.d.). Any disease affecting the heart or blood vessels is called cardiovascular disease. It includes coronary artery disease, arteriosclerosis, heart valve disease, arrhythmia, heart failure, hypertension, orthostatic hypotension, shock, endocarditic, diseases of the aorta and its branches, disorders of the peripheral vascular system, and congenital heart disease percentage.

The breakdown of death from cardiovascular disease is

- 54% Coronary Heart Disease
- 18% Stroke
- 13% Other
- 6% Congestive Heart Failure
- 5% High Blood Pressure
- 4% Diseases of the Arteries
- 0.4% Rheumatic Fever/Rheumatic Fever Disease
- 0.4% Congenital Cardiovascular Defects

Figure 1 shows an image of a coronary artery. The heart muscle, like every organ or tissue of the body, needs oxygen-rich blood to survive. The main blood supplier to a body is called the aorta. It branches off into two main coronary blood vessels, which are called arteries; one on the left and one on the right side. By these two arteries, blood travels to all heart muscles. The left side of the heart is larger and more muscular compared to the right side, because the right side only pumps

the blood to the lungs, but the left side pumps the blood to the rest of the body.

Coronary Artery Disease

Coronary artery disease appears when there is a narrowing or blockage of the coronary arteries (figure 2). These arteries provide blood for the heart muscle. When too many of the arteries are narrowed, or one crucial artery is blocked, the heart does not get enough oxygen. Often, a person with coronary artery disease will get chest pain, called angina. A heart attack (myocardial infarction) can happen when at least one of the coronary arteries is completely blocked. The heart attack can result in permanent damage to the heart.

There are currently two basic surgical methods used to unblock a coronary artery: Coronary Artery Bypass Graft (CABG), and Percutaneous Transluminal Coronary Angioplasty (PTCA) (Iezzoni et al., 1995).

Coronary Artery Bypass Graft (CABG)

Saphenous veins are taken from the leg, or the internal mammary artery is used to attach to the blocked artery (Figure 3).

Figure 1. Coronary arteries (Taken from http://en.wikipedia.org/wiki/File:Gray492.png)

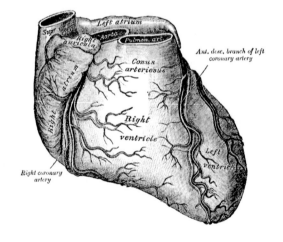

Figure 2. Narrowing of an artery (Taken from http://en.wikipedia.org/wiki/File:Endo_dysfunction_Athero. PNG)

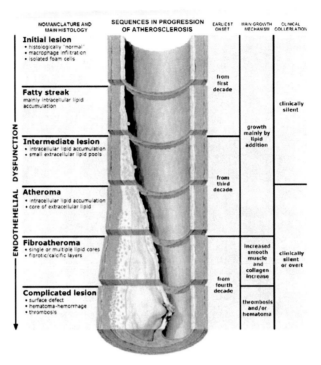

In this way, blood flow is diverted from the blockage through the attached vessel so that blood can flow freely to provide nutrients to the heart. This process is called revascularization. In order to perform this procedure, the heart must be stopped and the blood is pumped through the use of a bypass machine. More recently, an off-pump procedure has been developed.

Angioplasty (PTCA)

In this procedure, a cardiologist passes a wire from an artery in the groin area to the heart, through the diseased coronary artery to the blockage. Over this wire, a catheter (a hollow tube) with a small balloon at its tip is passed through the vessel and inflated. The purpose of this inflation is to compress the plaque that is causing the blockage. The result is to make the inner diameter of the blood vessel larger so that blood can flow more easily. Once the balloon has inflated, the catheter is removed (Figure 4).

Figure 3. Bypass graft (http://en.wikipedia.org/wiki/File:Heart_saphenous_coronary_grafts. jpg)

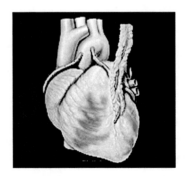

To prevent re-blocking, an expandable wire mesh tube (stent) is usually implanted in the vessel at the point of the blockage to maintain the openness of the artery from the inside (figure 5). Unfortunately, about 30% of all vessels tend to re-close after balloon angioplasty. The bare metal stents may prevent the artery from closing, but there is still re-blocking after six months in almost

Figure 4. Angioplasty (Taken from http://www.nhlbi.nih.gov/health/dci/Diseases/Angioplasty/Angioplasty_howdone.html)

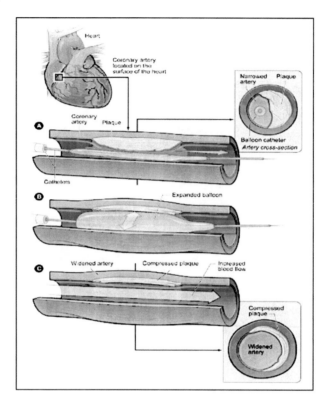

25% of cases, even with the stent (Austin, Alter, & Tu, 2003).

The reason for the re-blocking of an artery (re-stenosis) is not really known. However, there are a number of theories that have been presented. One theory is that re-stenosis, rather than a return of coronary artery disease, is a response of the body to what the body perceives as an injury to the vessel caused by the angioplasty, and is essentially a growth of smooth muscle cells that is actually similar to a scar forming at a wound site (Austin et al., 2003). A number of drugs have been tested that were known to interrupt re-stenosis. Stents were coated with these drugs, usually in a thin layer, for a timed release. To test the coated stent, clinical trials were conducted. These coated stents generally are called drug-eluting.

Drug-Eluting Stents

The Food and Drug Administration (FDA) approved the first drug-eluting stent for angioplasty on April 24, 2003 (Poses et al., 2000) . The new stent, permanently implanted in the artery, slowly releases a drug. The clinical studies showed that the released drug reduces the rate of re-blockage when compared randomly to treatment with the bare stents. (Burt Cohen, 2008) "Drug-eluting stents combine drugs with medical devices to provide more effective care for many patients with heart disease," said FDA Commissioner Mark McClellan, M.D., Ph.D (FDA news, 2003). Since one of the reasons for by-pass (CABG) surgery is the lower rate of re-stenosis, it is likely that more patients and physicians will opt for PTCA with an eluting-stent instead of CABG.

Figure 5. Coronary angioplasty with bare stent (Taken from http://www.nhlbi.nih.gov/health/dci/Diseases/Angioplasty/Angioplasty_howdone.html)

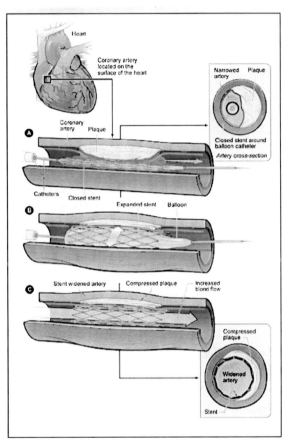

There are three major parts to the drug-eluting stent (Austin et al., 2003):

1. Choice of the type of stent
2. Method of drug-delivery of the coated drug to the artery wall
3. The choice of the drug itself.

The two drug-eluting stents, the Cordis CYPHER™ (approved in April, 2003) contains the drug, sirolimus, and the Boston Scientific TAXUS™ (approved, March, 2004) contains the drug, paclitaxel. A third eluting stent has been approved for sale in Europe (CE Mark). In addition, the Cook V-Flex Plus is available in Europe. Since approval, trials have shown that both the TAXUS and CYPHER stents reduce the occurrence of restenosis (P. Cerrito & J. C. Cerrito, 2006; Poses et al., 2000; Thomas, 1998).

Recently an analysis demonstrated that using both the sirolimus-eluting stent and the paclitaxel-eluting stent reduce the risk of target lesion revascularization by 74% compared to the bare metal stent (Sousa JE, Costa MA, Sousa AG, 2003). In the SIRIUS study performed in the US, 1058 patients were randomized either to the Cypher stent or to a standard metal stent (David J, ; Jeffrey W. Moses). The patients had large blockages of size 15mm to 30mm. Results were similar for both types of stents immediately following the angioplasty. After nine months of follow up, the patients who received the experimental stent had a significantly lower rate of repeat angioplasty compared to the patients who received the regular stent (4.2% versus 16.8%). In addition, patients treated with the drug-eluting stent had a lower re-stenosis rate of 8.9% compared to 36.3% for the regular stent. In total, the occurrence of repeat angioplasty, bypass surgery, heart attacks and death was 8.8% for the experimental stent compared to 21% for the regular stent (Jeffrey W. Moses, n.d.).

A smaller study of 238 patients was conducted outside of the US (the RAVEL study) (Fajadet J, Mar 18 2002). It evaluated patients with a smaller blockage. However, the results were similar with statistically significant reductions in the rate of re-stenosis (Dr. Paul Barrentt, 2002). In fact, the re-stenosis with the metal stent can be as much as 64 times higher compared to that with the drug-eluting stent (P. Cerrito & J. C. Cerrito, 2006).

Because of the promising results, more patients and physicians probably will opt for the newer, drug-eluting stent. Currently, about 90% of all stents used in the United States and Europe are drug-eluting stents (Lisa T. Newsome, MD, Michael A. Kutcher, MD, Sanjay K. Gandhi, MD, Richard C. Prielipp, MD, and Roger L. Royster, MD, 2008). However, it is also much more costly, resulting in higher immediate costs in performing angioplasty. More evidence is needed to see if the early promise of these results continues in the long-term, and to see whether drug-eluting stents improve a patient's quality of life. It is also important to see when and how physicians decided to switch from bare-metal stents to drug-eluting stents in the treatment of their patients.

In October 2003, the FDA issued a warning concerning sub-acute thrombosis (blood clotting) with the CYPHER stent. The initial warning indicated that the stent could cause a higher proportion of deaths compared to other stents. Further study demonstrated that the incidence of thrombosis is no greater compared to the bare metal stent (Austin et al., 2003).

It is expected that the drug-eluting stent will reduce the need for repeat angioplasties, saving payers $10,000 to $12,000 per procedure. These stents are also predicted to reduce the need for open-heart surgeries, which have a considerably higher cost compared to angioplasty (Thomas, 1998).

More than half of heart disease deaths are related to coronary heart disease. There are some alternative treatments for this disease, so from a societal perspective, it is important to see which treatments for coronary heart disease can maximize benefits while minimizing costs. The objective of this proposal is to examine information about patients with coronary artery disease who had invasive procedures (such as balloon angioplasty or stents) or coronary artery bypass surgery to investigate the economic impact of the drug- eluting stent as an advanced treatment for coronary artery disease. Without examining the eluting stent, most studies have confirmed that bypass surgery is more effective than angioplasty with the use of the standard, bare-metal stent because of the risk of re-blocking and the need for repeat procedures (Cynthia A. Yock, 2003).

A Canadian report was issued concerning the cost-effectiveness of the eluting stent. The conclusion was that the stent was not cost-effective because the cost of repeating the procedure was less compared to the cost of the stent. However, the report did not consider a reduction of bypass surgeries as a result of the use of the eluting stent. (Brophy & Erickson, 2004) We will examine and compare the effectiveness of the drug eluting stent versus bypass surgery. Similarly, a report by the British organization, National Institute for Health and Clinical Excellence issued a report that allowed the eluting stent in some instances a cost effective while denying it in others. However, neither study examined the potential for shifting away from bypass procedures.

Episode Grouping

For a long time, healthcare organizations considered the cost of a treatment of a disease as the total dollars spent for pharmacy services, procedures, treatment and other services, but there is a question as to whether the treatment is the most cost effective for the disease; that is, whether those dollars are delivering the best care in the most effective way (Manage Health Care Executive, n.d.).

Episode Grouping is a methodology that enables healthcare professionals to analyze patient treatments and evaluate the quality of the treatments and manage the related costs. That means that by examining the nature of a disease and the patients' overall health severity, the cost of treatment can be managed. Episode Grouping defines a group of inpatient, outpatient, professional, lab, x-ray and pharmaceutical claims into units, or episodes, of analysis that are clinically meaningful. An episode describes the complete condition of a particular patient treatment for a single disease at a single time, and its severity. Episode Grouping provides an effective means to define care and determines which treatment is more cost effective. Also, it allows a payer to compare physician performance. To better understand claims data and for a range of decision-support applications, healthcare organizations have started to use episode grouping (Manage Health Care Executive, n.d.). Episode grouping includes:

- "Evaluating return on disease management programs;
- Identifying high-risk patients;
- Assessing the extent to which medical and surgical treatments are appropriate;
- Analyzing cost and use;
- Comparing physician performance;
- Rating employer groups;
- Allocating resources more effectively; and
- Targeting clinical- and financial- improvement opportunities."

In addition, episode grouping is used for:

- Profiling providers, physicians and specialists in order to determine the appropriate treatment for a disease on the basis of severity level,
- Using provider language and disease staging to determine clinical validity, and
- Risk-adjusting on the basis of the severity of a patient's disease and comparing the risk to norms.

Qualified Episodes

A period of an episode starts when a patient seeks care and treatment, and visits a provider of healthcare; it ends when the treatment is completed. The cost of an episode is the total charge of all services that are provided by all doctors/ professional providers, pharmacy services, and all facilities related to that episode of care. Qualified episodes are completed; their costs are not extremely high or low compared to others of the same Medical Episode Group, Severity, or Comorbidity, and they are within the normal range of practice for the specialty or episode (Blue Cross Blue Shield of Texas, n.d.).

Medstat Episode Grouper (MEG)

MEG is the name of an episode grouper software provided by the commercial firm, Medstat. It is developed and marketed by David Schutt, MD, Associate Medical Director for healthcare-information ((MEG)). The Medstat episode grouper uses diagnosis codes only and does not consider account procedure codes. It uses the data from the entire Medicare population. MEG uses claims data and patient demographics and diagnoses in order to link inpatient, outpatient, and pharmacy services into disease-related episodes of care and then classifies the severity of disease inside the episode (Thomson Reuters, 2008).

A unit or episode of a disease treatment starts with a contact to a healthcare provider, physician office visit or hospitalization. Laboratory tests, x-rays, and pharmacy services can be joined to existing episodes, but cannot start an episode. The end point of an episode is when the treatment is completed. Since the end of an episode is not obvious, the clean period decision rule is used to establish the end point. It is a period of time for a patient not undergoing treatment for a disease or condition. The subsequent visits during a clean period are assumed to be a part of the episode, including the previous visit for that disease. Any contact with healthcare for a disease after a clean period should be considered as starting a new episode for the patient. It is common to have a non-specific primary diagnosis for a patient. For instance, an initial visit of a patient can be coded as abdominal pain, but later can be classified as appendicitis. MEG logically links the disease to a specific episode if the date of non-specified primary diagnosis is close to the date of a specific episode.

Patients with coronary artery disease usually may have different options of treatments to choose. The average cost, risk of re-blocking a sick artery, the level of severity of procedures, and the quality of life are not the same for the four procedures that were mentioned in this section. Logically, all patients would like to have the peace of mind to know that their choice about a treatment is the best one. Now, there is a new technology, episode grouper, which can give better information to healthcare providers, physicians and specialists to determine the appropriate treatment for a disease on the basis of severity level. Patients are able to consider the risks that are involved for a different or alternative treatment.

SETTING THE STAGE

Use of the Procedures over Time

The percentage of the patient population that selects the drug-eluting stent (DES) as a treatment for coronary artery disease is increasing. Every day, patients and their physicians know more about the improvement of technology and access to less invasive treatment. This causes them to choose the drug-eluting stent rather than an open heart bypass surgery, if it is a viable option. To project the cost saving of the shift from open heart bypass surgery to DES, we use time series analysis to examine the behavior of the four procedures through time, and the average cost of each procedure as well.

Time series is a set of ordered observations of a variable on a quantitative characteristic that is collected over time. Usually, the observations are successive and collected during the same time interval. For instance, the monthly total number of open heart bypass surgeries at a hospital is a time series with the time interval as monthly. There are two main goals of time series analysis: (1) identifying the pattern of a time series, and (2) forecasting or predicting the time series variable for the future. We can forecast a time series by extrapolation methods or by explanatory models. Extrapolation methods are some adapted techniques that simply project the series by smoothing observed data.

It has been explained that a patient with coronary artery disease usually has an option to choose one of the four procedures (angioplasty, bare-stent, open heart bypass surgery, and the drug-eluting stent) as a treatment for the disease. The drug-eluting stent is a new treatment compared to the other treatments. The primary goal of time series analysis is to examine the trend and behavior of the number of each procedure performed during a time period; that is, the patient's choices for treatment or their demands for the procedure. Our next goal is to examine the effect of the drug-eluting stent on the other three procedures, especially on open bypass surgery. Furthermore, we examine the behavior of the average charge of each treatment or procedure during a fixed time interval.

After data processing, we received access to the dataset, with each observation containing information about patient ID, conducted procedure (Bare-stent, angioplasty, drug-eluting stent, or open bypass surgery), date, and total charge . The dataset was de-identified according to HIPAA requirements. We then used Enterprise Guide software, a GUI interface component of SAS (SAS Institute, Inc; Cary, NC), to prepare the time series data based upon the number of performed procedures and semi monthly time intervals. Figure 6, time series plots, shows that the number of drug-eluting stents has an increasing trend and the number of the other three procedures has a decreasing trend after approving the drug-eluting stent by the FDA (Food and Drug administration, n.d.). The bare stent has the strongest decreasing trend. This implies that, as far as the demand for the drug-eluting stent as a treatment increases, the demand for the bare stent decreases.

Figure 6 shows the plot of the number of the four procedures based on the insurance company database. The semi-monthly numbers of procedures before August, 2002 and after October, 2005 are very small compared to other semi-months between them. The reason can be a lack of information about the number of procedures in the beginning and the end of the time interval that the data were collected. In order to avoid any misleading result from the dataset, we use a smaller subset of the time series that contains all observations within the interval [16 August, 2002 to 10 October, 2005]. Figure 7 shows the line plot of the frequency of procedures in the smaller time period.

The fluctuations in figure 7 do not confirm the existence of seasonality in the time series data. According to the main objectives, forecasting the demand of open heart bypass surgery and the drug-eluting stent, and to examine the effect of the drug-eluting stent on the demand of bypass surgery as it is an alternative treatment for coronary artery disease, we focus mostly on analyzing open bypass surgery and the drug-eluting stent. SAS software is used to estimate good models to forecast the number of bypass surgeries and the drug-eluting

Figure 6. Time series plot of total number of each procedure (time interval=semi monthly)

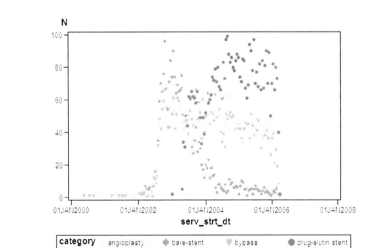

Figure 7. Line plot of the total number of each procedure in [16 august, 2002 to 10 october, 2005]

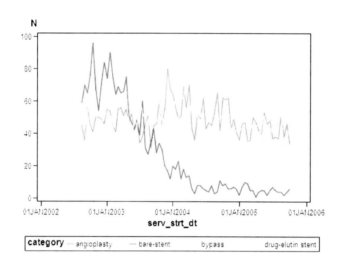

Figure 8. Simple exponential smoothing model for the average charge of open bypass surgery

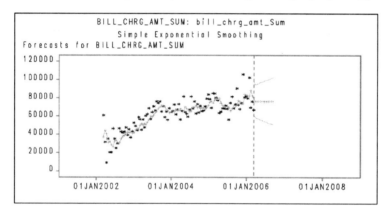

stent procedures and their average charges. A simple exponential smoothing model (ARIMA (0, 1, 1)) shown in figure 8, and a linear model shown in figure 9, have been estimated for the average total charges for open bypass surgery and the number of open bypass surgeries, respectively.

To check the accuracy of the estimated models, white noise and stationary tests are performed (Figures 10 and 11).

The white noise tests indicate failure to reject a null hypothesis of white noise for all alternative lags. The unit root tests indicate rejection of a null hypothesis of a unit root for all polynomials up to lag three.

The period of fit for average charges for the drug-eluting stent procedure and the number of procedures is from August 16, 2003 to October 1, 2005, and the unit of time is semimonthly. Figures 12 and 13 show the estimated models for the drug-eluting stent procedures.

To check the estimated models, the following test is performed to find the prediction error (Figures 14 and 15).

The autocorrelation functions in figure 14 indicate a failure to reject a null hypothesis of zero autocorrelation at all lags.

The white noise test and stationary test for the number of drug-eluting stents during the time

Figure 9. Linear model to forecast the number of open bypass surgeries

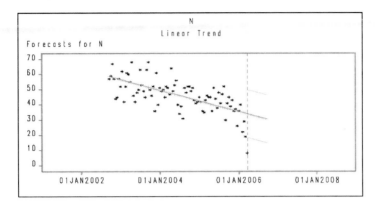

Figure 10. White noise & stationary test for the model in Figure 8

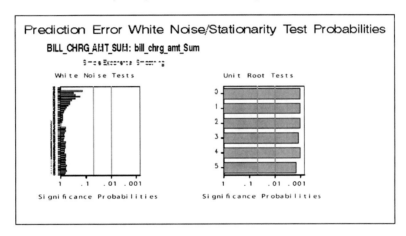

Figure 11. White noise & stationary test for the model in Figure 9

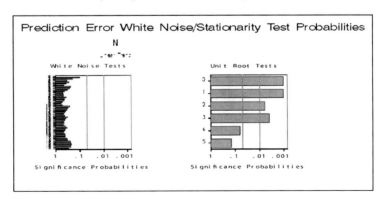

Figure 12. Simple exponential smoothing model for the number of drug-eluting stents

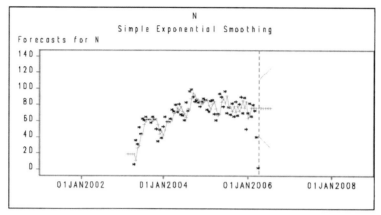

Figure 13. Simple exponential smoothing model for the average charge of drug-eluting stents

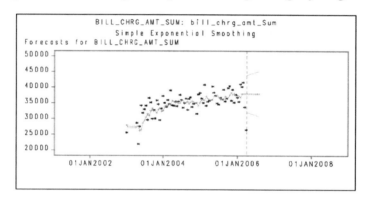

Figure 14. Prediction error for the estimated model for the average of total charges of drug-eluting stents

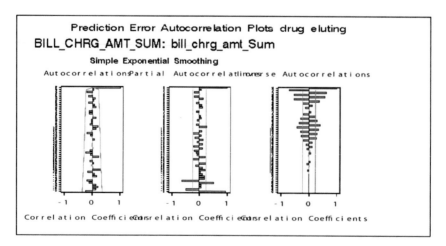

Figure 15. Prediction error autocorrelation for the number of drug-eluting stents

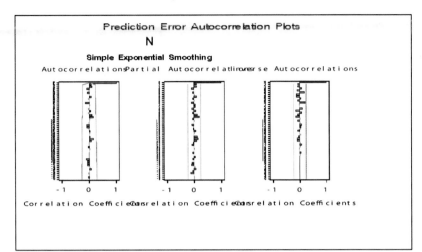

Figure 16. White noise and stationary probability test for average charge of drug-eluting stent

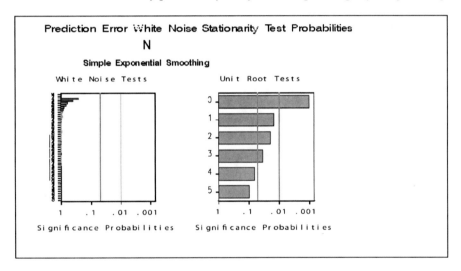

series has the same result as shown in figure 16.

The Food and Drug Administration (FDA) approved the use of the drug-eluting stent in April, 2003. To estimate the effect of this technology improvement on a patient's choice of having bypass surgery, an intervention step function is used. It is well known that the average cost of any kind of service affects the demand for the service; that is, the number of patients who have an open heart bypass surgery depends upon the average cost of the procedure if they have an alternative choice.

Using SAS software and the time series forecasting system, a model is estimated for the number of bypass surgeries using a combination of dynamic regressors and an intervention point. The independent variable or predictor is the semimonthly average cost for the open bypass procedure, and April, 2003 is chosen as a point for a ramp intervention variable.

Logically, the dependent variable will be affected by the next lag on a semimonthly basis, so we use lag =1 for the model. The size of the time series data is about 76 and we use a holdout sample of 10 elements to validate the model. The result is the function that is shown in figure 17. It confirms that the number of patients who have bypass surgery has a decreasing trend after April, 2003. That means that more patients will choose a drug-eluting stent instead of the open bypass surgery procedure in the future.

To evaluate the estimated model autocorrelation tests, error plots, white noise and stationary test were performed. Ignoring the lag zero value, we see that there are no significant autocorrelation values. Figures 18 and 19 are evidence for failing to reject the null hypotheses that the autocorrelation at each lag is zero.

Table 1 illustrates that the average charge for bypass (or price of open bypass surgery) has a very small effect, 0.0004, on the next period demand for open bypass surgery. This is a reasonable ef-

Figure 17. Estimated model for the number of open bypass surgeries, where April, 2003 is an intervention point and the total average cost is an independent variable

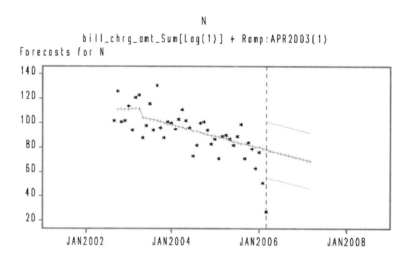

Figure 18. Prediction error autocorrelation for the number of open bypass surgery procedures

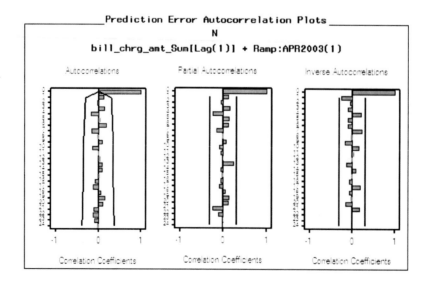

fect, because the patients are shielded from cost, and also, there is a small difference between the stent and bypass surgery. The slope of the model, -7.53834, confirms a decreasing trend during the time after April, 2003 (Figure 20).

This residual plotting does not confirm any significant change in the residual distribution over the whole period of fit, and does not show any pattern or seasonality over time. Therefore, there is no evidence for existence of a seasonality factor in the time series data that affects the model. The mean error is close to zero; that is, the forecast is unbiased.

The time series that is used to model the demand of the bare stent is semimonthly. The dependent series or response variable is the number of bare stent procedures in the dataset; the independent variable is the average charge, and approval of the drug-eluting stent in April, 2003 is an intervention that changes the pattern of the dependent series. Since the dataset is semi-monthly, the May, 2003 date is considered the starting point when the demand for the bare stent is affected by the drug-eluting stent. The model in figure 21 fits the data better than all other models that were checked (relatively). The combination of trend curve by log transformation and an intervention has been used.

Table 2 shows the estimated parameter for the forecasting model for the bare stent procedure.

The p-values in Table 2 show that the estimated parameters are significant at a more than 90% confidence level except for the trend.

Figure 19. White noise /stationary test probability for the number of open bypass surgery procedures

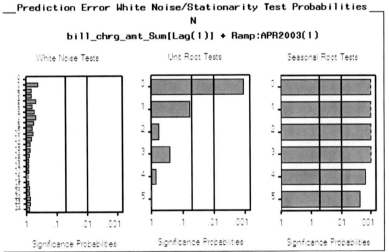

Table 1. Estimated parameters of the number of open bypass surgery procedures for bill_chrg_amt_sum[Lag(1)]+Ramp:APR2003(1)

Model Parameter	Estimate	Standard Error	T-Statistic
Intercept	109.63203	16.6684	6.5772
Bill Charge Amount Sum (Lag(1)	0.0000418	0.000346	0.1206
Ramp:APR2003(1)	-7.53834	8.3216	-0.9059
Ramp:APR2003(1) Num1	-6.73279	8.3382	-0.8075
Model Variance (sigma squared)	135.38885	.	.

Figure 20. Error of the estimated model for the number of open bypass surgery procedures

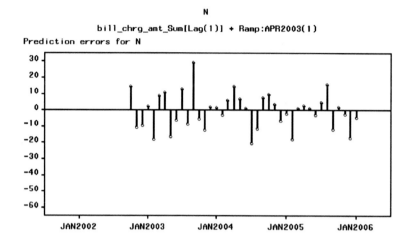

Figure 21. Forecasting model for the demand of the bare stent

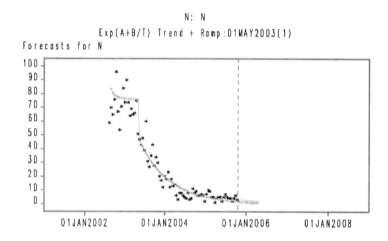

- Mean Square Error =

$$MSE = \frac{1}{n} \sum_{t=1}^{n} (y_t - \hat{y}_t)^2$$

- Root Mean Square Error =
  RMSE = $\sqrt{MSE}$
- Mean Absolute Percent Error =

  (MAPE) = $\frac{100}{n} \sum_{t=1}^{n} \left| (y_t - \hat{y}_t) / y_t \right|$

- Mean Absolute Error = $\frac{1}{n} \sum_{t=1}^{n} \left| y_t - \hat{y}_t \right|$
- R-Square =

$$R^2 = 1 - \frac{\sum_{t=1}^{n} (y_t - \hat{y}_t)^2}{\sum_{t=1}^{n} (y_t - \overline{y})^2}$$

The Statistic fitness values listed in Table 3 that are usually used to compare different models seems to be small and good compared to other models that were checked, but the R-Square still is negative, and this implies that the model does not fit the time series data well.

The HPF procedure in SAS is an automatic and quick way to forecast a time series for transactional data. If the series can be organized into separate variables by group in a dataset, then the procedure can forecast many series at a

Table 2. Estimation parameter for the bare stent on the base of curve trend and an intervention

Model Parameter	Estimate	Std. Error	T	Prob>|T|
Intercept	4.22088	0.1719	24.5605	<.0001
Exp(A+B/T) Trend	0.22620	0.9214	0.2455	0.8158
Ramp:01MAY2003(1)	-0.50145	0.1879	-2.6681	0.0445
Ramp:01MAY2003(1) Num1	-0.44532	0.1901	-2.3431	0.0661
Model Variance (sigma squared)	0.19121	.	.	.

Table 3. Different measure of error for forecasting the model for the number of bare stents: statistics of fit for Exp(A=B/T) Trend+Ramp:01MAY2003(1)

Statistics of Fit	Value
Mean Square Error	6.6
Root Mean Square Error	2.5
Mean Absolute Percent Error	45.6
Mean Absolute Error	2.2
R-Square	-2

Table 4. RMSE for different forecasting models for variable bypass surgery

Model Selection Criterion = RMSE		
Model	Statistic	Selected
Simple Exponential Smoothing	7.5769119	
Double Exponential Smoothing	7.5811678	
Linear Exponential Smoothing	7.2602693	Yes
Damped-Trend Exponential Smoothing	7.2813443	

time in one step. All estimated parameters for a forecast model are optimized based on the data. The HPF system can use a holdout sample and select the appropriate smoothing model based on one of several model selection criteria. A holdout sample is a subset at the end of a series that is not used to estimate the parameters of the forecasting model, but it is used to test the accuracy level of the forecast model. One of the advantages of the High Performance Forecasting procedure is that it can forecast both time series data, with equally spaced intervals defined by a specific time interval (e.g., daily, weekly,…), or transactional data, with observations that are

not spaced by any particular time interval. Also, the HPF system can perform trend and seasonal analysis on transactional data.

Table 4 shows the results for the prediction model of the demand of bypass surgery when the time interval is semimonthly and the series accumulates by total; that is, HPF predicts the series on the basis of the total number of each procedure, N, at each time interval. According to the HPF procedure, the best prediction model for the number of bypass surgeries (demand for bypass procedure) is a linear exponential smoothing model. Table 5 shows the estimated parameters for the model.

Table 5. Linear exponential smoothing parameter estimation for the bypass surgery

Linear Exponential Smoothing Parameter Estimates				
Parameter	Estimate	Standard Error	t Value	Approx Pr > |t|
Level Weight	0.02203	0.01191	1.85	0.0685
Trend Weight	0.0010000	0.0087189	0.11	0.9090

By replacing 0.022 and 0.001 for ω *and* γ in a Linear Exponential Smoothing Model, we get the following model:

$$L_t = .022Y_t + .97(L_{t-1} + T_{t-1}),$$
$$T_t = .001(L_t - L_{t-1}) + .999T_{t-1},$$
$$\hat{Y}_{t+k} = L_t + kT_t$$

On the basis of the HPF procedure, the best model to forecast the number of drug-eluting stents is also a linear exponential smoothing model. In Tables 6a, 6b, and 6c, we see the summary of estimating a forecast model for the number of drug eluting stents that is performed by the HPF procedure.

Table 6c confirms that in order to make a smooth forecasting model for the demand of the drug-eluting stent, almost 64% of the weight is given to the most recent data; that is, $\omega = 0.63922 \cong 0.64$. However, the trend weight is very small, 0.001, and its effect is small to make the model smooth with respect to the trend.

Similarly, the HPF procedure is performed to find the best forecasting models for both vari-ables, the number of bare stents and angioplasty. The result shows that damped-Trend exponential smoothing models are the best for both of them. Tables 7 and 8 show the estimated parameters for the bare-stent and angioplasty, respectively.

According to table 7, the level weight is about 0.1. That means that only 10% of the weight is given to the most recent observation in order to forecast. The most effective weight is trend weight; that is, about 1. The damping weight is about 0.92 to reduce the amount of growth extrapolated into the future.

The forecasting models of the demand (the number of procedures) of the four procedures that are performed by HPF, are visualized in figure 22.

Figure 22 confirms that as long as the demand of the drug-eluting stent increases, the demand for the bare-stent decreases rapidly. Also, the demand for bypass procedures decreases, but not as much as the demand for the bare stent. The estimated trend weight by the HPF procedure for the forecasted models of the bare-stent and bypass procedures are 0.999 and 0.001, respectively. That means

Table 6a. Basic information about the used data (Category=Drug-Eluting Stent)

Variable Information	
Name	N
Label	N
First	09JAN2003
Last	15OCT2005
Number of Observations Read	4106

Table 6b. RMSE statistic value for the different models

Model Selection Criterion = RMSE		
Model	Statistic	Selected
Simple Exponential Smoothing	11.139271	
Double Exponential Smoothing	11.526255	
Linear Exponential Smoothing	10.968200	Yes
Damped-Trend Exponential Smoothing	10.971356	

Table 6c. The estimated parameters for a linear exponential smoothing model for (DES)

Linear Exponential Smoothing Parameter Estimates				
Parameter	Estimate	Standard Error	t Value	Approx Pr > |t|
Level Weight	0.63922	0.08649	7.39	<.0001
Trend Weight	0.0010000	0.01624	0.06	

Table 7. Estimated parameters for the selected forecasting model for bare-stent

Damped-Trend Exponential Smoothing Parameter Estimates				
Parameter	Estimate	Standard Error	t Value	Approx Pr > |t|
Level Weight	0.10527	0.06311	1.67	0.0996
Trend Weight	0.99900	0.78311	1.28	0.2061
Damping Weight	0.91859	0.04119	22.30	<.0001

Table 8. Estimated parameters for the selected forecasting model for angioplasty

Damped-Trend Exponential Smoothing Parameter Estimates				
Parameter	Estimate	Standard Error	t Value	Approx Pr > |t|
Level Weight	0.24346	41.62007	0.01	0.9953
Trend Weight	0.0010000	6.84275E-8	14614.0	.
Damping Weight	0.0010000	170693.0	0.00	1.0000

that the demand for the bare-stent changes faster over time. There is a question as to whether the drug-eluting stent causes the reduction of demand for the bare-stent, or whether other factors are involved. The risk of re-blocking a coronary artery or average cost of the procedure may affect the demand of the bare-stent.

Average Cost of the Four Procedures

Figure 23 is the result of performing the HPF procedure to select the best models that fit the data and forecast the average charge of the four procedures. According to the HPF procedure, the best selected models for a response variable, average charge series, for the bare-stent is a linear

Figure 22. Forecasting result for the demand of four procedures performed by HPF

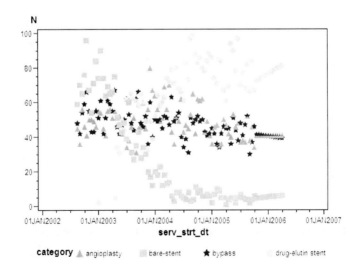

Figure 23. Average charge series of the four procedures

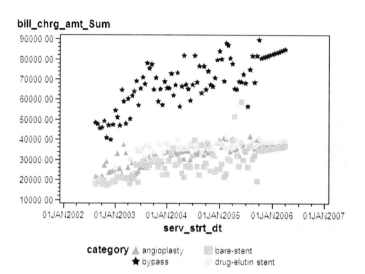

exponential smoothing model. The drug-eluting stent uses a damped-trend exponential smoothing model. Trend weights for the bare-stent and the drug-eluting stent are 0.001 and 0.99, respectively. This implies that the rate of change for average charges for the bare-stent is not so high that it has a big effect on the demand for the bare-stent procedure. Also, the average charge of the drug-eluting stent is not far from the average charge of the bare-stent. Therefore, it seems that the difference of the re-blocking risk of the two procedures causes a shift of demand from the bare-stent to the drug-eluting stent.

To forecast the total number of all procedures together with respect to the semimonthly time interval, the HPF procedure is used. A Damped –Trend Exponential Smoothing model, figure 24, is selected as a best model.

The prediction in figure 24 shows a decreasing trend on demand for the total number of procedures for those who were insured by a health insurance company. Figure 25 shows the error distribution of the estimated model in figure 24; it does not confirm any special pattern.

Using the database that is provided by a health insurance company, the demand for the procedures does not increase. However, the demand for the

drug-eluting stent increases while the demand for the bare stent decreases sharply and the demand for bypass surgery decreases slowly. The average charges for the bare-stent and drug-eluting stent do not change very much with time. If an inflation factor is added, the amount actually decreases. Therefore, the existence of the trend is not caused by the price of the procedures. It seems that a patient with coronary artery disease prefers the drug-eluting stent procedure rather than a bare-stent for other reasons.

According to all estimated forecasting models, the hypothesis that the drug-eluting stent is an alternative treatment for open heart bypass surgery is still an open question. Next, we will discuss the patient's condition and their choice of a procedure as a treatment. Also, we will discuss the risk of re-blocking an artery of a patient after each procedure.

CASE DESCRIPTION

When patients with coronary artery disease face different alternative treatments, what is the most important factor to affect their decision?

Figure 24. Forecasting model for the total number of procedures

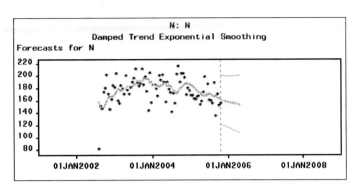

Figure 25. Error distribution of the forecasting model, Figure 19

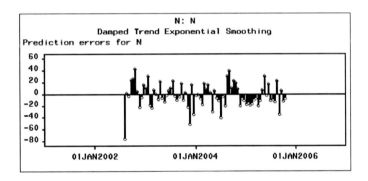

Re-Blocking an Artery

There are 16 different DRG codes in the database that can be classified as one of the four procedure categories named angioplasty, bare-stent, drug-eluting stent, and open bypass surgery as a treatment. Sometimes, a procedure is not a final treatment for a patient, and after months or years, the patient may have to have another procedure. The reason for the second procedure is a re-blocking of the previous sick artery or possibly the blockage of another artery.

Since the result of this research is based on the database that was provided by an insurance company, we assume that; 1) All the clients who were diagnosed to one of the DRG codes related to coronary artery disease in the database had been insured by the company at least for the time

period that the database was collected. 2) The cause of having another procedure or repetition of a procedure is re-blocking of arteries. 3) The rate of failing a procedure (patient expiration during a procedure) is very small and it is ignored.

Re-blocking an artery after a procedure has a negative effect on the quality of life of a patient. Therefore, the risk of re-blocking an artery with respect to each procedure is a very important factor that the patients should know before deciding which procedure is an optimal treatment. Another important factor that may affect a decision of a patient is the short and long term monetary cost of each procedure. Risk of a procedure includes the risk of failure and the risk of a need for another procedure during a patient's life-time. The risk of failure or the risk of going through another procedure can be defined as a probability of failure or the probability of facing another procedure. Obviously, a procedure with the higher risk has a negative effect on a patient decision.

In order to analyze these values, we must first define an episode of care for each patient. After considerable data processing, a patient is diagnosed to one of the four categories (Bypass surgery, drug-eluting stent, bare-stent, and angioplasty). The total observations in the dataset are 18,166 but related to only 13,304 patients. Therefore, some patients received some treatments or services on different days. The first question is how we can distinguish billed charges (cost) for each patient. That means that the correspondence between the set of patients and service dates is not a one-to-one function. Consequently, the relation between patients and cost (bill charges) is not a one-to-one function. There are some clients who have multiple billed charges. This implies that some patients received treatment on different days. The SAS code 1 has been used to create a column, n_day, in the dataset. The variable, n_day = 1 means that the observation is related to the first day of a treatment for a client, and n_day = 2 means that the observation is related to the second day of a treatment for a patient, and so on.

Code 1. Codes to Add a New Column, n_day, to the Dataset

```
proc sort data=sasuser.clm_category4;
by patient_id serv_strt_dt;
run;
data sasuser.cat4_count_day;
set sasuser.clm_category4;
by Patient_id;
if FIRST.Patient_id THEN N_DAY=1;
```

The DRG code is one of the factors that can be used to differentiate the costs related to different treatments. It works if a patient has gone through the different procedures (diagnosed with different DRG codes). If a patient undergoes a procedure for two or more times, all of them will be diagnosed with the same DRG code. If we consider the total cost of all the records related to a patient who is diagnosed with the same DRG code as the procedure cost, it is an incorrect conclusion. It is rare that a patient with coronary disease needs a procedure for the second time in less than a 10-day period. Therefore, we assume that the observations with the same ID number and the same DRG code are related to the same procedure if their service date is less than 10 days apart. Otherwise, they are related to different procedures or treatments.

With this assumption, there is a need of another variable named diff. In each observation, the variable, diff, explains the difference of the service date with the previous service date of a patient. For example, assume there are three observations related to a patient with the same DRG codes, and diff equals 0, 1, and 3 respectively. That means that the patient received some services on the first day, second day, and fifth day for a procedure. Now, assume that there are three observations with the same ID number and the same DRG code such that the variable, diff, is 0, 1, and 120 respectively. Diff set equal to 0 and to 1 imply that the first and second observations are related to the same procedure and the third observation is related to the second procedure for the patient. That means that the patient had to undergo the procedure for a second time. For this purpose, the SAS code 2 is used.

Code 2. Codes to Add a Diff Column

```
DATA sasuser.cat4_count_day_diffserv;
set sasuser.cat4_count_day;by patient_id
serv_strt_dt;
diff=DIF(serv_strt_dt);
```

In Figure 26, diff = 0 means that the observation is related to the first day of treatment for a patient. The observations of rows 63 through 68 explain that the billed charges are related to only one day of treatment for each patient. In contrast, the observations of rows 69 through 74 are all related to the same patient. The corresponding entries of the column, diff, are 0, 162, 1, 174, 1, and 518 respectively. These imply that the patient had an angioplasty on Aug, 2003 and 162 days (almost five and half months) later, the same patient had a drug-eluting stent procedure. Again, this patient had another drug-eluting stent procedure after 174 days or almost 6 months. Finally, after 518 days or (almost one and a half years), the patient had an open heart bypass surgery.

We assume that the repetition of a procedure or having another procedure most often happens in more than 9 days. Therefore, in the data analysis, if the variable, diff, is less than 10, it means that the observation is linked to the procedure in the previous observation. This implies that the cost of each row with diff less than 10 needs to be added to the previous row. This process is completed by the Excel software, and Figure 27 shows the partial result of it.

How can we compute the risk of different procedures of coronary artery disease? After data processing, we use the fact that each observation has information about the patient ID, date of service, total charge, category, procedure, diff (diff= 0 means the record shows the first procedure for a patient, and diff= k, where k is nonzero means the observation is related to the previous patient

who had another procedure that happened k days after the previous one), and N (the order of procedures).

In order to demonstrate all the procedures that each patient had, SAS code 3 is used. The result is a transpose of the column named procedure for the patients, where the variables, Date of services, and diff (difference between the procedures for each patient) are kept in the table.

Code 3. SAS Code to Transpose the Column Procedure

```
proc transpose data=sasuser.cat4_final_
code out=sasuser.transpose1 prefix=proc;
by patient_id;
COPY serv_strt_dt diff;
VAR procedure;
```

In Figure 28, a column labeled $proc_i$, where $i \in \{1,2,3,\ldots,11\}$, shows the procedure for all patients in the dataset. For instance, column, $proc_2$, shows the second procedure for each patient if there exists any. The frequencies of the column, $proc_1$, provide the information about the number of each procedure that has been chosen as a first treatment by the patients with coronary artery disease. Table 9 shows the frequency of the column,

Figure 26. A Partial result of the Code 2

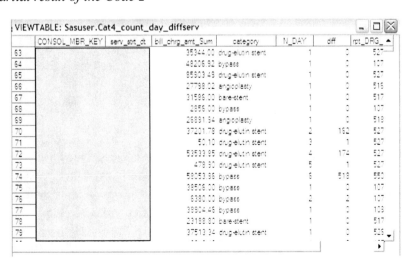

Figure 27. Partial part of the data set showing the total billed charges for each procedure with respect to a patient

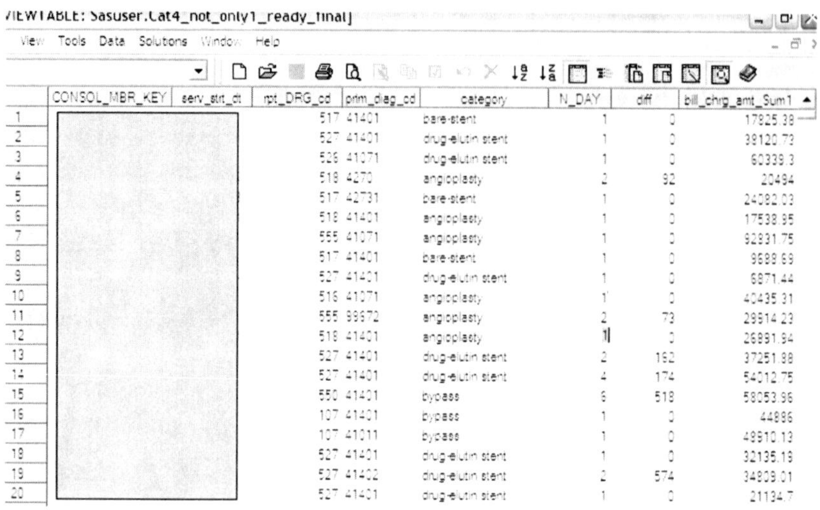

Figure 28. A Partial of Transposed Data

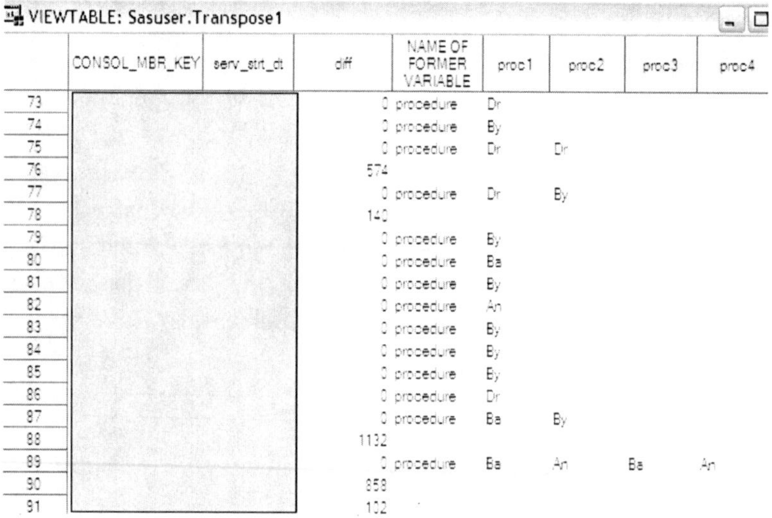

$proc_1$. It confirms that most of the patients, about 30 percent, had a drug-eluting stent as a treatment for the first time and less than 15 percent of the patients chose the bare stent procedure as a treatment for coronary artery disease.

The definition of the probability of an event is

$$\Pr obabilty\ of\ an\ event = p(event) = \frac{the\ number\ of\ the\ event}{the\ total\ number\ of\ events}$$

Figure 29 is derived from table 9, and it shows the probabilities of angioplasty, bare stent, bypass surgery, and drug-eluting stent as the first treatment for a patient with coronary artery disease.

Outcomes Research in Cardiovascular Procedures

Table 9. The number of the procedures as a first procedure or treatment for the patients

Proc1	Frequency	Percent	Cumulative Frequency	Cumulative Percent
An	3521	26.69	3521	26.69
Ba	1930	14.63	5451	41.32
By	3836	29.08	9287	70.39
Dr	3906	29.61	13193	100.00

Figure 29. The probabilities of the first treatment choice

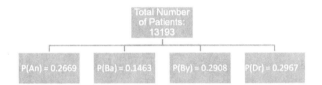

Some patients need to undergo more than one procedure, because of re-blocking the sick artery. That means re-blocking can happen for the second, third, fourth, and even for more than the fifth time. Therefore, the risk of re-blocking after a procedure (or probability of re-blocking) can be computed based on the chain of procedures from the dataset "transpose" until the last procedure.

For this purpose, Enterprise Guide and SAS software were used for the dataset named "Transpose" in many steps. The columns named "$proc_i$" are characteristic columns, and they include only the four values, An, Ba, By, and Dr, where these abbreviations stand for the procedures angioplasty, bare-stent, bypass surgery, and drug-eluting stent. For instance, $proc_1$ = An means that the first procedure for the patient is angioplasty and similarly, $proc_2$ = By implies that the second procedure for the patient is bypass surgery. Consequently, if $proc_i$ = null = "empty cell" for any i, it means that the patient did not have any procedure for the ith time. Therefore, by computing the frequency or using a pie chart for the column $proc_1$, we get the total number and percentage of each type of the procedure as the first treatment for the patients.

The results summary is shown in table 9 and figure 29. There is a chance for re-blocking after each procedure. To estimate the risk of re-blocking of the sick artery for the second time with respect to the type of the first procedure, the dataset named transpose is separated by filtering to the following four subsets: transpose_1an, transpose_1ba, transpose_1dr, and transpose_1by. All observations in each subset have the same procedure in the column $proc_1$ (or the first procedure). For instance, the subset named transpose_1dr includes all clients who had the drug-eluting stent as a first treatment. Accordingly, in each mentioned subset, by performing a frequency count for the column named $proc_2$, we can get the total number and consequently, the probability of having a second procedure with respect to the given first procedure. The SAS code 4 is used for the frequency of $proc_2$ when "$proc_1$=Dr".

Code 4. SAS Code for Frequency $proc_2$ when $proc_1$=Dr

```
proc freq data=sasuser.transpose_1dr
order=internal;
```

71

Table 10. Frequency of proc$_2$ when proc$_1$=Dr

proc2	Frequency	Percent	Cumulative Frequency	Cumulative Percent
An	91	17.11	91	17.11
Ba	30	5.64	121	22.74
By	38	7.14	159	29.89
Dr	373	70.11	532	100.00

```
tables proc2;
run;
```

The result of code 4 is table 10.

By using the information of figure 31, table 10, and the probability formula, we computed the probabilities of having a second procedure for the patients who had a drug-eluting stent as a first procedure with respect to the different types of procedures. We need to compute the probabilities of having second procedures for each patient who had a drug-eluting stent as a first procedure. Note that the percentages given in table 10 are not the same as the conditional probability.

Figure 30 shows the summary of the result. Each number inside the parenthesis in the second row stands for the total number of the first procedures, and in the third row, they stand for the total number of the second procedures when the drug-eluting stent is given as the first procedure. Also, the probability of any event is in the form of p(e), where e is an event. For instance, p(DrBy)=0.01 is a conditional probability; that is, the probability

of bypass as a second procedure given the drug-eluting stent as a first procedure is 0.01.

Note: We can compute the conditional probability of event B when event A is given by using the following formula:

$$p(A \text{ } given \text{ } B) = \frac{p(A \cap B)}{p(B)} = \frac{n(A \cap B)}{n(B)}.$$

Therefore,

$p(DrBy) =$ *the probability of having By as the second procedure when the first treatment is Dr*

$= \dfrac{\text{the number of the patients that use Dr as the first procedure and By surgery as the second one}}{\text{the total number of the patients who use Dr as the first treatment}}$

To find the probability of having a third procedure by a patient who had a drug-eluting stent as a first one, we should consider all the possibilities of conditional events for each previous conditional probability. There are four possibilities for each box in the last branch. Figure 33 illustrates the conditional probabilities of third procedures given the drug-eluting stent and bare stent as

Figure 30. Probabilities of having first procedures and conditional probabilities of second procedure when the drug-eluting stent is given as a first procedure

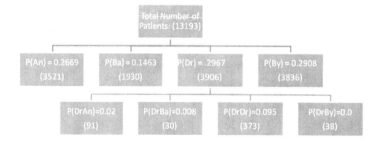

Figure 31. Conditional probability of third procedures given drug-eluting stent and bare stent as the first and second procedure respectively

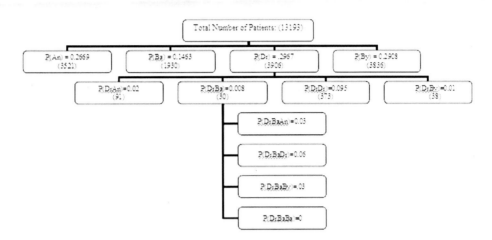

the first and second procedures respectively; that is, p(DrBaDr), p(DrBaBy), p(DrBaBa), and p(DrBaAn).

To find these probabilities, we filter table transpose_1dr with respect to the "$proc_2$ = Ba", and the results table is called transpose_1dr2ba. In this table, all entries of the column $proc_1$ are Dr and for the column, $proc_2$ are Ba. Now, by applying a frequency for the column $proc_3$, we have the total number of each procedure as the third one. Using the probability formula, we compute the conditional probabilities for the third procedures. By the same routine, the probabilities of all possible outcomes are calculated. In the database, there were some patients who had more than three procedures, but the probabilities of those events were sufficiently small to ignore them. We had four possible options for the first, second, and third time procedures. That means we have used 64 steps of filtering and frequency to calculate all probabilities for at most three procedures for each patient.

The results of the conditional probabilities of re-blocking an artery after bypass surgery, drug-eluting stent, and bare stent are shown in Figures 32, 33, and 34.

The risk of re-blocking or the probability of a need for a second procedure after an open bypass surgery, ignoring the type of second procedure, is less than 0.07, (.01+.035+.004+.02=.069). On the basis of the conditional probability, the risk of the need for the third procedure, ignoring the type of the procedure, is

0.01(0.11+0+0+0.03)+0.035(0+0.095+0.007+ 0.14)+0.004(0+.2+.07+.07)+.02(0+.01+.03+ .06)= .0088

According to the information of figure 33, ignoring the type of the second or third procedure, we compute the risk of re-blocking an artery for the second and third time after the drug-eluting stent procedure.

The risk of re-blocking an artery after using the drug-eluting stent as a first treatment is equal to the probability of having another procedure after using the drug-eluting stent twice = (.01+.095+.008+.02)=.133~13%. The risk of re-blocking an artery after undergoing a drug-eluting stent for the second time = .095(.01+.09+.03) = .012~1%, and the risk of re-blocking for the third time, ignoring the type of the second procedure, = 0.0167.

Similarly, using the information in figure 34, we compute the risk of re-blocking of an artery for the second and third time when the first procedure

Figure 32. Conditional probabilities until the third procedures given bypass as a first procedure

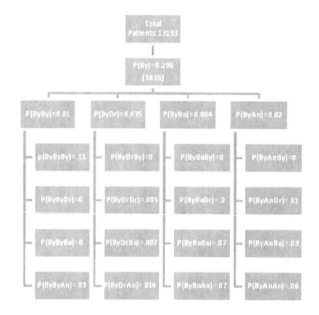

Figure 33. Conditional probabilities until the third procedure given the drug-eluting stent as a first procedure

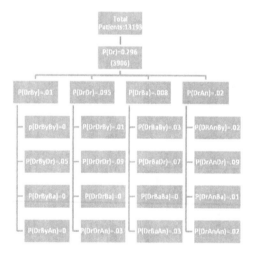

is using a bare stent. The risk of re-blocking is 03+.07+.07+.065=0.235, and the risk of re-blocking for the third time is equal to 0.065.

Comparing the three types of procedures; bypass surgery, drug-eluting stent, and bare stent, shows that the risk of re-blocking an artery after a bare stent is almost 24%, and by using the drug-eluting stent, this risk decreases to almost 13%, and the bypass surgery procedure probability of the re-blocking rate is lower still at less than 7%.

CURRENT AND FUTURE CHALLENGES THAT FACE THE ORGANIZATION

Since the database was not a clinical trial, it was hard to determine the patient conditions precisely, and we had to make some assumptions related to the database, which may increase the error of the result.

Figure 34. Conditional probabilities until the third procedures given the bare stent as a first procedure

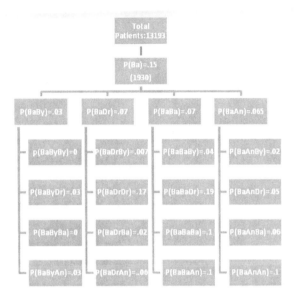

- The total cost in the database was based on the bills that the Insurance Company received from hospitals and physicians before any discount and reduction.
- In this study, we assumed that all patients with coronary artery disease were candidates for the three different procedures, Bypass Surgery, drug-eluting stent, and bare stent. This assumption may not be justified.
- In the database, the DRG codes are used to classify the patients who had different procedures, and it does not include any information about the number or the length of the stent.
- Different drugs inserted with the stent may have a different effect. In this study, we had to consider them only as the drug-eluting stent.
- The cost of different procedures may depend on the rank of hospitals, and we did not have any information to consider the effect of the hospital rank in the cost-effectiveness result.

According to the results of this research, the time series analysis demonstrated that the drug-eluting stent innovation decreases the demand for the bare stent sharply and its effect on bypass surgery is much less than our expectation. That means that this question still is open about whether the drug-eluting stent is an alternative procedure for an open bypass surgery or not. The Drug-eluting stent reduces the rate of re-blocking an artery to 46% compared to the bare stent. This is the main reason for shifting from the bare stent to the drug-eluting stent and makes the drug-eluting stent more effective. The database shows that the rate of re-blocking after the drug-eluting stent is still about 6% more than the rate of re-blocking after an open bypass surgery.

The main question remaining is how the higher rate of re-blocking after the drug-eluting stent compared to open bypass surgery affects the Cost-Effectiveness analysis between the two treatments.

REFERENCES

Anonymous-NICE. (2008). *Drug Eluting Stents for the Treatment of coronary artery disease.* London: National Institute for Health and Clinical Excellence.

Austin, P. C., Alter, D. A., & Tu, J. V. (2003). The use of fixed- and random-effects models for classifying hospitals as mortality outliers: a monte carlos assessment. *Medical Decision Making, 23,* 526–539. doi:10.1177/0272989X03258443

Barrentt, P. (2002, March 11).*W. i. C.-E. A.* Retrieved from http://www.here.research.med. va.gov/FAQ_AL.htm

Blue Cross Blue Shield of Texas. (n.d.). *W. I. t. R. A. C.* Retrieved from http://www.bcbstx.com/provider/bluechoice_solutions_tool_raci.htm.

Brophy, J., & Erickson, L. (2004). An economic analysis of drug eluting coronary stents: a Quebec perspective. *AETMIS, 4*(4), 38.

Brophy, J., & Erickson, L. (2005). *Cost Effectiveness of Drug Eluting Coronary Stents A Quebec Perspective.* Cambridge, UK: Cambridge University Press.

Cerrito, P., & Cerrito, J. C. (2006). Data and Text Mining the Electronic Medical Record to Improve Care and to Lower Costs [Electronic Version]. *SUGI 31 Proceedings, 31.* Retrieved January 2007, from http://www2.sas.com/proceedings/sugi31/077-31.pdf.

Circulation, American Heart Association. (2006) *Heart disease and Strok Statistics.* Retrieved from http://circ.ahajournals.org/cgi/reprint/113/6/e85. pdf.

Cohen, B. (2008). *Drug-Eluting Stent overview.* Retrieved from http://www.ptca.org/stent.html

Cohen, D. J., Bakhai, A., Shi, C., Githiora, L., Lavelle, T., & Berezin, R. H. (2004). *Cost-Effectiveness of Sirolimus-Eluting Stents for Treatment of Complex Coronary Stenoses.* Boston: Harvard Clinical Research Institute.

Fajadet, J. P. M., Hayashi, E. B., et al. (2002, March 18) *American College of Cardiology 51st Annual Scientific Session* (Presentation #0032-1). Retrieved from http://www.stjohns.com/doctorclark/AnswerPage.aspx?drclark_id=22

FDA. (2003, April). *Food and Drug administration news, Media Inquiries: 301-827-6242, Consumer Inquiries: 888-INFO-FDA.* Retrieved from http://www.fda.gov/bbs/topics/NEWS/2003/NEW00896.html

Gillette, B. (2005, September). *Manage Health Care Executive.* Retrieved from http://www.managedhealthcareexecytive.com/mhe/article

Iezzoni, L. I., Ash, A. S., Shwartz, M., Daley, J., Hughes, J. S., & Mackleman, Y. D. (1995). Predicting who dies depends on how severity is measured: implications for evaluating patient outcomes. *Annals of Internal Medicine, 123*(10), 763–770.

Igor Singer, M. (n.d.). *FRACP, FACP, FACC, FACA, Executive Medical Director, Cardiovascular Services, Methodist Medical Center.* Retrieved from http://week.com/health_med/health_med. asp?id=4495

Loren, K. (n.d.). *Heart Disease: Number One Killer.* Retrieved from http://www.heart-disease-bypass-surgery.com/data/footnotes/f5.htm

Mc, L. T. C., & Allaster, D. L. (n.d.). *B. U. o. S. E. S. t. F. a. T. S.* Fort Lee, VA . *Us Army Logistics Management Collage.*

Moses, J. W., & Leon, M. B. (n.d.). *Lenox Hill Hospital, U.S. SIRIUS Study, Cardiovascular Research Foundation:1,058 Patients.* Retrieved from http://www.investor.jnj.com/releaseDetail.cfm?ReleaseID=90711&year=2002

National HeartLung and Blood Institute. (n.d.). *D. a. C. I., Angioplasty.* Retrieved from http://www.nhlbi.nih.gov/health/dci/Diseases/Angioplasty/Angioplasty_WhatIs

Newsome, L. T., Kutcher, M. A., Gandhi, S. K., Prielipp, R. C., & Royster, R. L. (2008). *A Protocol for the Perioperative Management of Patients With Intracoronary Drug-Eluting Stents.* Winston-Salem, NC: Wake Forest University School of Medicine.

Pear, R. (2007, August 19). Medicare Says It Won't Cover Hospital Errors. *New York Times.*

Poses, R. M., McClish, D. K., Smith, W. R., Huber, E. C., Clomo, F. L., & Schmitt, B. P. (2000). Results of report cards for patients with congestive heart failure depend on the method used to adjust for severity. *Annals of Internal Medicine, 133,* 10–20.

Reuters, T. (2008). *Health Care, Medical Episode Grouper - Government.* Retrieved from http://research.thomsonhealthcare.com/Products/view/?id=227

SAS. (n.d.). *Introduction to Time Series Forecasting Using SAS/ETS Software Course Notes, C. b. S. I. I.* Cary, NC . *SAS Publishing.*

Sousa, J. E., Costa, M. A., & Sousa, A. G. (2003). Two-year angio-graphic and intravascular ultrasound follow-up after implantation of sirolimus-eluting stents in human coronary arteries. *Circulation, 107,* 381–383. doi:10.1161/01.CIR.0000051720.59095.6D

Texas Heart Institute. H. I. C. (n.d.). *Coronary Artery Bypass, at St.Lukes'Episcopal Hospital.* Retrieved from http://texasheart.org/HIC/Topics/Proced/cab.cfm

Thomas, J. W. (1998). Research evidence on the validity of adjusted mortality rate as a measure of hospital quality of care. *Medical Care Research and Review, 55*(4), 371–404. doi:10.1177/107755879805500401

Yock, C.-A. M., Boothroyd, D. B., Owens, D. K., Garber, A. M., & Hlatky, M. A. (2003). *Cost-effectiveness of Btpass Surgery versus Stenting in Patients with Multivessele Coronary Artery Disease.* Boston: Harvard Clinical Research Institute.

ADDITIONAL READING

Anonymous-NICE. (2008). *Drug Eluting Stents for the Treatment of coronary artery disease.* London: National Institute for Health and Clinical Excellence. Retrieved from http://www.nice.org.uk/nicemedia/pdf/TA152Guidance.pdf.

Brophy, J., & Erickson, L. (2004). An economic analysis of drug eluting coronary stents: a Quebec perspective. *AETMIS, 04*(04), 38. Retrieved from http://www.aetmis.gouv.qc.ca/site/download.php?f=059cca28f196fb38f30873d34a39efb7.

Cerrito, P. B. (2009a). *Data Mining Healthcare and Clinical Databases.* Cary, NC: SAS Press, Inc.

Cerrito, P. B. (2009b). *Text Mining Techniques for Healthcare Provider Quality Determination: Methods for Rank Comparisons.* Hershey, PA: IGI Publishing.

Kashan, F. (n.d.). Cost-shifting of the Drug-eluting Stent (PhD Dissertation). Retrieved from http://www.lulu.com/content/compact_disc/dissertations_on_data_mining_healthcare/2165369

Chapter 4
Outcomes Research in the Treatment of Asthma

Ram C. Neupane
College of Georgia, USA

Jason Turner
University of Louisville, USA

ABSTRACT

Asthma is a common chronic disease in the United States, with increasing prevalence. Many patients do not realize therapeutic goals because of poor disease management. The purpose of this study is to examine the costs of the commonly used drugs used to treat asthma. We examined the contribution of individual, government and private agencies for medication payment. We next compared the prescription cost to the cost of emergency room visits. The data are taken from the Medical Expenditure Panel Survey. SAS Enterprise Guide was used for preprocessing and data visualization. It was found that prednisone is the cheapest drug and the drug, albuterol, is the most common, even if it is more expensive. The contribution of the government is higher than the amount paid by individuals and other agencies. We examined data from the National Inpatient Sample to investigate trends in asthma as well.

BACKGROUND

Asthma is a chronic disease that affects the human respiratory system. Because of asthma, the airways in the lungs become narrower. Consequently, there is less airflow through the lungs. Its main symptoms are trouble in breathing, coughing and chest tightness. Asthma cannot be cured, but most people with asthma can control it so that they have few symptoms and can live a normal and active life. When the symptoms of asthma become worse than usual, this is called an asthma attack. In a severe case, the airways might narrow so much that oxygen cannot circulate to the vital organs of the body. As a result, people may die from severe asthma attacks.

Asthma is a worldwide public health problem affecting approximately 300 million people. Most of them are living in the developing countries. Despite the existence of effective medications and international medical guidelines, the continuous high cost of asthma medications becomes a major problem for most of the developing countries. (Ait-Khaled,

DOI: 10.4018/978-1-61520-723-7.ch004

Copyright © 2010, IGI Global. Copying or distributing in print or electronic forms without written permission of IGI Global is prohibited.

Enarson, Bissell, & Billo, 2007) According to the National Center for Health Statistics, there are at least 21 million patients with asthma in the United States. Among them are about 6 million children under 18 years of age. In 2000, there were 1.9 million emergency department visits for asthma leading to 465,000 hospital admissions overall, with 214,000 for children 1 to 17 years of age. (Conboy-Ellis, 2006)

According to the American Lung Association, in the year 2007, there were 22.2 million Americans suffering from asthma, including 6.5 million children of 5 to 17 years of age. Also, in 2005, there were 488,594 asthma related hospitalizations, 1.8 million emergency department visits and 3,780 deaths in 2004. The annual cost in 2007 was $ 19.7 billion. (Anonymous-asthma, 2007)

The main causes of asthma are allergens such as skin, hair and feathers of animals, pollen from trees, cockroaches, dust mites, irritants such as air pollution, cigarette smoke, strong odors, cold air and strong emotional expressions, and viral infections. Working closely with a doctor, avoiding things that create asthma symptoms, using asthma medicines, monitoring asthma symptoms and responding quickly to prevent an asthma attack are the main procedures used to treatment asthma. (Anonymous-NIH asthma, 2008)

There are many factors that influence the level of asthma control. Mainly, they are classified as physiologic, environmental and behavioral. Physiologic factors include circadian fluctuations, hormonal status, pregnancy, obesity, airway remodeling, and airway hyper responsiveness. Environmental factors include viral infections, allergens, air pollution, seasonal variation, tobacco and behavioral factors that include patient understanding of asthma, adherence to asthma therapy regimen, knowledge and/or avoidance of asthma triggers, and recognition of worsening symptoms. One physiologic factor is gender. The number of males with asthma is more than the number of females in childhood, while we get the opposite result in adulthood. Air pollution such as ozone

sulfuric oxide creates the problem in lung function. Behavioral factors are related to the perception of asthma severity and the proper response to escape symptoms. (Chipps & Spahn, 2006)

Because of different causes and different levels of severity of asthma, the treatment of asthma varies from person to person. There are three basic types of medications to control asthma, long-term control medications, quick relief medications and medications for allergy-induced asthma. The drugs, fluticasone, budesonide, triamcinolone, flunisolide, qvar, montelukast, and beta-2 agonists such as salmeteral and formoterol are used to treat persistent asthma. These medications reduce bronchal inflation and open the airways. The drugs, cromolyn and nedocromil, are used to decrease the allergic reaction, and Theophylline is a daily pill that opens airways and relaxes the muscles around them. Quick-relief medications are used during an asthma attack. A short-acting, beta-2 agonist such as albuterol is given for easy breathing by temporarily relaxing airway muscles. The drug, iprotropium, is also given for immediate relief to allow breathing. Moreover, the drugs, prednisone and methylprednisolone, are given to treat acute asthma attacks, but those drugs may cause serious side effects if they are used in the long term. Anti-igE monoclonal antibodies such as xolair reduce the patient's immune system's reactions to allergens. It is given by injections every two to four weeks. (Anonymous-Mayoasthma, 2008)

Besides drug treatment, behavioral modification is another most important aspect for asthma management. The National Institutes of Health (NIH) established five general goals for asthma management. They include no missed school or work days, no sleep disruptions, and maintenance of normal activity levels. A minimal or absent need for emergency department visits or hospitalizations and maintenance of normal lung functions are also goals for treatment.

However, achieving these goals remains incomplete. Low rates of patient adherence to treatment, or failure to follow a prescribed treatment plan are the major hindrances to affective asthma management. There is often a communication gap between physicians and patients. Primary care physicians are not effectively communicating the important messages about treatment to their patients diagnosed with asthma and then in creating the treatment goals to accomplish, although most primary care physicians are aware of and follow the NIH asthma treatment guidelines. In actual practice, however, treatments recommended by guidelines are often under-utilized. The low adherence rates among asthma patients can be improved by educational programs. Interactive physician programs can improve guideline implementation and physician communication skills. Effective physician-patient communication can be the most important factor for improving guideline implementation and patient treatment, resulting in the decrease of asthma-related mortality. (Brown, 2001)

According to the 2002 National Health and Blood Institute (NHLBI)'s Asthma Education and Prevention Program, the treatment of asthma has four components: (i) use of objective measures of lung function to access the severity of asthma and to monitor results of therapy; (ii) implementation of environmental control measures designed to avoid or eliminate factors (allergens and irritants) that contribute to asthma severity; (iii) use of pharmacologic therapy that treats asthma exacerbations, and modulates on a long term basis the airways inflation that is an intrinsic component of the disease; (iv) implementation of patient education programs with the purpose of educating patients and their families, and also to establish a partnership between the healthcare provider and both patient and family for asthma management. The goals of asthma therapy are to (i) control symptoms of asthma and to prevent exacerbations; (ii) maintain normal activity levels, including exercise; (iii) maintain pulmonary function as close to normal as possible; (iv) minimize the adverse drug treatment effects. (Conboy-Ellis, 2006)

The purpose of this study is to investigate asthma and its outcomes. We will find cheaper and frequently used drugs to treat asthma. There are three types of payments such as self, private and government payments. We will compare the costs of those payments. We will then observe the frequency of emergency visits of patients. After that, we will compare doctors' payments, doctors' charges and facilities payments and charges. Then, we will compare the costs of each prescription with the costs of emergency visits made by each patient.

SETTING THE STAGE

From the Medical Expenditure Panel Survey (MEPS)

We downloaded the MEPS HC-094A datafile defined as the 2005 prescribed medicine files and HC-094E defined as the 2005 emergency room visits. (Anonymous-MEPS, 2007) There were 16,347 asthma related prescriptions and 187 emergency room visits. Kernel density estimation was used to examine the data. The kernel density estimations of charges and payments show that as value increases, the probabilities of paying those amounts drop sharply. It has been found that the payments for facilities is approximately five times more than the payments for physicians, and the total costs of emergency room visits is about three times the total cost of prescribed medicines. Though the visits to the emergency department seem occasional, they are more expensive then the prescribed medicines.

In this project, we used Enterprise Guide from SAS and data from the Medical Expenditure Panel Survey. First, we downloaded MEPS HC-094A defined as the 2005 prescribed medicines file. (Anonymous-MEPS, 2007) We next created a SAS data file from the data. There are 317,587 observations containing all prescriptions from a population cohort of approximately 30,000 individuals. Here, we are interested only in asthma related medications. Therefore, we next filtered the data to a specific list of medications.

After filtering those observations from the whole data set, we were left with a total of 16,347 asthma-related observations; each observation is a prescription for an asthma medication. Then, since there are many brand names for each generic drug, we used one generic name to refer to a specific group of asthma medications. Drugs included in the survey are advair, albuterol, budesonide, cromolyn, decadron, elixophyllin, flunisolide, formoterol, ipratropium, mometasone, montelukast, pibuterol, prednisone, qvar, terbutaline, xolair, and xopenex. We examine the cost per patient for using each particular drug. We then downloaded MEPS HC-094E defined as the 2005 emergency room visits files. There are 6446 observations in total in that dataset.

After using filter and query commands, we had a total of 187 emergency room visits related to asthma. Then, we counted the frequencies, and observed the charges and payments made by the patients.

We use statistical summaries and kernel density estimation to investigate the data. Kernel density estimation is a non-parametric way of estimating the probability density function of a random variable. For instance, given some data about a sample of a population, kernel density estimation makes it possible to extrapolate the data to the entire population.

From the National Inpatient Sample (NIS)

The Healthcare Cost Utilization Project (HCUP) is a state and federal collective effort that maintains several health care related databases and software. The purpose of HCUP is to provide the ability to perform health care related research on authentic data. One of the databases maintained by HCUP is the National Inpatient Sample. (Anonymous-NIS,

2007) Four of the 175 data attributes that the NIS database contains are the month that the patient was admitted, the length of their stay in the hospital, and total cost of their stay. In this experiment, an analysis was performed on the overall data as well as on the dataset of patients who had asthma and the patients who did not have asthma.

Time series analysis can be utilized to analyze the NIS database, which will allow the cost and length of an inpatient stay to be predicted based on past occurrences. The method of time series to be used is the autoregressive integrated moving average (ARIMA) model. Linear models can aide in determining some of the effects that some of the variables in the dataset have on the length of stay and total charges.

The results of this experiment showed that the months of June and July have the highest average length of stay and total charges for both the asthma and non-asthma patients. Based on this, it can be determined that in subsequent years, June and July will continue to be peak months in hospital stays and expenses, and that expenses will continue to rise. The linear model analysis on the total charges showed that out of the length of stay, patient age, asthma diagnosis, race, gender, and two-way interaction combinations, only the age and asthma diagnosis have no statistical significant effects. The linear model analysis on the length of stay showed that only the asthma diagnosis and the two-way interaction of age and gender diagnosis have no statistical significant effects. The results of the analysis showed relationships between length of stay and total charges for the overall dataset. The length of stay and total charges for the asthma patients all followed a very similar pattern, which was also true for the non-asthma patients. The combination of asthma diagnosis and age have no significant effect on the total charges, while the asthma diagnosis and the combination of age and gender have no effect on the length of stay.

In this project, we will examine, the length of stay and total charges of the patients for

Table 1. Number of prescriptions of each medication

RXNAME_cleanup	Frequency	Percent	Cumulative Frequency	Cumulative Percent
Advair	2573	15.75	2573	15.75
Albuterol	5307	32.48	7880	48.22
Budesonide	397	2.43	8277	50.65
Cromolyn	66	0.40	8343	51.06
Decadron	137	0.84	8480	51.89
Elixophyllin	499	3.05	8979	54.95
Flunisolide	984	6.02	9963	60.97
Formoterol	401	2.45	10364	63.42
Ipratropium	485	2.97	10849	66.39
Mometasone	419	2.56	11268	68.96
Montelukast	2614	16.00	13882	84.95
Pirbuterol	55	0.34	13937	85.29
Prednisone	2005	12.27	15942	97.56
Qvar	110	0.67	16052	98.23
Terbutaline	6	0.04	16058	98.27
Xolair	1	0.01	16059	98.27
Xopenex	282	1.73	16341	100.00

the months of admission in the 2004 and 2005 National Inpatient Sample so that the outcome variables can be predicted based on the events that already occurred (Anonymous-NIS, 2008). We consider the patients who only had an asthma condition and compare them to the patients who did not have asthma. The data analysis used was the autoregressive integrated moving average model. The time interval used in this time series analysis was one month.

Initially, the month admitted field was an integer (1-12) format, representing calendar months. In order for SAS to be able to perform any time series analysis, the length of stay field was modified to a date data-type. This was performed on both the 2004 and 2005 datasets, after which the two datasets were combined.

The data were then divided into two additional datasets; the first one containing the records of the original dataset (with the date modification) that contained patients who had an asthma condi-

tion, and the other containing the patients who did not have an asthma condition. The "codeasthma" variable signifies if a patient has asthma or not (0 = non-asthma, 1 = asthma). This was performed by using the SQL procedure in SAS.

CASE DESCRIPTION

MEPS

Table 1 gives the frequency count of each of the medications used in the study.

The drug, albuterol, which is for treating emergency asthma attacks, has the highest percentage, followed by the drugs, montelukast, advair and prednisone. There is a drug, xolair, that was used by only one patient in the cohort.

Table 2 shows the relationship of payment to medication. The variable we used was total payment for the medication for each individual

Table 2. Costs of each medication

RXNAME_cleanup	No. obs.	Mean
Prednisone	2005	8.4369
decadron	137	13.8778
abuterol	5307	28.6143
mometasone	419	31.6294
terbutaline	6	35.8733
elixophyllin	499	56.5120
cromolyn	66	60.0931
qvar	110	68.3018
ipratropium	485	69.2292
flunisolide	984	85.3969
xopenex	282	86.9964
montelukast	2614	98.1711
pirbuterol	55	100.7365
formoterol	401	127.7927
advair	2573	142.3074
budesonide	397	156.3184
xolair	1	9088.27

prescription. This payment was the combined reimbursement paid by the patient, insurance, and government agencies.

Table 2 shows that prednisone is the cheapest drug used by patients. The total cost per person averages to $ 8.4369. Few people used the more expensive drugs such as mometasone, terbutaline, cromolyn and qvar. On the other hand, many patients took the drugs, advair and montelukast, which are also more expensive. The drug, xolair, is the most expensive drug that is taken by only one patient. Table 3 gives a breakdown in payment by each entity.

Table 3 shows that out of seventeen drugs, the payment made by the government for nine of the drugs is more than the self payment and the private payment by insurers. If we observe the costs of the main four drugs used by most patients, the government payment is more for the drugs, montelukast and albuterol, than for the remaining two medications. For the drug, advair,

Table 3. Government, private and self payments for each medication

RXNAME_cleanup	No. Obs	GOV. Support	Private payment	Self payment	Mean total
xolair	1	8954.65	0	133.62	9088.27
budesonide	397	81.1581	48.5353	26.6249	156.3183
formoterol	401	67.8322	37.3270	22.6334	127.7926
flunisolide	984	48.7426	25.2620	11.5922	85.5968
xopenex	282	47.8215	9.7941	29.3807	86.9963
elixophyllin	499	35.4523	5.3119	15.7477	56.5119
advair	2573	51.8269	61.3545	39.1259	142.3073
pirbuterol	55	23.9820	27.1347	49.6198	100.8365
montelukast	2614	38.9108	38.3314	20.9288	98.1710
ipratropium	485	31.5156	9.4354	28.2782	69.2292
qvar	110	20.8341	22.7368	24.7308	68.3017
cromolyn	66	24.1469	1.4544	34.4918	60.0931
terbutaline	6	10.8750	19.9650	5.0333	35.8733
mometasone	419	11.2099	7.4868	12.9326	31.6293
albuterol	5307	11.7776	6.6177	10.2189	28.6142
decadron	137	3.1249	3.2178	7.5360	13.8787
prednisone	2005	2.2934	0.8955	5.2479	8.4368

private payment is the most and the self payment is the most for the drug, prednisone.

Kernel Density Estimation allows us to visualize subgroup comparisons because graphs can be over-laid. Figure 1 gives the probability density for total pay.

Figure 1 shows that the payment for the drug, prednisone, has the highest probability of pay-

Figure 1. Kernel density for total pay

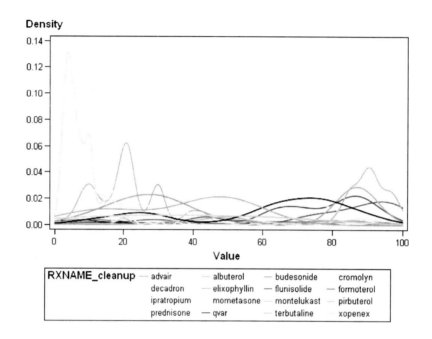

Figure 2. Kernel density for insurance pay

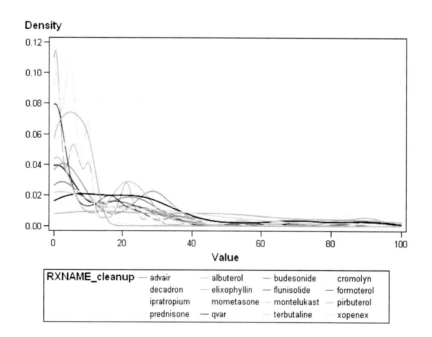

ing up to $ 3.75 per prescription followed by the drug, decadron, with $ 8.25. The payment for the drug, montelukast, has a still higher probability of paying $ 90.50 than most of the drugs even if it is more expensive.

Figure 2 shows that the payment for the drug, albuterol, has the highest probability of paying up to $ 5.00 per prescription followed by the drug, prednisone, with payment up to $ 4.50.

Figure 3 shows that the payment for the drug, decadron, has the highest probability of paying a small cost. This is followed by the drug. albuterol.

Figure 4 shows that the amount of payment for the drug, mometasone, has the highest probability of Medicaid paying up to $ 2 followed by the drug, albuterol, which has payment up to $ 2.50 by Medicaid. We also investigated the total

Figure 3. Kernel density for self pay

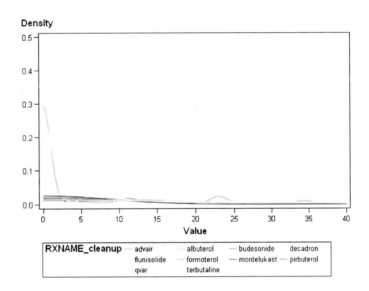

Figure 4. Kernel density for medicaid pay

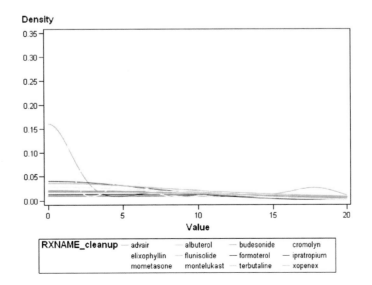

amount that patients and other agencies paid for the drugs over a year. We compute the summary values.

Figure 5 shows that the payment for the drug, prednisone, has the highest probability of paying $ 5.25 in total followed by the drug, decadron, paying $ 10.50 and the drug, terbutaline, paying $ 47.50.

Figure 6 shows that the amount of payment for the drug, terbulaline, has the highest probability of $ 4.75 followed by the drug, prednisone, paying $ 3.75 and the drug, mometasone, with $ 2.75.

Figure 7 shows that the payment for the drug, mometasone, has the highest probability of paying a negligible amount followed by the drug, decadron.

Figure 5. Kernel density for yearly total pay

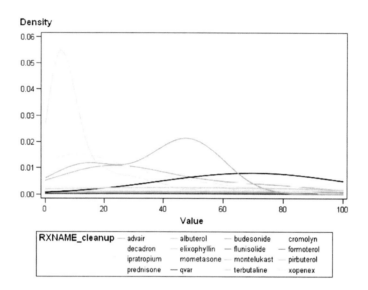

Figure 6. Kernel density for yearly self pay

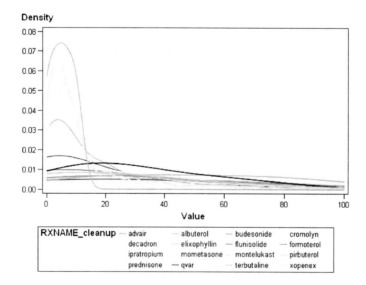

Figure 7. Kernel density for yearly private pay

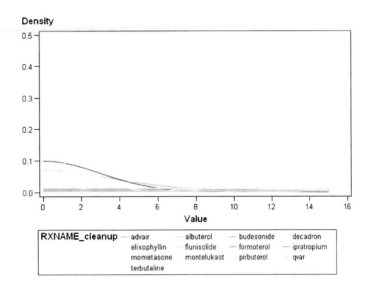

Figure 8. Kernel density for yearly medicare pay

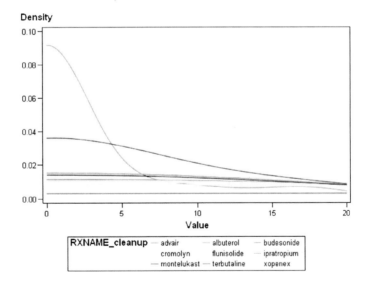

Figure 8 shows that payment for the drug, albuteral, has the highest probability of costing up to $ 4.25. The remaining drugs are highly variable in their costs. We next observed the emergency room visits of patients of asthma during a year. Here, we want to examine the frequencies of visits so that we can investigate asthma to determine whether it is controlled or not.

Table 4 shows that there are 91 patients who had only one emergency visit in the year. There is also a patient who visited thirteen times in the year. There is a facilities charge and a physician charge. Those charges are always less than the actual amount of payments made by the patients.

Table 5 shows that the mean amount of the facility sum payment per year per patient is $ 567.00,

Table 4. Frequency of emergency visits

# of Visits	Frequency	Percent	Cumulative Frequency	Cumulative Percent
1	91	74.59	91	74.59
2	19	15.57	110	90.16
3	4	3.28	114	93.44
4	5	4.10	119	97.54
5	1	0.82	120	98.36
8	1	0.82	121	99.18
13	1	0.82	122	100.00

Table 5. Costs for emergency visit

Variable	Mean	Std Dev	Minimum	Maximum
Total Expense	672.9641	1025.28	0	6422.18
Total Charge	1595.2100	1954.09	0	14648.54
Facility Payments	567.0050	909.5494712	0	5794.98
Facility Charge	1273.5100	1559.27	0	7901.71
Physician Payments	105.9590	203.3631966	0	1764.88
Physician Charge	321.6997	676.1784334	0	7015.66

Variable	Lower Quartile	Median	Upper Quartile	
Total Expense	135.06	312.8650	715.04	
Total Charge	535.60	976.1100	1861.00	
Facility Payments	80.92	272.3650	633.85	
Facility Charge	307.00	750.7500	1700.30	
Physician Payments	0	42.3000	121.22	
Physician Charge	0	205.0000	415.00	

while the mean amount of total facility charge is $ 1273.51. The mean amount of total physician payment per year per patient is $ 105.96. The mean amount of total doctor charge is $ 321.70.

Figure 9 shows that there is a high probability of paying around $ 120 to the facility. This probability drops so that the probability of paying $ 600 is negligible.

Figure 10 shows that charging around $400 is the main probability for the facility. As this charge increases, the probability falls very quickly.

Figure 11 shows that there is a high probability of paying around $10 for the Doctor Sum payments.

Figure 12 shows that there is a high probability of the doctor charging $ 55.

Figure 13 shows that there is a high probability of expending around $ 180 for facility and Doctor Payment combined.

Figure 14 shows that there is a high probability of charging around $ 630 for total charge.

Here, we concentrate on showing the relationship between the emergency room visits and medications.

In figure 15, values 1 and 2 show the costs of emergency visits and the cost of prescriptions, respectively. The next component is the density of these costs. We see that there is a small variance between these two costs.

The relationship between two variables can be observed by plotting these values in the two dimensional graph.

Figure 9. Kernel density for facility sum payments

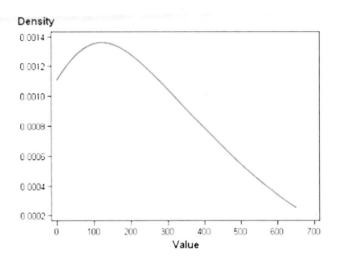

Figure 10. Kernel density for total facility charge

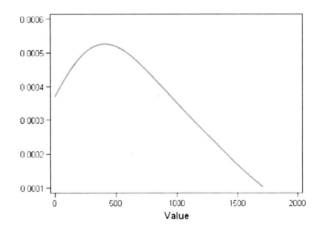

Figure 11. Kernel density for doctor sum payments

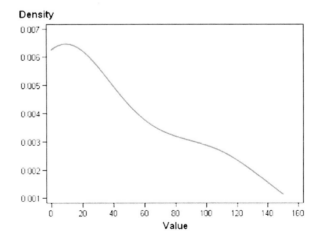

Figure 12. Kernel density for total doctor charge

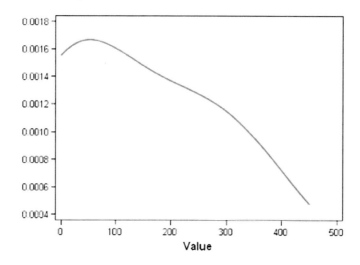

Figure 13. Kernel density for total expenditure

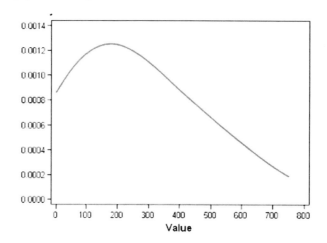

Figure 14. Kernel density for total charge

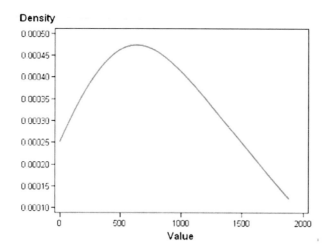

Figure 15. Bivariate graph of total prescription costs and costs of emergency visits.

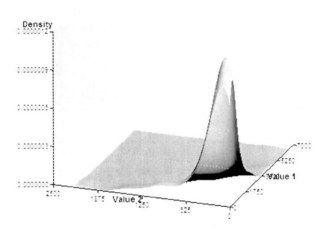

Figure 16. Linear relationships

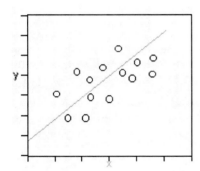

$$Y= b_0+b_1 X \qquad (1)$$

where,

Y= the Y axis variable
X= the X axis variable
b_0= the value of the Y variable when X=0
b_1=the slope of the line.

Most of the plotted points are not on the line. So, we add one term "e" (called the error term) to the equation (1) so that the resulting equation can represent the pattern of the whole distribution. Hence, we get a equation of the form:

$$Y=b_0 ++b_1 X+e \qquad (2)$$

where the term e is called the error term, which is the vertical distance from the straight line to each point. The equation (2) is a Linear Model for two variables.

We can extend the two-variables Linear Model to the General Linear Model by using a set of variables instead of a single variable. Thus, the General Linear Model can be written as:

$$Y= b_0+b_1 X+e \qquad (3)$$

Figure 16 shows the bivariate plot of two variables. The pattern of this plot shows that as the value of the one variable increases, the value of the other also increases, and vice versa. The straight line through the bivariate plot describes the pattern of the data even if most of the points do not lie on this straight line. When a given set of x, y variables is fitted on a straight line, we are using what is called a linear model. The term, "Linear," implies that the data are fitted on a line and the term, "Model," implies the equation that summarizes the line that estimates the data. This line is called a regression line.

The equation of the line in the figure can be written as:

Table 7. Coefficients of independent variables and standard errors

Parameter	Estimate		Standard Error	t Value	Pr > |t|
Intercept	367.7848750	B	169.8169449	2.17	0.0314
The sum of total costs for prescriptions for one individual	-0.0848869		0.1070829	-0.79	0.4288
advair	70.7930157	B	198.7837978	0.36	0.7221
albuterol	7.9497661	B	176.5577303	0.05	0.9641
budesonide	-84.2336707	B	256.3683712	-0.33	0.7428
cromolyn	98.8191489	B	531.4792788	0.19	0.8527
decadron	-262.8244388	B	531.8378849	-0.49	0.6217
elixophyllin	237.4795811	B	253.9976418	0.93	0.3508
flunisolide	84.0614891	B	205.8163149	0.41	0.6833
formoterol	723.3662073	B	310.3941559	2.33	0.0207
ipratropium	61.4969816	B	305.2734270	0.20	0.8405
mometasone	803.8250529	B	394.0516661	2.04	0.0425
montelukast	168.4429614	B	192.3699906	0.88	0.3822
prednisone	125.8886429	B	190.3513420	0.66	0.5091
qvar	78.8800603	B	303.1654385	0.26	0.7950
xopenex	0.0000000	B	.	.	.

where,

Y = a set of outcome variables

X = a set of covariates

b_0 = the set of intercepts (i.e.; the values of each y at each x=0)

b = a set of X coefficients.

The generalized linear model is a generalization of the general linear model. It can be expressed as the relationship between a dependent variable Y and the set of predictor variables, X's, such that

$$Y = b_0 + b_1 X_1 + b_2 X_2 + \ldots\ldots\ldots + b_k X_k \qquad (4)$$

where, b_0 is the regression coefficient for the intercept and b_i, (i= 1, 2,……, k) are called the regression coefficients that can be calculated from the data. The error term can be identified as normal, as in the general linear model; or it can be from a different distribution such as gamma or exponential, which are usually the distributions of healthcare costs.

There are some variables that have a linear relationship. For instance, height, weight and gender are linearly related. We can predict a person's weight on the basis of the distribution of height and gender. In this case, we can use the general linear model for prediction. On the other hand, there are some variables that have a nonlinear relationship. For example, the relationship between age and health status of a person is nonlinear. In this case, we have to use the generalized linear model for prediction.

Here, the study is concentrated on the healthcare costs. For the treatment of asthma, some patients used prescription medications and/or emergency room visits. Emergency treatment seems more expensive than treatment by using prescriptions. In this model, emergency cost is used as a dependent variables and the type of prescription is used as an independent variable.

Table 7 shows that the coefficient for the drug, decadron, is -626.82, which is a minimum among these fourteen drugs. When patients used this drug for treatment, the emergency cost also was a minimum. This implies that this drug worked effectively to cure asthma. The coefficient for the drug, advair, is 70.79 and for the drug, albuterol, is 7.95. When patients used these drugs, emergency costs increased respectively. On the other hand, the coefficient for the drug, mometasone, is 803.83, which is a maximum. Consequently, the emergency cost became maximal when patients used the drug, mometasone. This indicates that use of the drug, mometasone, seems to be less effective to control asthma.

National Inpatient Sample

Before any time series techniques were performed, basic descriptive statistical analyses were performed on the overall dataset. The descriptive statistics for the length of stay and total charges are in Table 8.

From Table 8, it can be determined that the mean length of stay was 3.47 days with a standard deviation of 6.09 days. The median length of stay was 2.00 days, which means that half of the dataset had a length of stay below 2.00 days and half of

the dataset had a length of stay above 2.00 days. The mean total charges were $14,686.18 with a standard deviation of $30,164.05 and a median of $7,649.00. Basic descriptive statistical analyses were also performed on the asthma and non-asthma datasets, which are in Tables 9 and 10.

From Table 9, it can be determined that the mean length of stay for the patents with asthma was 3.09 days with a standard deviation of 4.76 days. The median length of stay was 2.00 days, which means that half of the dataset had a length of stay below 2.00 days and half of the dataset had a length of stay above 2.00 days. The mean total charges were $12,195.70 with a standard deviation of $22,198.04 and a median of $6,916.00.

From Table 10, it can be determined that the mean length of stay for the patents without asthma was 3.84 days with a standard deviation of 7.16 days. The median length of stay was 2.00 days. The mean total charges were $17,161.79 with a standard deviation of $36,224.47 and a median of $8,505.00.

SAS Enterprise Guide's ARIMA procedure from SAS/ETS was then utilized to generate three

Table 8. Overall descriptive statistics (length of stay and total charges)

Variable	Label	Mean	Std Dev	Median	Minimum	Maximum
TOTCHG	Total charges	14686.18	30164.05	7649.00	25.00	995531.00
LOS	Length of stay	3.4655689	6.0949293	2.00000	0	348.00

Table 9. Asthma dataset descriptive statistics (length of stay and total charges)

Variable	Label	Mean	Std Dev	Median	Minimum	Maximum
TOTCHG	Total charges	12195.70	22198.04	6916.00	25.00	992088.00
LOS	Length of stay	3.0889186	4.7614756	2.00000	0	300.00

Table 10. Non-Asthma dataset descriptive statistics (length of stay and total charges)

Variable	Label	Mean	Std Dev	Median	Minimum	Maximum
TOTCHG	Total charges	17151.79	36224.47	8585.00	25.00	995531.00
LOS	Length of stay	3.8391759	7.1573549	2.00	0	348.00

graphs (Figures 17, 18, and 19) representing the moving average for both the length of stay and total charges for each of the months in the year 2005.

Based on Figure 17, it can be determined that the months January (≈3.46 days), June (≈3.52 days), and July (≈3.48 days) had the peak patient length of stays in 2004. The month of October, 2004 had the lowest patient length of stay (≈3.24

days). In the year 2005, the months of January, June, and July had similar average lengths of stay, which were also the highest (≈3.66 days). The month of November in 2005 had the lowest average length of stay (≈3.34 days).

Based on Figure 18, it can be determined that in the year 2004, the months of June (≈$15,200) and July (≈$15,000) had the highest average total charges. The months of January and March in 2004

Figure 17. ARIMA model for length of stay

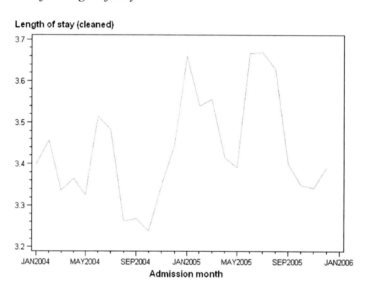

Figure 18. ARIMA Model for total charges

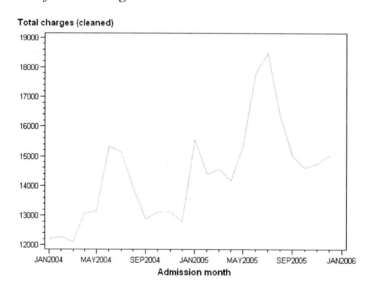

had the lowest average total charges (≈$12,200). In the year 2005, the months June (≈$18,000) and July (≈$18,600) had the highest average total charges. The months of April (≈$14,200) and October (≈$14,600) in 2005, had the lowest average total charges.

The same time series techniques were performed on the asthma and non-asthma datasets. Figure 19 shows the ARIMA model for the length of stay.

Figure 19 demonstrates that in 2004, the non-asthma patients had the highest average length of stay in December (≈3.92 days) and the lowest in

April (≈3.52 days) and August (≈3.50 days). In 2005, the months of January (≈4.00 days), July (≈4.06 days), and November (≈4.05 days) had the highest average length of stay and the lowest average length of stay was in April (≈3.76 days) and December (≈3.74 days). With asthma patients in 2004, the months of June (≈3.30 days) had the highest average length of stay and September (≈2.88 days) had the lowest average length of stay. For the asthma patients in 2005, the month of July (≈3.32 days) had the highest average length of stay, while October (≈2.86 days) had the lowest average length of stay.

Figure 19. ARIMA model for the length of stay for non-asthma patients and asthma patients

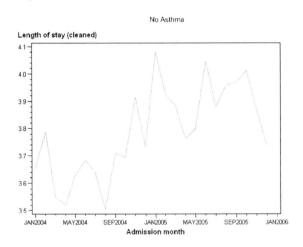
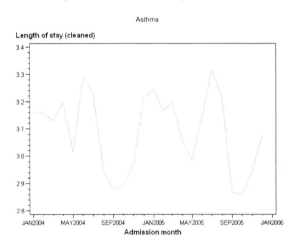

Figure 20. ARIMA model for the total cost for non-asthma and asthma patients

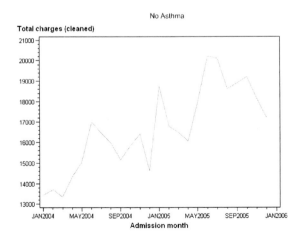
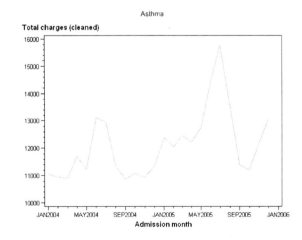

Figure 20 demonstrates that in 2004, the non-asthma patients had the highest average total charges in June ($\approx$$17,200) and the lowest average total charges in January ($\approx$$13,400) and in March ($\approx$$13,200). In 2005, the month of June ($\approx$$20,200) had the highest average length of stay and the lowest average total charges occurred in April ($\approx$3.76 days). With asthma patients in 2004, the month of June ($\approx$$13,200) had the highest average total charges. The months of March ($\approx$$11,000), September ($\approx$$11,000), and November ($\approx$$11,000) had the lowest average total charges. For the asthma patients in 2005, the month of July ($\approx$$15,600) had the highest average total charges, while October ($\approx$$11,300), had the lowest average total charges.

SAS Enterprise Guide's ANOVA Linear Model analysis was performed on the length of stays and total charges variables. Based on the ANOVA tables for both variables (Tables 11 and 12), with an α-level of 0.5, both models generated are statistically significant. Based on the R-Square values, the model accounts for 49.9% of the variability for the total charges and 44.6% of the variability for the length of stay variable.

The Type III sum of squares for the total charges (Table 13) showed that the patient's age, length of

stay, asthma diagnosis, gender, ethnicity, and all two-way combinations are statistically significant effects on the length of stay, with the exception of the two-way interaction of age and asthma diagnosis. The p-value of the two-way interaction of age and asthma diagnosis is equal to 0.6758, which is greater than the α-level of 0.05.

The Type III sum of squares for the length of stay (Table 14) showed that the patient's age, total charges, gender, ethnicity, and all two-way combinations are statistically significant effects on the length of stay, with the exception of the asthma diagnosis and the two-way interaction of age and gender. The p-values of the asthma diagnosis and the two-way interaction of age and gender (0.4817 and 0.3914 respectively) are greater than the α-level of 0.05.

CURRENT AND FUTURE CHALLENGES FACING THE ORGANIZATION

There are seventeen drugs used to treat asthma. Among those drugs, the drug, prednisone, is the cheapest used by many patients. The government contribution or payment for asthma medication is

Table 11. ANOVA (total charges)

Source	DF	Sum of Squares	Mean Square	F Value	Pr>F
Model	36	1.2255221E14	3.404228E12	6471.15	<.0001
Error	159399	8.3853836E13	526062497.8		
Uncorrected Total	159435	2.0640605E14			

R-Square	Coeff Var		Root MSE		TOTCHG Mean
0.499426	146.8545		22936.05		15618.22

Table 12. ANOVA (length of stay)

Source	DF	Sum of Squares	Mean Square	F Value	Pr>F
Model	36	4755671.167	132101.977	6095.82	<.0001
Error	159399	3454321.833	22.671		
Uncorrected Total	159435	8209993.000			

Table 13. Type III sum of squares (total charges)

Source	DF	Type I SS	Mean Square	F Value	Pr > F
Intercept	1	3.8890784E13	3.8890784E13	73928.1	<.0001
AGE	1	642018185389	642018185389	1220.42	<.0001
LOS	1	7.1802115E13	7.1802115E13	136490	<.0001
codeasthma	1	284119472633	284119472633	540.09	<.0001
FEMALE	1	90168242549	90168242549	171.40	<.0001
RACE	5	245515111449	49103022290	93.34	<.0001
AGE*LOS	1	6.7170892E12	6.7170892E12	12768.6	<.0001
AGE*codeasthma	1	92031559.656	92031559.656	0.17	0.6758
AGE*FEMALE	1	166172389778	166172389778	315.88	<.0001
AGE*RACE	5	24845500849	4969100169.8	9.45	<.0001
LOS*codeasthma	1	634420176503	634420176503	1205.98	<.0001
LOS*FEMALE	1	184839475387	184839475387	351.36	<.0001
LOS*RACE	5	2.8308064E12	566161278237	1076.22	<.0001
codeasthma*FEMALE	1	9683912810.4	9683912810.4	18.41	<.0001
codeasthma*RACE	5	11193365393	2238673078.6	4.26	0.0007
FEMALE*RACE	5	18346671007	3669334201.5	6.98	<.0001

Table 14. Type III sum of squares (length of stay)

Source	DF	Type I SS	Mean Square	F Value	Pr > F
Intercept	1	1976405.488	1976405.488	91200.8	<.0001
TOTCHG	1	2694719.670	2694719.670	124347	<.0001
AGE	1	7035.632	7035.632	324.66	<.0001
FEMALE	1	168.017	168.017	7.75	0.0054
RACE	5	6388.899	1277.780	58.96	<.0001
codeasthma	1	10.729	10.729	0.50	0.4817
TOTCHG*AGE	1	5220.645	5220.645	240.91	<.0001
TOTCHG*FEMALE	1	13739.221	13739.221	633.99	<.0001
TOTCHG*RACE	5	41872.474	8374.495	386.44	<.0001
TOTCHG*codeasthma	1	5631.570	5631.570	259.87	<.0001
AGE*FEMALE	1	15.742	15.742	0.73	0.3941
AGE*RACE	5	2127.514	425.503	19.63	<.0001
AGE*codeasthma	1	230.060	230.060	10.62	<.0001
FEMALE*RACE	5	368.592	73.718	3.40	0.0045
FEMALE*codeasthma	1	325.691	325.691	15.03	<.0001
RACE*codeasthma	5	1411.222	282.244	13.02	<.0001

considerably higher compared with the self payment and private payment. After observing the emergency visit frequency table, we can conclude that the condition of asthma results in occasional visits to the emergency department. Charges are always greater than the actual payment in the emergency visits. Kernel Density Estimation of charges and payments implies that as values increase, the probabilities of paying those amounts decrease very rapidly. When we observe the costs, total charge is much higher compared to the actual payment, and facilities payment is more than payment for physicians. The cost of emergency visits is approximately three times more than the cost of medicines.

The results of the length of stay modeled using ARIMA procedures for the overall, asthma, and non-asthma datasets showed that there are peaks in both the length of stay and total charges during the months of June and July, whereas the non-peak months are less predictable. The patients who do not have asthma have higher average length of stays and total charges compared to the patients who have asthma. It is also noticeable that the average total charges from 2004 to 2005 increased for all patients. These properties should then reappear in subsequent years.

The results of the linear model analysis showed that the two-way interaction of the age and asthma diagnosis had no effect on the total charges, while the patient's age, length of stay, asthma diagnosis, gender, ethnicity, and all other two-way combinations do. As for the length of stay, the asthma diagnosis and the two-way interaction of age and gender had no effect, unlike the patient's age, total charges, gender, ethnicity, and all other two-way combinations which do have statistically significant effect.

In the future, multiple datasets such as those used here will be used to examine some of the consequences of patient treatment choices. Medication choices can be monitored to investigate patient compliance, inpatient and outpatient treatments, and the need for emergency treatment.

REFERENCES

Ait-Khaled, N., Enarson, D., Bissell, K., & Billo, N. (2007). Access to inhaled corticosteroids is key to improving quality of care for asthma in developing countries. *Allergy, 62*(3), 230–236. doi:10.1111/j.1398-9995.2007.01326.x

Anonymous-asthma. (2007). *Trends in asthma morbidity and mortality*. Retrieved September, 2008, from http://www.lungusa.org/site/c. dvLUK9O0E/b.22884/k.7CE3/Asthma_Research__Studies.htm

Anonymous-Mayoasthma. (2008). *Asthma*. Retrieved September, 2008, from http://www.mayoclinic.com/health/asthma/DS00021/DSECTION=treatments-and-drugs

Anonymous-MEPS. (2007). *Medical Expenditure Panel Survey* [Electronic Version]. Retrieved December, 2007, from http://www.meps.ahrq.gov/mepsweb/.

Anonymous-NIHasthma. (2008). *What is Asthma?* Retrieved September, 2008, from http://www.nhlbi.nih.gov/health/dci/Diseases/Asthma/Asthma_WhatIs.html

Anonymous-NIS. (2008). *Introduction to the HCUP Nationwide Inpatient Sample (NIS)*. Retrieved 2005, from http://www.hcup-us.ahrq.gov/db/nation/nis/NIS_Introduction_2005.jsp

Brown, R. (2001). Behavioral issues in asthma management. *Pediatric Pulmonology, 21*(Supplement), 26–30. doi:10.1002/ppul.2003

Chipps, B., & Spahn, J. (2006). What are the determinates of asthma control? *The Journal of Asthma, 43*(8), 567–572. doi:10.1080/02770900600619782

Conboy-Ellis, K. (2006). Asthma pathogenesis and management. *The Nurse Practitioner, 31*, 24–44. doi:10.1097/00006205-200611000-00006

ADDITIONAL READING

Brandt, P. T., & Taylor, J. (2006). *Multiple Time Series Models*. Thousand Oaks, CA: Sage Publications.

Cerrito, P. (2010). *Clinical Data Mining for Physician Decision Making and Investigating Health Outcomes*. Hershey, PA: IGI Publishing.

Cromwell, J. B., Labys, W. C., & Terraza, M.Univariate Tests for Time Series Models. Thousand Oaks, CA:Sage Publications.

Raddish, M., Horn, S. D., & Sharkey, P. D. (1999). Continuity of care: is it cost effective? *The American Journal of Managed Care, 5*(6), 727–734.

Shih, Y. C., Mauskopf, J., Borker, R., Shih, Y.-C. T., Mauskopf, J., & Borker, R. (2007). A cost-effectiveness analysis of first-line controller therapies for persistent asthma. [Research Support, Non-U.S. Gov't Review]. *PharmacoEconomics, 25*(7), 577–590. doi:10.2165/00019053-200725070-00004

Staff, M. C. (2009). Asthma: Treatment and Drugs, Retrieved 2009, from http://www.mayoclinic.com/health/asthma/DS00021/DSECTION=treatments-and-drugs

van Grunsven, P. M., van Schayck, C. P., van Deuveren, M., van Herwaarden, C. L., Akkermans, R. P., & van Weel, C. (2000). Compliance during long-term treatment with fluticasone propionate in subjects with early signs of asthma or chronic obstructive pulmonary disease (COPD): results of the Detection, Intervention, and Monitoring Program of COPD and Asthma (DIMCA) Study. Research Support, Non-U.S. Gov't]. *The Journal of Asthma, 37*(3), 225–234. doi:10.3109/02770900009055445

Chapter 5
Analysis of Breast Cancer and Surgery as Treatment Options

Beatrice Ugiliweneza
University of Louisville, USA

ABSTRACT

In this case, we analyze breast cancer cases from the Thomson Medstat Market Scan® data using SAS and Enterprise Guide 4. First, we find breast cancer cases using ICD9 codes. We are interested in the age distribution, in the total charges of the entire treatment sequence and in the length of stay at the hospital during treatment. Then, we study two major surgery treatments: Mastectomy and Lumpectomy. For each one of them, we analyze the total charges and the length of stay. Then, we compare these two treatments in terms of total charges, length of stay and the association of the choice of treatment with age. Finally, we analyze other treatment options. The objective is to understand the methods used to obtain some useful information about breast cancer and also to explore how to use SAS and SAS Enterprise Guide 4 to examine specific healthcare problems.

BACKGROUND

Breast cancer can be defined as a malignant tumor that develops in the breast. There are many types of treatment options including surgery, chemotherapy, radiation therapy, and hormonal therapy. The medical team and the patient analyze the options together and decide the best treatment. However, surgery is so far defined as the best therapeutic option for breast cancer. There are mainly two types of surgery options: mastectomy and lumpectomy. Lumpectomy is a breast conserving procedure that consists of removing the 'tumor' and a margin of tissue surrounding it to make sure all breast cancer has been removed. Mastectomy is the surgery that removes the whole breast.

A considerable number of studies have been made to compare Mastectomy and Lumpectomy. Fisher, Bernard; Anderson, Stewart, Redmond, Carol K at all (1995) conclude that there are no significant differences found between the patients who underwent total mastectomy and those treated by

DOI: 10.4018/978-1-61520-723-7.ch005

Copyright © 2010, IGI Global. Copying or distributing in print or electronic forms without written permission of IGI Global is prohibited.

lumpectomy alone or by lumpectomy plus breast irradiation. Lumpectomy is a breast conserving procedure and is more modern. Mastectomy is more "traditional". Mastectomy was for long believed to be the best treatment option. Now, with new techniques, the greater concern is on knowing which one is better and which one fits better the needs of the patient, and also which one works. It is in this view that many analyses were made and they all seem to agree on the fact that these two treatments deliver the results. Fisher, Bernard; Anderson, Stewart and Bryant, John at all (2002) found that no significant differences were observed among the three groups of women with respect to disease-free survival, distant-disease free survival, or overall survival. In the same spirit, Obedian Edwards; Fischer Diana B.and Haffty, Bruce G. (2000) discovered that there seems to be no increased risk of second malignancies in patients undergoing Lumpectomy and Radiation Therapy using modern techniques, compared with Mastectomy. Their studies did not yield statistical differences.

It is clear that these two surgical procedures do not statistically differ in treatment outcomes. In agreement with this fact, we put our interest, during this case study, on the comparison of these two treatment options with respect to Length of Stay at the hospital during treatment and the total charges for the whole treatment sequence.

SETTING THE STAGE

For the analysis in this whole chapter, we use SAS software and the SAS Enterprise Guide 4.1. SAS is software that is used for explaining statistically the data or for predicting results.

Enterprise Guide 4 is a point and click interface that uses SAS in-built functions. It helps the user to explore the power of SAS without writing the codes. Throughout this chapter, SAS and Enterprise Guide 4 are used to produce the results. We divide our study into three parts: Analysis of breast cancer, analysis of mastectomy and lumpectomy as breast cancer treatments and other frequent treatments used for breast cancer.

MEPS and NIS

This project examined the breast cancer cost and treatment of mastectomy versus lumpectomy. Mastectomy is the surgical procedure in which the entire breast is removed and lumpectomy, also called wide local excision, is a conservative surgery in which only the cancer, along with a border of healthy tissue around it is removed. We used two datasets incomplete in themselves: the National Inpatient Survey (NIS) and the Medical Expenditure Panel Survey (MEPS). (Anonymous-MEPS, 2007; Anonymous-NIS, 2007)

The NIS data are used to complete the MEPS data using predictive modeling. Data Mining can be defined as the process to extract the implicit, previously unknown, and potentially useful information from data. It includes the general technique of predictive modeling. Predictive modeling is the process by which a statistical model is created or chosen to find the best predictor of an outcome.

First, mastectomy and lumpectomy were studied using a suitable model, and then the result was scored to the MEPS data that were then analyzed with more traditional statistical tools. Mastectomy is higher in cost and hospital length of stay, and is more likely to be used as a treatment than lumpectomy. Once the MEPS data are scored, we can examine differences in follow up treatments when comparing the two procedures.

The data used were from the NIS and MEPS. These data were first filtered for breast cancer cases only. The MEPS data were downloaded from the MEPS website: www.meps.ahrq.org. For these data, four sets of files were chosen: inpatient, outpatient, physician visits, and the medication dataset. To execute the entire task for this research, we used SAS Enterprise Guide 4.1. We wanted to study the treatment procedures of breast cancer, the follow up and different complications.

The NIS data are very detailed on the kind of procedure performed, but are not complete for the follow up because they do not contain any links to patients across observations. The MEPS data are not precise on the procedure because of the HIPAA de-identification of the information. We used these two incomplete datasets to get one complete dataset that would satisfy our requirements for further research while still respecting the privacy policy.

First, we worked with the NIS data. We extracted the surgical cases among others using the procedure codes. The code for lumpectomy is 85.21. The procedure codes for the different types of mastectomies are 85.41, 85.43, 85.44, 85.34, 85.33, 85.36, 85.47, 85.48, 85.23, 85.45, and 85.46.

Then, we created a code variable with 1= mastectomy and 2= lumpectomy. These two were merged into one sorted table. In this new dataset, we considered both the total charges reported and the length of Stay (LOS) as the variables to predict procedure. In order to have an idea of the distribution of these two variables, we used kernel density estimation, Proc KDE in SAS. The SAS code that we used for our two variables, Length of Stay (LOS) and Total Charges is

```
data meps3.kde_mastectomy_lumpectomy;
set meps3.mastectomy_lumpectomy;
proc kde data=meps2.mastectomy_lumpectomy
gridl=0 gridu=10 method=SNR out=kdeLOS;
var LOS;
by codation;
run;
proc kde data=meps3.mastectomy_lumpec-
tomy gridl=0 gridu=131172 method=SNR
out=kdeTotal_charges;
var Total_charges;
by codation;
run;
```

Kernel Density Estimation is a way of estimating the probability function of a random variable.

If $x_1,x_2,....,x_N$ are independent and identically distributed random variables, then the kernel density approximation of their probability density function is

$$f_h(x)=(1/Nh)\sum_{i=1,N} K((x-X_i)/h),$$

Where K is some probability density function and h is the bandwidth (smoothing parameter). Quite often, K is taken to be a standard normal distribution function with mean zero and variance one. PROC KDE uses

$$K(x) = (1/\sqrt{2})\exp((-1/2)x^2).$$

After using the kernel density estimation on our data, we used predictive modeling with a logistic regression model. What we obtain was scored to the MEPS data in order to complete the observations.

With each set of files in the MEPS data, we first merged all the files into one table. Then, we extracted the cases of breast cancer using the ICD9 diagnosis code, 174, a three digit code for breast cancer. Code translations are available online at http://icd9cm.chrisendres.com/. Among these cases, we extracted those with an ICD9 procedure code of surgery, 85. Then, we used information from the NIS to score the surgical procedures and examine the distributions of the resulting datasets.

Thomson Medstat

A second set of data used for analysis is the Thomson MedStat Market Scan data. (Anonymous-Medstat, 2007) The Market Scan data are healthcare data. They are complete and detailed for analysis. The Market Scan data contain all claims for all individuals enrolled by 100 different insurance providers. For our study, we will use the inpatient data files. For the analysis in this whole chapter, we use SAS software and the SAS Enterprise Guide 4. SAS is a software that is used for explaining statistically the data or for predicting results.

We first extract breast cancer cases among all other inpatient events; we look at the age distribution and then we analyze the stratified data with respect to age. Finally, we study the total charges of treatment and the length of stay at the hospital during treatment.

To extract breast cancer cases, we use the ICD9-CM diagnosis codes. ICD9-CM stands for "the International Classification of Disease, 9th division, Clinical Modification". There are two types of CD9 codes: diagnosis and procedure codes. These codes and their translations are available online at http://icd9cm.chrisendres.com/. The diagnosis codes we use are:

174.0: Nipple and Areola
174.1: Central portion
174.2: Upper Inner quadrant
174.3: Lower Inner quadrant
174.4: Upper Outer quadrant
174.5: Lower Outer quadrant
174.6: Axillary tail
174.8: Other specified sites of female breast
174.9: Breast unspecified
199.0: Disseminated (cancer unspecified site)
199.1: Other (cancer unspecified site)
233.0: Breast

In the data, these codes are written without the decimal point; they are four digit numbers. They are recorded in fifteen variable columns: dx1 thru dx15. To extract breast cancer cases, we use the following code.

Code 1. Extract breast cancer cases from the dataset

```
data sasuser.inpatientfiles1;
set sasuser.inpatient_files;
diagnoses=catx('', dx1, dx2, dx3, dx3,
dx4, dx5, dx6, dx7, dx8,dx9, dx10, dx11,
dx12, dx13, dx14, dx15;
```

```
if ((rxmatch ('1740',diagnoses)>0)
or (rxmatch('1741',diagnoses)>0) or
(rxmatch('1742',diagnoses)>0)
or (rxmatch('1743',diagnoses)>0) or
(rxmatch('1744',diagnoses)>0) or
(rxmatch('1745',diagnoses)>0)
or (rxmathc('1746',diagnoses)>0) or
(rxmatch('1747',diagnoses)>0) or
(rxmatch('1748',diagnoses)>0)
or (rxmatch('1749',diagnoses)>0) or
(rxmatch('1990',diagnoses)>0) or
(rxmatch('1991',diagnoses)>0)
or (rxmatch('2330',diagnoses)>0)) then
code=1;
else code=0;
data sasuser.inpatient_files_breastcan-
cer;
set sasuser.inpatientfiles1;
where code=1;
run;
```

Breast cancer is diagnosed in women of different ages, but we want to know if, according to these data, there is a particular age for diagnosis. For this, we take the breast cancer data set and we try to estimate the distribution of the variable age using the kernel density estimation (kde). The kernel density estimation is a non-parametric way of estimating the probability density function of a variable that is usually continuous. The kernel density estimation can be used in SAS though the proc kde procedure. We use proc kde on our data, and then we plot the density to see what it looks like.

Code 2. Estimate the density function

```
proc kde data=M2008.breastcancer
out=book.bcagedensity;
var age;
run;
```

Code 3. Plot the density function

```
proc gplot data=book.bcagedensity;
title1 'The density distribution of age';
title2 'in breast cancer data';
plot density*age;
symbol color=green i=spline w=3 v=none;
run;
```

Another way to study breast cancer with respect to age is to analyze the stratified data.

We next stratify the age into 6 groups:

Group1: From 0 to 30 years old
Group2: From 31 to 40 years old
Group3: From 41 to 50 years old
Group4: From 51 to 60 years old
Group5: From 61 to 70 years old
Group6: From 71 to 80 years old

In the MedStat data, the age is recorded in a variable called age. To stratify, we use the following code.

Code 4. Stratify the age

```
data book.stratifiedbreastcancer;
set book.mastlump;
if (age lt 30) then group=1;
else if (31 lt age lt 40) then group=2;
else if (41 lt age lt 50) then group=3;
else if (51 lt age lt 60) then group=4;
else if (61 lt age lt 70) then group=5;
else if (71 lt age lt 80) then group=6;
run;
```

With these stratified data, we produce a summary table that gives us the exact number of patients in each group, a bar chart that shows us the frequency of each group in the data, and a pie chart that gives us the percentage of each group in the data. The summary table, the bar chart and the pie chart are produced with the built-in commands in Enterprise Guide 4.

It is important to note that the data we have available cover only one year. So, the results

we will get here may not represent the total charges for the whole treatment sequence for just one year.

We look at the data regardless of the specific treatment. Later in the chapter, we will analyze the specific treatments. In our data, the total charges are registered in the variabke, TOTPAY, which stands for total pay and represents the cost of treatment in the whole year. We use the summary statistics built in Enterprise Guide 4 to get the description of the TOTPAY variable. In the data, the Length of Stay is recorded in a variable named DAYS. Again here, we use the summary statistics from Enterprise Guide 4.

In this part, we analyze lumpectomy and mastectomy individually in terms of total charges and length of stay. Then, we compare these two treatments in terms of total charges and length of stay. Finally, we test to see if there is any association between the choice of treatment and age. In the MarketScan data, the procedures are recorded in the variables PROC1 thru PROC15. We use these variables to extract Mastectomy and Lumpectomy datasets. We use the following ICD9 procedure codes:

- Lumpectomy
  - 85.21: Local excision of lesion of breast (Lumpectomy)
- Mastectomy
  - 85.23: subtotal mastectomy
  - 85.33: Unilateral subcutaneous mammectomy with synchronous implant
  - 85.34: Other unilateral subcutaneous mammectomy
  - 85.36: Other bilateral subcutaneous mammectomy
  - 85.41: Unilateral simple mastectomy
  - 85.43: Unilateral extended simple mastectomy
  - 85.44: Bilateral extended simple mastectomy
  - 85.45: Unilateral radical mastectomy
  - 85.46: Bilateral radical mastectomy

- ○ 85.47: Unilateral extended radical mastectomy
- ○ 85.48: Bilateral extended radical mastectomy

To extract the two datasets Mastectomy and Lumpectomy, we use the following SAS code:

Code 5. Extract Mastectomy and Lumpectomy datasets among breast cancer cases

```
libname Book "F:\Book";
libname M2008 "F:\M2008";
/*Extract the mastectomy and the lumpec-
tomy cases*/
data book.mastlump;
set M2008.BREASTCANCER;
procedures= catx("", proc1, proc2, proc3,
proc4, proc5, proc6, proc7,proc8, proc9,
proc10, proc11, proc12, proc13, proc14,
proc15);
if ((rxmatch('8541', procedures)>0)
or (rxmatch('8543', procedures)>0) or
(rxmatch('8544',procedures)>0)
or (rxmatch('8534',procedures)>0) or
(rxmatch('8533',procedures)>0) or
(rxmatch('8536',procedures)>0)
or (rxmatch('8547',procedures)>0) or
(rxmatch('8548',procedures)>0) or
(rxmatch('8545',procedures)>0)
or (rxmatch('8546',procedures)>0) or
(rxmatch('8523',procedures)>0) or (rx-
match ('8521', procedures)>0))
then code=1;
else if (rxmatch ('8521', procedures)>0)
then code=2;
else code=0;
run;
data Book.mastectomy;
set book.mastlump;
where code=1;
run;
data Book.lumpectomy;
set book.mastlump;
```

```
where code=2;
run;
```

With the datasets obtained, we are interested in the total charges and length of stay for each patient. After the individual analyses, we compare mastectomy and lumpectomy use. First, we compare the two treatments with respect to total pay. For this, we first estimate the density of this variable in both datasets using the kernel density estimation in SAS. We use the following proc kde procedure code.

Code 6. Compute the densities of total pay in both datasets

```
/*densities of total pay*/
data mast1;
set book.mastectomy;
keep totpay;
run;
proc kde data=mast1 out=book.mast_totden-
sity;
var totpay;
run;
data lump1;
set book.lumpectomy;
keep totpay;
run;
proc kde data=lump1 out=book.lump_totden-
sity;
var totpay;
run;
```

After computing the two densities, we merge the two resulting tables and we plot them on the same graph.

Code 7. Merge and plot the densities for total pay

```
/*Combine the two tables with the two
densities*/
data book.mastlump_densities;
```

```
set book.mast_totdensity
(rename=(totpay=mast_totpay density=mast_
totdensity count=mast_totcount));
set book.lump_totdensity
(rename=(totpay=lump_totpay density=lump_
totdensity count=lump_totcount));
merge book.mast_totdensity book.lump_tot-
density;
run;
/*Plot the two total pay densities in the
same coordinate system*/
title1 'Comparison of the total pay';
title2 'in Mastectomy and Lumpectomy';
proc gplot data=book.mastlump_densities;
symbol1 color=red i=spline w=3 v=none;
symbol2 color=blue i=spline w=3 v=none;
/*red=mastectomy blue=lumpectomy*/
plot mast_totdensity*mast_totpay lump_
totdensity*lump_totpay/overlay haxis=0 to
30000 by 5000;;
label mast_density='density'
mast_totpay='total pay'
lump_density='density'
lump_totpay='total pay';
run;
```

Second, we compare mastectomy and lumpectomy in terms of days spent at the hospital. We use the same procedures as in the comparison of the charges.

Code 8. Compute the densities of days in both datasets

```
/*densities of days of stay*/
data mast2;
set book.mastectomy;
keep days;
run;
proc kde data=mast2 out=book.mast_days-
density;
var days;
run;
data lump2;
```

```
set book.lumpectomy;
keep days;
run;
proc kde data=lump2 out=book.lump_days-
density;
var days;
run;
```

Code 9. Merge and plot the densities for length of stay

```
/*Combine the two tables with the two
densities*/
data book.mastlump_densities;
set book.mast_daysdensity
(rename=(days=mast_days density=mast_day-
sdensity count=mast_dayscount));
set book.lump_daysdensity
(rename=(days=lump_days density=lump_day-
sdensity count=lump_dayscount));
merge book.mast_daysdensity book.lump_
daysdensity;
run;
/*Plot the two days of stay densities in
the same coordinate system*/
title1 'Comparison of the days of stay';
title2 'in Mastectomy and Lumpectomy';
proc gplot data=book.mastlump_densities;
symbol1 color=red i=spline w=3 v=none;
symbol2 color=blue i=spline w=3 v=none;
/*red=mastectomy blue=lumpectomy*/
plot mast_daysdensity*mast_days lump_
daysdensity*lump_days/overlay haxis=0 to
10 by 2;
label mast_density='density'
mast_totpay='total pay'
lump_density='density'
lump_totpay='total pay';
run;
```

Finally, we want to know if there is any association between the choice of treatment and the patient's age. For this, we first produce a table with

R rows and C columns with groups of age as row entries and procedures as column entries using the FREQ procedure in Enterprise Guide 4. Then, we use the R*C contingency table procedure.

Code 10. Test of association between procedure and age

```
data book.count;
input code group count;
cards;
1 1 29
1 2 318
1 3 1383
1 4 2424
1 5 942
1 6 2
2 1 3
2 2 23
2 3 152
2 4 120
2 5 47
2 6 0
;
run;
proc freq data=book.count;
table code*group/chisq expected nopercent
fisher;
weight count;
run;
```

First, we look at the five most frequent treatments per procedure. For this, we use the summary tables in Enterprise Guide 4 to produce the list of procedure codes ordered in descending order for each of the 15 procedure variables (PROC1-PROC15). Then, we gather the first 5 appearing procedure codes for each procedure in descending order.

From the table obtained, we record all the procedure codes present in this table and we order them in descending order of their frequency.

CASE DESCRIPTION

MEPS and NIS Data

The NIS data contain various surgical treatment procedures for breast cancer. After filtering the cases of mastectomy and lumpectomy, the number of observations was considerably reduced. The analysis was performed on 315 observations for the variable, LOS (Length Of Stay) and 301 observations for the Total Charges. Table 1 gives the summary statistics.

The Kernel Density Estimation helps visualize the density function and test for normality. PROC KDE for Length of Stay is a way of examining the procedures in detail.

Figure 1 shows that the LOS is normally distributed for both mastectomy and lumpectomy. This is very important because many statistical tests require data to be normally distributed. This graph shows that the patients having a mastectomy stay longer than those having a lumpectomy. Figure 2 gives the kernel density for Total Charges.

Table 1. Summary of NIS data

	Mastectomy		Lumpectomy	
	Length Of Stay	**Total Charges**	**Length Of Stay**	**Total Charges**
Number Of Observations	289	277	26	24
Mean	2.45	19,564	1.23	11,912
Variance	7.89	2.57E8	0.42	7.04E7
Standard deviation	2.81	16038	0.65	8391

The total charges variable is also normally distributed for both mastectomy and lumpectomy. This facilitates the research because all statistical tests can be performed on these data. This graph points out that the total cost of mastectomy has a higher probability of a higher cost compared to the cost of lumpectomy.

The MEPS data are not precise on different treatments, especially on surgical treatments of breast cancer. In order to get a complete data set, the previous results were scored to this data set. The different data sets (inpatient, outpatient and physician visit) obtained after conversion to time series were merged together and then attached to the data set of mastectomy and lumpectomy from NIS. In order to do this, the variables, Total charges, Patient ID, LOS, and Procedures were extracted from both datasets with the procedure value left blank for the MEPS data.

Before merging, we created a new variable in each table called number. To define the variable, number, we let 1=mastectomy_lumpectomy, 2=inpatient, 3=outpatient, 4=physician visit. We merged the tables with respect to this variable number.

Logistic regression, as a predictive modeling procedure, is applied to the result. The basic lo-

Figure 1. Kernel density estimation for LOS for mastectomy and lumpectomy in the NIS data

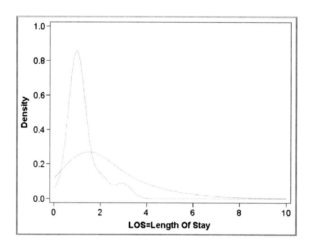

Figure 2. Kernel density estimation for total charges for mastectomy and lumpectomy in the NIS data

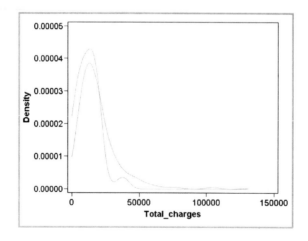

gistic regression model is performed by the PROC GENMOD. We apply the logistic regression to the result using SAS Enterprise Guide 4. The code used by Enterprise Guide is:

```
Input Data: SASUSER.APPEND_TABLE_0011
Server: Local
----------------------------------------
------------------------ */
PROC SQL;
%_SASTASK_DROPDS(SASUSER.PREDLogRegPre-
dictionsAPPEND_TABL);
%_SASTASK_DROPDS(WORK.SORTTempTableSort-
ed);
%_SASTASK_DROPDS(WORK.TMP1TempTableFor-
Plots);
QUIT;
/* -----------------------------------
----------------------------
Data set SASUSER.APPEND_TABLE_0011 does
not need to be sorted.
----------------------------------------
------------------------ */
PROC SQL;
CREATE VIEW WORK.SORTTempTableSorted
AS SELECT * FROM SASUSER.APPEND_TA-
BLE_0011;
QUIT;
TITLE;
TITLE1 "Logistic Regression Results";
FOOTNOTE;
FOOTNOTE1 "Generated by the SAS Sys-
tem (&_SASSERVERNAME, &SYSSCPL)
on %SYSFUNC(DATE(), EURDFDE9.) at
%SYSFUNC(TIME(), TIMEAMPM8.)";
PROC LOGISTIC DATA=WORK.SORTTempTable-
Sorted
;
MODEL procedures1= /
SELECTION=NONE
LINK=LOGIT
;
OUTPUT OUT=SASUSER.PREDLogRegPrediction-
sAPPEND_TABL(LABEL="Logistic regression
```

```
predictions and statistics for SASUSER.
APPEND_TABLE_0011")
PREDPROBS=INDIVIDUAL;
RUN;
QUIT;
TITLE;
TITLE1 "Regression Analysis Predictions";
PROC PRINT NOOBS DATA=SASUSER.PREDLogReg-
PredictionsAPPEND_TABL
;
RUN;
/* -------------------------------------
----------------------------
End of task code.
----------------------------------------
------------------------ */
RUN; QUIT;
PROC SQL;
%_SASTASK_DROPDS(WORK.SORTTempTableSort-
ed);
%_SASTASK_DROPDS(WORK.TMP1TempTableFor-
Plots);
QUIT;
```

By doing this, we use the model of NIS procedures to score the MEPS procedures. After this step, we separated the MEPS data from the NIS data. This is one of the first steps to preprocess the MEPS data for further analysis. The summary statistics of the MEPS data are given in Table 2.

The outpatient number of observations is too small to give a significant output. The LOS has an average of one day for both inpatient and physician visits.

We applied Kernel Density Estimation to the total charges of each data set, inpatient and physician visits. Figure 3 compares the MEPS to NIS for total charges in the inpatient data set; Figure 4 compares it in the physician visit data set.

Figures 3 and 4 show that the resulting Total Charges for Mastectomy in the MEPS data are skewed and normally distributed compared to the Mastectomy in NIS, which is fairly normally distributed. For this reason, after merging the

Table 2. Summary of MEPS data

	Total Charges	
	Inpatient	**Physician visit**
Number of observations	5	185
Mean	2773	271
Variance	5.54E6	822,601
Standard deviation	2353	907

Figure 3. Kernel density estimation for total charges for mastectomy in MEPS inpatient data set compared to NIS dataset

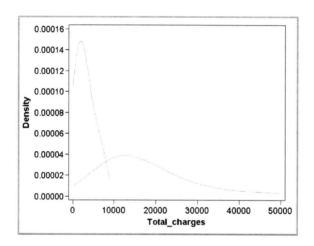

Figure 4. Kernel density estimation for total charges for mastectomy in MEPS physician visits data set compared to NIS dataset

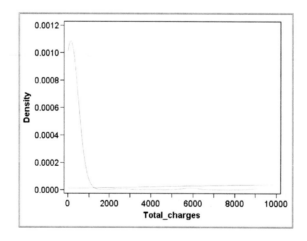

physician visit data and the inpatient data, miner changes are needed for this variable before proceeding in the analysis.

From the two incomplete NIS and MEPS datasets, we are able to construct a complete MEPS dataset. The diagnosis codes in the MEPS are now complete and we can differentiate mastectomy from lumpectomy. The dataset is ready to be used for longitudinal analysis

In the treatment of breast cancer, the chance of having a mastectomy is significantly higher. The cost of this treatment is high, too, but the length of stay is similar for each procedure.

Thomson Medstat Data

From our breast cancer data, we get the age distribution shown in Figure 5.

From this graph, we see that the probability of getting breast cancer is close to zero from 0 to almost 30 years old; the probability gets higher as the age increases to a peak at 50-55 years of age. Then, the probability gets closer to zero from 70 years old and older. Looking at this graph, we have a clear idea of which age is more at risk of breast cancer. However, we want to dig deeper into age classes. We look at the stratified data (Table 3).

We can see that the group 4 (51 to 60 years old) has the largest number of patients, followed by group 3 (41 to 50 years old). This alone is enough to confirm the results we obtained with the age distribution. Another way to look at it is to analyze the bar chart (Figure 6).

Here, group 4 has the highest frequency followed by group 3. This is a visual way to look at what the summary table described.

This shows us the association of breast cancer with age. However, we must note that there are

Table 3. Summary table of the stratified breast cancer data

group	N
1	785
2	4032
3	12570
4	22536
5	8445
6	87

Figure 5. The distribution of age in breast cancer data

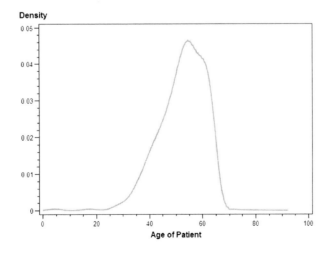

The density distribution of age
in breast cancer data

many other factors, not considered here, that elevate the probability of getting breast cancer.

We next look at the patient outcomes of charges. Table 4 gives the basic summary information.

The charges can go as high as $626,058, but the mean is $16,733. This gives an idea of how much the treatment can cost. Concerning the time spent at the hospital, it can be up to one whole year, but on average, it is about five days and at least 1 day.

Here, we looked at the breast cancer data without taking into consideration any particular

treatment. In the following part, we are going to study two particular surgery treatments: Mastectomy and Lumpectomy.

In Table 5, we summarize the data concerning the total pay and the length of stay for lumpectomy and for mastectomy.

The maximum charge is $28,275 and the mean is $10,219. The maximum number of days a patient can stay at the hospital is 11 and the average number of days is 1 (Table 6).

The maximum charge is $97,242 and the average is $11,319. The maximum number of days is

Figure 6. Bar chart of the stratified breast cancer data

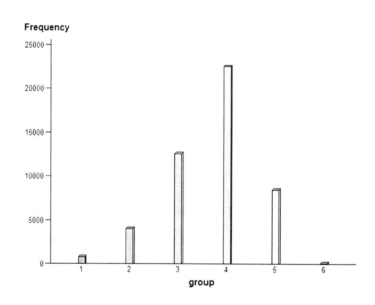

Table 4. Summary statistics of total pay and length of stay in breast cancer data

Analysis variables	Mean	Std dev	Min	Max	N
TOTPAY (Total payments)	16733.30	28085.28	0	626058.00	60394
DAYS (Length of Stay)	5.43	8.65	1	367	6312

Table 5. Summary statistics for total pay and length of stay in lumpectomy

Analysis variables	Mean	Std dev	Min	Max	N
TOTPAY (Total payments)	10219.76	8178.27	0	28275.00	471
DAYS (Length of Stay)	5.43	8.65	1	367	172

Table 6. Summary statistics for total pay and length of stay in mastectomy

Analysis variables	Mean	Std dev	Min	Max	N
TOTPAY (Total payments)	11319.61	11052.25	0	97242.00	6568
DAYS (Length of Stay)	2.2166772	1.6941708	1	25	1583

Figure 7. Compared densities for total pay

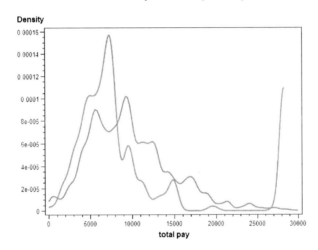

25 and the average is 1. Next, we compare these two surgical treatments in terms of total pay and length of stay. First, we compare their respective cost (Figure 7).

This graph shows us that in both treatments, the probability of paying around $10,000 is high, but it is higher for lumpectomy than mastectomy. Also, we can see that there is a higher probability of a higher cost for lumpectomy. Second, we compare their respective length of stay (Figure 8).

There is higher probability of a longer stay when treated by mastectomy.

These two treatments are the most used for breast cancer. Since breast cancer is associated with age, we test for an association between mastectomy, lumpectomy and age. In other words, we want to know if age is a factor in determining which treatment to use. We use the age distribution by procedure (Figure 9).

There are spikes in age at 43 and 50 years of age; the likelihood of a lumpectomy decreases after the age of 50 (Figure 10).

For a mastectomy, the highest spike occurs at age 53, declining in rate beyond 53, and declining to virtually zero after age 65. This decline to zero occurs because the Thomson Medstat dataset does not include sufficient data for Medicare recipients.

The results are significant, which means that the choice of treatment does depend on age (Table 7). However, we must note that there are other, stronger factors that affect the choice of treatment.

These two surgical treatments (Mastectomy and Lumpectomy) are the most frequent major

Figure 8. Compared densities for days

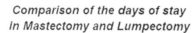

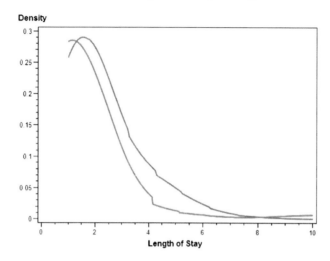

Figure 9. The distribution of age in the lumpectomy data

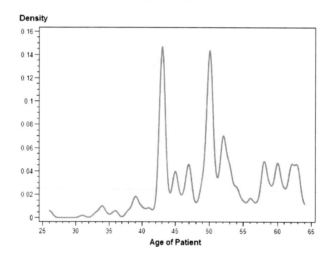

procedures. Beside these procedures, there are other treatments for breast cancer. In the following part of the chapter, we are going to try to see what those treatments are (Table 8).

This table shows the most frequent treatments, in descending order, received by breast cancer patients on top of the mastectomy or lumpectomy.

CURRENT AND FUTURE CHALLENGES FACING THE ORGANIZATION

This research shows that data mining can be used to complete one dataset using another one that also has incomplete information. The MEPS dataset,

Figure 10. The distribution of age in the mastectomy data

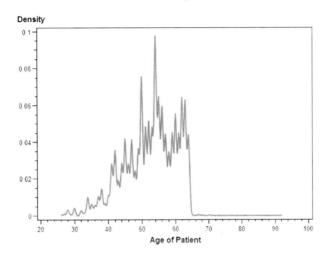

The density distribution of age
in mastectomy data

Table 7. Statistics for the test of the association of age and procedures (mastectomy and lumpectomy)

Statistic	DF	Value	Probability
Chi-Square	5	49.0250	<0.0001
Likelihood Ratio Chi-Square	5	45.9789	<0.0001
Mantel-Haenszel Chi-Square	1	25.3967	<0.0001
Phi Coefficient		0.0949	
Contingency Coefficient		0.0945	
Carmer's V		0.0949	
Table Probability (P)			7.136E-15
Pr<P			4.480E-09

p.value=e.e8E-o9<<<<.05.

which is incomplete on the procedures because of the HIPAA de-identification, is completed by the NIS dataset using predictive modeling and scoring. We found the variable, Total charges, is normally distributed and the LOS (Length Of Stay) is mostly one day. All this helped us to do the first preparation of the MEPS data. Further analysis will be done with an ARIMA (Auto regressive Integrated Moving Average) model.

Breast cancer is a terrible disease for women. According the website, www.home.thomsonhealthcare.com, more than 25% of cancer cases diagnosed are breast cancer. It is important for women to take care of themselves and report any changes in their breasts. But also, it is important to be informed about the realities surrounding breast cancer. This chapter roughly answers some questions: If I have breast cancer, what are my treatment options? How much is the treatment going to cost me? How long will I be staying at the treatment center during treatment? In answering these questions, this chapter also shows how to get general important information about a particular case from a very large dataset

Table 8. Most frequent procedure codes in descending order

99.23	Injection of steroid
99.25	Injection or infusion of chemotherapeutic substance
99.22	Injection of other anti-injective
71	Operations on vulva and perineum
88	Other related diagnosis radiology and related techniques
93	Physical therapy, respiratory therapy, rehabilitation, and related procedures
72	Forceps, vacuum and breech delivery
70	Operations on vagina and cul-de-sac
34.91	Theracentesis
33.27	Closed endoscopic biopsy of lung
01.59	Other excision or destruction of lesion or tissue of tissue of brain

using a statistical tool such as SAS and Enterprise Guide 4. However, the disease of breast cancer is large and many questions and opportunities are not explored in this chapter; for example, there are many other risk factors of breast cancer and there are many things that should be considered to determine the optimal treatment. A treatment sequence can contain more than one treatment... These are interesting challenges to consider in a further analysis.

REFERENCES

Fisher, B., Anderson, S., & Bryant, J. (2002). Twenty-Year Follow-Up of a Randomized Trial Comparing Total Mastectomy, Lumpectomy, and Lumpectomy plus Irradiation for the Treatment of Invasive Breast Cancer. *The New England Journal of Medicine, 347*(16), 1233–1241. doi:10.1056/NEJMoa022152

Fisher, B., Anderson, S., & Redmond, C. K. (1995). Reanalysis and Results after 12 years of Follow up in a Randomized Clinical Trial Comparing Total Mastectomy with Lumpectomy with or without Irradiation in the Treatment of Breast Cancer. *The New England Journal of Medicine, 333*(22), 1456–1461. doi:10.1056/NEJM199511303332203

Obedian, E., & Fischer, D. B., Haffty, & B. G. (2000). Second malignancies After Treatment of Early-Stage Breast Cancer: Lumpectomy and Radiation Therapy Verus Mastectomy. *Journal of Clinical Oncology, 18*(12), 2406–2412.

ADDITIONAL READING

Cerrito, P. B. (2009a). *Data Mining Healthcare and Clinical Databases*. Cary, NC: SAS Press, Inc.

Cerrito, P. B. (2009b). *Text Mining Techniques for Healthcare Provider Quality Determination: Methods for Rank Comparisons*. Hershey, PA: IGI Publishing.

Gold, H., & Do, H. (2007). Evaluation of three algorithms to identify incident breast cancer in Medicare claims data. *Health Services Research, 42*(5), 2056–2069. doi:10.1111/j.1475-6773.2007.00705.x

Little, R. C., Milliken, G. A., Stroup, W. W., Wolfinger, R. D., & Schabenberber, O. (2006). *SAS for Mixed Models* (2nd ed.). Cary, NC: SAS Press.

Preminger, B. A., Pusic, A. L., McCarthy, C. M., Verma, N., Worku, A., & Cordeiro, P. G. (2008). How should quality-of-life data be incorporated into a cost analysis of breast reconstruction? A consideration of implant versus free TRAM flap procedures. [Comparative Study]. *Plastic and Reconstructive Surgery, 121*(4), 1075–1082. doi:10.1097/01.prs.0000304246.66477.cd

Ugiliweneza, B. (2008). Mastectomy Versus Lumpectomy in Breast Cancer Treatment. In *Proceedings of MWSUG*. Retrieved from www.mwsug.org

Chapter 6
Data Mining and Analysis of Lung Cancer

Guoxin Tang
University of Louisville, USA

ABSTRACT

Lung cancer is the leading cause of cancer death in the United States and the world, with more than 1.3 million deaths worldwide per year. However, because of a lack of effective tools to diagnose lung cancer, more than half of all cases are diagnosed at an advanced stage, when surgical resection is unlikely to be feasible. The purpose of this study is to examine the relationship between patient outcomes and conditions of the patients undergoing different treatments for lung cancer and to develop models to estimate the population burden, the cost of cancer, and to help physicians and patients determine appropriate treatment in clinical decision-making. We use a national database, and also claim data to investigate treatments for lung cancer.

BACKGROUND

Lung Cancer

Lung cancer is a disease of uncontrolled cell growth in tissues of the lung. This growth may lead to metastasis, which is an invasion of adjacent tissue and infiltration beyond the lungs. It is usually suspected in individuals who have abnormal chest radiograph findings or have symptoms caused by either local or systemic effects of the tumor. There are two main types of lung carcinoma categorized by the size and appearance of the malignant cells seen by a histopathologist under a microscope: non-small cell lung carcinoma (NSCLC) (80.4%) and small-cell lung carcinoma (SCLC) (16.8%) (Travis, WD, 1995).

At the end of the 20th century, lung cancer had become one of the world's leading causes of preventable death. It was a rare disease at the start of that century, but exposures to new etiologic agents and an increasing lifespan combined to make lung cancer a scourge of the 20th century. Table 1 shows the estimated numbers of cases and deaths for 26 different

DOI: 10.4018/978-1-61520-723-7.ch006

Copyright © 2010, IGI Global. Copying or distributing in print or electronic forms without written permission of IGI Global is prohibited.

types of cancer in men and women, together with the standardized incidence and mortality rates and the cumulative risk (%) between ages 0 and 64. There are some differences in the profile of cancers worldwide, depending on whether the incidence or mortality is the focus of interest. Lung cancer is the main cancer in the world today, whether

considered in terms of number of cases (1.35 million) or deaths (1.18 million), because of the high case fatality (ratio of mortality to incidence, 0.87) (Parkin, D, 2005).

There were 1.35 million new cases, representing 12.4% of all new cancers. Lung cancer is also the most common cause of death from cancer,

Table 1. Incidence and mortality by sex and cancer site worldwide, 2002

	Incidence				Mortality			
	Males		Females		Males		Females	
	Cases	Cumulative risk (age 0-64)	Cases	Cumulative risk (age 0-64)	Deaths	Cumulative risk (age 0-64)	Deaths	Cumulative risk (age 0-64)
Oral Cavity	175,916	0.4	98,373	0.2	80,736	0.2	46,723	0.1
Nasopharynx	55,796	0.1	24,247	0.1	34,913	0.1	15,419	0.0
Other pharynx	106,219	0.3	24,077	0.1	67,964	0.2	16,029	0.0
Esophagus	315,394	0.6	146,723	0.3	261,162	0.5	124,730	0.2
Stomach	603,419	1.2	330,518	0.5	446,052	0.8	254,297	0.4
Colon/rectum	550,465	0.9	472,687	0.7	278,446	0.4	250,532	0.3
Liver	442,119	1.0	184,043	0.3	416,882	0.9	181,439	0.3
Pancreas	124,841	0.2	107,465	0.1	119,544	0.2	107,479	0.1
Larynx	139,230	0.3	20,011	0	78,629	0.2	11,327	0
Lung	965,241	1.7	386,891	0.6	848,132	1.4	330,786	0.5
Melanoma of Skin	79,043	0.2	81,134	0.2	21,952	0	18,829	0
Breast			1,151,298	2.6			410,712	0.9
Cervix uteri			493,243	1.3			273,505	0.7
Corpus uteri			198,783	0.4			50,327	0.1
Ovary			204,499	0.5			124,860	0.2
Prostate	679,023	0.8			221,002	0.1		
Testis	48,613	0.1			8,878	0		
Kidney	129,223	0.3	79,257	0.1	62,696	0.1	39,199	0.1
Bladder	273,858	0.4	82,699	0.1	108,310	0.1	36,699	0
Brain,nervous system	108,221	0.2	81,264	0.2	80,034	0.2	61,616	0.1
Thyroid	37,424	0.1	103,589	0.2	11,297	0	24,078	0
Non-Hodgkin lymphoma	175,123	0.3	125,448	0.2	98,865	0.2	72,955	0.1
Hodgkin Disease	38,218	0.1	24,111	0.1	14,460	0	8,352	0
Multiple my-eloma	46,512	0.1	39,192	0.1	32,696	0.1	29,839	0
Leukemia	171,037	0.3	129,485	0.2	125,142	0.2	97,364	0.2

with 1.18 million deaths, or 17.6% of the world total. Almost half (49.9%) of the cases occur in the developing countries of the world; this is a big change since 1980, when it was estimated that 69% were in developed countries. Worldwide, it is by far the most common cancer of men, with the highest rates observed in North America and Europe (especially Eastern Europe). Moderately high rates are also seen in Australia and New Zealand, and eastern Asia (China and Japan). In women, incidence rates are lower (globally, the rate is 12.1 per 100,000 women compared with 35.5 per 100,000 in men). The highest rates are in North America and Northern Europe. It is of note that the incidence in China is rather high (approximately 19.0 per 100,000); this rate is similar to that in, for example, Australia and New Zealand at 17.4 per 100,000 (Parkin, D, 2005).

Lung cancer remains a highly lethal disease. Survival at 5 years measured by the Surveillance, Epidemiology and End Results (SEER) program in the United States is 15%, the best recorded at the population level. The average survival in Europe is 10%, not much better than the 8.9% observed in developing countries (Alberg, Anthony J, 2003).

Because of the high case and fatality rate of lung cancer, the incidence and mortality rates are nearly equivalent, and, consequently, routinely collected vital statistics provide a long record of the occurrence of lung cancer. Figure 1 shows the epidemic of lung cancer that dates to the mid-20th century (Wingo, Phyllis A, 2003).

Lung cancer was rare until the disease began a sharp rise around 1930 that culminated by mid-century with lung cancer becoming the leading cause of cancer death among men. The epidemic among women followed that among men, with a sharp rise in rates from the 1960s to the present, propelling lung cancer to become the most frequent cause of female cancer mortality. The epidemic among women not only occurred later, but would not peak at as high a level as that among men. Note that the level for men is declining; women have a static rate but not yet a decline.

The Causes of Lung Cancer

Cigarette smoking is a well-established cause of lung cancer. In fact, an estimated 87% of all lung cancers can be attributed to cigarette smoking alone. Although it is by far the leading cause of lung cancer, the disease has several other causes (Figure 2). Lung cancers are still directly or indirectly related to tobacco use from cigars, pipes, and secondhand cigarette smoke, but several other risk factors act independently or synergistically with tobacco to cause lung cancer. Occupational

Figure 1. Lung cancer mortality rates for the United States from 1930 to 1998, age-standardized to the 1970 US population

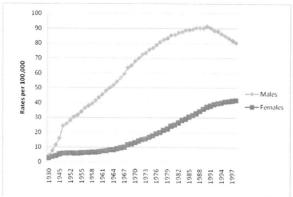

Figure 2. A breakdown of lung cancer's major causes

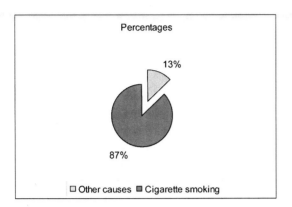

and environmental exposures, such as asbestos, arsenic, secondhand smoke, and radon, also increase the risk of lung cancer. (Earle and Earle, 2004)

Diagnosis and Staging of Lung Cancer

The method of diagnosis of suspected lung cancer depends on the type of lung cancer, the size and location of the primary tumor, the presence of metastasis, and the overall clinical status of the patient. Achieving a diagnosis and staging are usually done in concert because the most efficient way to make a diagnosis often is dictated by the stage of the cancer. The best sequence of studies and interventions in a particular patient involves careful judgment of the probable reliability of a number of presumptive diagnostic issues, so as to maximize the sensitivity and to avoid performing multiple or unnecessary invasive procedures.

The first step in lung cancer detection and diagnosis is a routine history and physical examination by a primary care physician. Learning about the patient's symptoms and observing possible indicators such as difficulty in breathing, bluish skin or nail bed clubbing may alert the physician to the possibility of lung disease. There are specific tests to diagnose lung cancer that we define below (Thompson Cancer Survival Center, 2008).

a) Diagnostic Imaging: The first step in determining if a mass is cancer or benign is a diagnostic image. One or several of these may be used:

○ *X-Ray.* The first diagnostic step is a chest X-ray. A chest X-ray can detect suspicious lung masses, but cannot be used to determine if they are cancerous or benign. Patients are exposed to small amounts of radiation during the X-ray procedure.

○ *CT Scan.* A computerized tomography (or CT or Cat) scan can provide a more-detailed image of the lung. CT scans are a series of X-rays combined by a computer in a cross-sectional view. They can be performed with injected contrast material to highlight lung tissue and suspicious masses. Since the basic imaging mechanism of a CT scan is X-rays, patients receive a low dose of radiation during the procedure. The radiation dosage is significantly lower with low-dose helical CT scans, but masses detected with this technology must be reexamined.

○ *MRI.* Magnetic resonance imaging (or MRI) scans use magnetism, radio waves and computer image manipulation to produce an extremely detailed image without radiation. Because of the extremely powerful magnetism of MRI scanners, they cannot be used on patients with any metal implants or pacemakers.

○ *PET Scan.* Positron-emission tomography (or PET) scans are three-dimensional images of the metabolic functioning of body tissues. PET scans can be used to determine the type of cells in a mass and to detect whether or not a tumor is growing. Patients receiving PET scans are injected with a radioactive drug with about as much radiation as two chest X-rays.

b) Biopsies: Biopsies are procedures in which a small amount of a suspicious mass is removed for examination by a pathologist. There are three main types of biopsy for suspected lung masses:

- *Surgical.* A surgical biopsy is a procedure in which the patient's chest is opened to gain access to a small sample of a suspected mass. The sample is analyzed by a pathologist while the surgery is proceeding, and all, or as much as possible, of the mass is usually removed during the operation, called a thoractomy. A thoractomy is a major surgical procedure performed under anesthetic in a hospital operating room.

- *Bronchoscopy.* In bronchoscopy, a fiber-optic tube, called a bronchoscope, is inserted through the patient's mouth or nose and passed through the trachea and bronchial tubes to the suspected area. The tube has a lens and light source that allow the physician to examine the lung mass. Frequently, the bronchoscope has a sampling device to retrieve a small section of the suspected mass for analysis. A bronchoscopy can be performed in an outpatient suite or a hospital operating room and requires a sedative and anesthetic.

- *Needle Aspiration or Core Biopsy.* In needle aspiration (often called core biopsy), a thin needle is inserted into the suspected mass and a small sample withdrawn for analysis. Needle aspiration is performed on an outpatient basis and requires a local anesthetic.

c) Sputum cytology: In sputum cytology, a pathologist examines the patient's sputum under a microscope. The cells of centrally-located tumors are often present in sputum, and if they are, the pathologist can diagnose the condition by simple visual examination.

d) Lung Cancer Staging. Staging is the evaluation of the extent to which a lung cancer tumor has grown and/or spread. Different lung cancer treatments are specifically for various stages of the disease. The stages of non-small cell and small cell cancers are:

- NSCLC stage I: The cancer is only in the lung.
- NSCLC stage II: The cancer is confined to the chest area.
- NSCLC stage III: The cancer is confined to the chest, but the tumors are larger and more invasive.
- NSCLC stage IV: The cancer has spread beyond the chest to other parts of the body.
- Limited-stage SCLC: The cancer is confined to the chest.
- Extensive-stage SCLC: The cancer has spread beyond the chest to other parts of the body.

Treatment of Lung Cancer

Lung cancer treatment is either curative (to eliminate the cancer) or palliative (to reduce pain and discomfort for patients whose cancer cannot be cured). In either case surgery, radiation, chemotherapy or a combination of two of the treatment types may be used.

- Surgery: Surgery is most often used to remove stage I non-small cell lung cancer tumors and some NSCLC stage II tumors. Surgery for lung cancer may involve removal of part of a lobe (wedge resection), removal of an entire lobe (lobectomy) or removal of an entire lung (pulmonectomy). Surgery is seldom performed on small cell lung cancer because the disease has usually

Figure 3. Lung cancer survival by stage

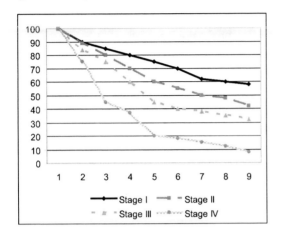

spread beyond the lung by the time it is detected and diagnosed.

- External Radiation Therapy: External radiation therapy is used in both curative and palliative treatment, alone and in combination with chemotherapy. In external radiation therapy, a map of the tumor's location is created with a CT scan, either before the treatment is planned or, with TomoTherapy, at the time of treatment, and then on subsequent visits, the tumor is radiated from different angles to maximize the dose delivered to the tumor with minimum impact on surrounding healthy tissue.
- HDR brachytherapy: In high-dose-rate brachytherapy, radioactive pellets are implanted into the tumor. The benefits of the technology are significant. Treatment time is reduced; affected areas receive a maximum dose and surrounding healthy tissue is spared.
- Chemotherapy: Both non-small cell and small cell lung cancer are treated with chemotherapy. This chemical treatment is especially effective in treating small cell lung cancer, and can increase patients' expected survival by four or five times what it would be otherwise. The latest chemotherapy drugs are tested in clinical trials.

- Photodynamic therapy: The treatment is usually performed on an outpatient basis, has limited side effects and preserves healthy lung tissue. However, it cannot penetrate deeply into the lung tissue and has limited use for lung cancer.

The Distribution of Lung Cancer in US

Lung cancer is a devastating disease. Not only is it the most common cancer in the United States and in Kentucky, it also claims more lives than any other cancer. Kentucky's lung cancer mortality rate is the highest of all states in the nation. The American Cancer Society estimated that in the year 2000, lung cancer accounted for 14% of all newly diagnosed cancers and 28% of all cancer deaths, killing more than 150,000 people. In Kentucky alone, more than 3,000 people die from lung cancer every year.

Kentucky has distinct geographic and lifestyle regions (e.g., western Kentucky differs substantially from eastern Kentucky, just as the state's rural areas tend to differ from its urban ones), each of which has different lung cancer rates. (Hopenhayn-Rich, 2001)

ICD9 Codes

ICD9 codes are provided in The International Statistical Classification of Diseases and Related Health Problems (most commonly known by the abbreviation ICD) to classify diseases and a wide variety of signs, symptoms, abnormal findings, complaints, social circumstances and external causes of injury or disease. Every health condition can be assigned to a unique category and assigned a code up to six characters long. Such categories can include a set of similar diseases that can be converted to a diagnosis.

The ICD 9 code of 162 means malignant neoplasm of trachea, bronchus, and lung. Below are all of the 4-digit codes associated with lung diseases:

162.0 Trachea (Cartilage of trachea, Mucosa of
    trachea)

162.2 Main bronchus (Carina, Hilus of lung)

162.3 Upper lobe, bronchus or lung

162.4 Middle lobe, bronchus or lung

162.5 Lower lobe, bronchus or lung

162.8 Other parts of bronchus or lung (Malignant
    neoplasm of contiguous or overlapping
    sites of bronchus or lung whose point of
    origin cannot be determined)

162.9 Bronchus and lung, unspecified

Overview of NIS Data

The National Inpatient Sample (NIS) is a unique and powerful database of hospital inpatient stays. Researchers and policymakers use the NIS to identify, track, and analyze national trends in health care utilization, access, charges, quality, and outcomes. It is part of the Healthcare Cost and Utilization Project (HCUP), sponsored by the Agency for Healthcare Research and Quality (AHRQ), formerly the Agency for Health Care Policy and Research. (Anonymous-NIS, 2007).

It is the largest all-payer inpatient care database in the United States. It contains data from approximately 8 million hospital stays each year from about 1,000 hospitals sampled to approximate a 20-percent stratified sample of U.S. community hospitals.

NIS data are available for a 19-year time period, from 1988 to 2006, allowing an analysis of trends over time. The number of States in the NIS has grown from 8 in the first year to 38 at present. The NIS is the only national hospital database containing charge information on all patients, regardless of payer, including persons covered by Medicare, Medicaid, private insurance, and the uninsured. Its large sample size enables analyses of rare conditions, such as congenital anomalies; uncommon treatments, such as organ transplantation, and special patient populations, such as the uninsured. For most States, the NIS can be linked to hospital-level data from the American Hospital Association's Annual Survey of Hospitals and county-level data from the Bureau of Health Professions' Area Resource File, except in those states that do not allow the release of hospital identifiers.

The NIS contains clinical and resource use information included in a typical discharge abstract, with safeguards to protect the privacy of individual patients, physicians, and hospitals (as required by data sources). The NIS can be weighted to produce national estimates. Beginning in 1998, the NIS changed from previous NIS releases: some data elements were dropped, some were added; for some data elements, the coding was changed, and the sampling and weighting strategy was revised to improve the representativeness of the data. Beginning with the 2002 NIS, severity adjustment data elements, including APR-DRGs, APS-DRGs, Disease Staging, and AHRQ Co-morbidity Indicators, are available. A new feature, beginning with the 2005 NIS, is the addition of Diagnosis and Procedure Groups Files. These discharge-level files contain data elements from AHRQ software tools designed to facilitate the use of the ICD9 diagnostic and procedure information in the HCUP databases. Access to the NIS is open to users who sign data use agreements. Uses are limited to research and aggregate statistical reporting. The data are available for a small charge at http://www.ahrq.gov.

The NIS is a uniform, multi-State database that promotes comparative studies of health care services and will support health care policy research on a variety of topics, including:

- Use and cost of hospital services
- Medical practice variation
- Health care cost inflation
- Hospital financial distress
- Analyses of States and communities
- Medical treatment effectiveness
- Quality of care
- Impact of health policy changes
- Access to care

- Diffusion of medical technology
- Utilization of health services by special populations.

The NIS includes more than 100 clinical and nonclinical data elements for each hospital stay. These include:

- Primary and secondary diagnoses
- Primary and secondary procedures
- Admission and discharge status
- Patient demographics (e.g., gender, age, race, median income for ZIP Code)
- Expected payment source
- Total charges
- Length of stay
- Hospital characteristics (e.g., ownership, size, teaching status).

Some of the variables we will work with in the NIS data include patient demographics:

- Age (in years)
- Female (0=male, 1=female)
- Race(1=White, 2=Black, 3=Hispanic, 4=Asian/Pacific Islander, 5=Native American, 6=Other)
- DRG
- Patient diagnoses in ICD9 codes (DX1-DX15, fifteen columns)
- Patient procedures in ICD9 codes (PR1-PR15, fifteen columns)
- TOTCHG (Total Charges)
- LOS (Length of Stay)

In order to work with these variables, there are some preprocessing issues, especially to work with 15 columns of diagnosis and procedure codes.

SETTING THE STAGE

The lung cancer data are from the NIS, and we had five years of data, 2000 to 2004. Here, we first

put all of the five years of data into one data set and created a binary variable to label lung cancer according to diagnosis codes. In order to simplify the process of discovery, we first concatenate all 15 columns of variables into one text string using the CATX statement in SAS. This code put all possible diagnosis codes into one text string, and defined a second string containing all possible procedure codes using the CATX statement. To find those patients with Lung Cancer, the RXMATCH function was used. The RXMATCH looked for the initial code of '162' that found all patients with a diagnosis code related to lung disease. Because '162' can occur in other codes that are not related to lung cancer, such as '216.2', we use four digits of code rather than three to avoid catching '216.2'. The code used was the following:

```
data nis.lungcancer_nis_00to04;
set nis. nis_00to04;
lungcancer=0;
diagnoses=catx(' ',dx1, dx2, dx3, dx4,
dx5, dx6, dx7, dx8, dx9, dx10, dx11,
dx12, dx13, dx14, dx15);
procedures=catx(' ',pr1, pr2, pr3, pr4,
pr5, pr6, pr7, pr8, pr9, pr10, pr11,
pr12, pr13, pr14, pr15) ;
if (rxmatch('1620',diagnoses)>0) then
lungcancer=1;
if (rxmatch('1621',diagnoses)>0) then
lungcancer=1;
if (rxmatch('1622',diagnoses)>0) then
lungcancer=1;
if (rxmatch('1622',diagnoses)>0) then
lungcancer=1;
if (rxmatch('1623',diagnoses)>0) then
lungcancer=1;
if (rxmatch('1624',diagnoses)>0) then
lungcancer=1;
if (rxmatch('1625',diagnoses)>0) then
lungcancer=1;
if (rxmatch('1626',diagnoses)>0) then
lungcancer=1;
if (rxmatch('1627',diagnoses)>0) then
```

```
lungcancer=1;
if (rxmatch('1628',diagnoses)>0) then
lungcancer=1;
if (rxmatch('1629',diagnoses)>0) then
lungcancer=1;
run;
```

Once we have isolated the lung cancer cases, we can investigate outcomes in relationship to procedures and co-morbidities.

Overview of MarketScan Databases

The MarketScan Databases capture person specific clinical utilization, expenditures, and enrollment across inpatient, outpatient, prescription drug, and carve-out (A program separate from the primary group health plan designed to provide a specialized type of care, such as a mental health carve-out. Also, it uses a method of integrating Medicare with an employer's retiree health plan (making the employer plan secondary), which tends to produce the lowest employer cost services from approximately 45 large employers, health plans, and government and public organizations. (Anonymous-Medstat, 2007)

The MarketScan databases reflect the healthcare experience of employees and dependents covered by the health benefit programs of large employers. These claims data are collected from approximately 100 different insurance companies, Blue Cross/Blue Shield plans, and third party administrators. These data represent the medical experience of insured employees and their dependents for active employees, early retirees, and Medicare-eligible retirees with employer-provided Medicare Supplemental plans.

The Inpatient Admissions Table contains records that summarize information about a hospital admission. Medstat constructs this table after identifying all of the encounters or claims (service records) associated with an admission (e.g. hospital claims, physician claims, surgeon claims and claims from independent labs). Facility and professional payment information is then summarized for all services. The admission record also includes data that can only be identified after all claims for an admission have been identified. These additional data include the principal procedure, principal diagnosis, Major Diagnostic Category (MDC), and Diagnosis Related Group (DRG).

CASE DESCRIPTION

National Inpatient Sample

There are a total of 40,363 observations for the five years of data related to lung disease out of 3,833,637 records in the NIS. Note that approximately 1.04% of the inpatient population has a diagnosis of lung disease (shown in Table 2 and Figure 4). It is clear that lung cancer is a small sample of patients with the occurrence compared with the entire data set.

The data summary of some of the variables is given in the Table 3. Note that the average age for patients with lung cancer is about 68, about 21 years more than the average age for those without lung cancer. Males have a higher probability of having lung cancer compared with females. The patients with lung cancer have a higher probability of staying about 7 days in the hospital compared

Table 2. The frequency of lung cancer

Lung Cancer	Frequency	Percent	Cumulative Frequency	Cumulative Percent
No	3833637	98.96	3833637	98.96
Yes	40363	1.04	3874000	100.00

Figure 4. The pie chart for the proportion of lung cancer

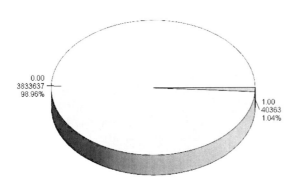

First, we use PROC KDE in SAS to examine the variables in relationship to the data with kernel density. The main advantage of using kernel density estimation is that the graphs can be overlayed for more direct comparisons. For example, we consider the relationship of lung cancer to Age, Length of Stay and Costs (also see Figures 5, 6, and 7).

```
proc sort data=medstat.inpatientadm
out=work.sortedinpatientadm;
by lungcancer;
proc kde data=work.sortedinpatientadm;
univar age/gridl=0 gridu=100
out=medstat.kdeinpatientadmage;
by lungcancer;
run;
proc kde data=work.sortedinpatientadm;
univar days/gridl=0 gridu=500
out=medstat.kdeinpatientadmdays;
by lungcancer;
run;
proc kde data=work.sortedinpatientadm;
univar totpay/gridl=-100000 gridu=300000
out=medstat.kdeinpatientadmtotpay;
by lungcancer;
run;
```

to those with conditions not related to lung cancer. Obviously, they also have higher costs.

Data visualization can be used to extract useful knowledge from large and complex datasets. The visualization can be used to build a narrative concerning the data. Kernel density estimation provides information about the entire population distribution rather than to rely on means and variances. Then Kernel Density Estimation (KDE procedure) was used to examine the lung disease by Age, Length of Stay and Total Charges, which showed the relationships among these outcomes by using data visualization.

Table 3. Summary of age, gender, length of stay and total charge

Lung Cancer=0						
Variable	**Label**	**Mean**	**Standard Deviation**	**Minimum**	**Maximum**	**N**
AGE	Age in years at admission	47.13	28.21	0	123	3831194
FEMALE	Indicator of Sex	0.59	0.49	0	1	3827460
LOS	Length of Stay	4.58	6.73	0	365	383334
TOTCHG	Total Charges	17227.54	32582.70	25	1000000	3720854
Lung Cancer=1						
Variable	**Label**	**Mean**	**Standard Deviation**	**Minimum**	**Maximum**	**N**
AGE	Age in years at admission	67.97	11.34	1	105	40361
FEMALE	Indicator of Sex	0.45	0.50	0	1	40254
LOS	Length of Stay	7.10	7.59	0	316	40359
TOTCHG	Total Charges	26425.10	38341.20	40	1000000	39371

Figure 5. The kernel density of lung cancers by age using kernel density estimation

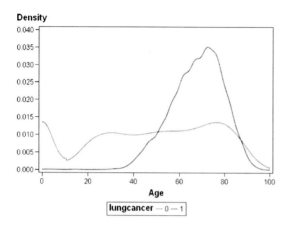

Figure 7. The density of lung cancer by total charge using kernel density estimation

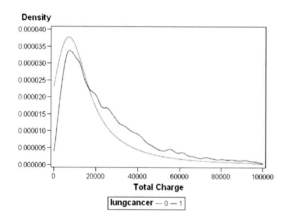

Note that the patients without lung cancer have a relatively constant likelihood of an inpatient event regardless of age (except for the interval of 0 to 20 and 60 to 80, where there is a slight change. However, the number of inpatient events increases starting at age 38, accelerating at age 45, and decreasing at age 78 for patients with lung cancer.

Those with lung cancer have a higher probability of a stay of 6 or more days, and a lower

Figure 6. The density of lung cancer by LOS (length of stay) using kernel density estimation

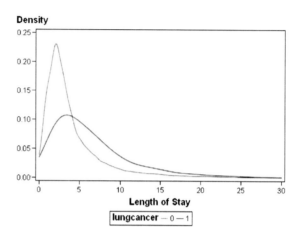

probability of staying 5 or fewer days compared to patients without lung cancer.

Note that there is an intersection point of costs for patients at around $19,000, indicating that there is a higher probability of higher cost if the patient has lung cancer. From the summary table, we know that the average cost for patients with lung cancer is around $26,425.

Next, we considered the diagnosis codes and examined more in-depth the types of complications that patients have in relationship to lung cancer. Recall that there are 8,216 patients with a diagnosis of lung cancer. Patients can be represented in multiple categories. Here, Text Miner in Enterprise Miner was used to examine the data according to text strings of patient conditions. In order to perform text analysis on the lung cancer data, the Text Miner node in Enterprise Miner was used to examine the data according to text strings of patient conditions. Cluster analysis was used to find the categories of documents. To define text clusters, we limit the number of terms to ten to describe the clusters. We use the standard defaults of Expectation Maximization and Singular Value Decomposition. For example, the text analysis defined seven different clusters in the data that are given in Table 4. In order to compare outcomes by text clusters, we merge the cluster descriptions and the cluster numbers into the original dataset. We use kernel density estimation to make a comparison of age, length of stay and cost by clusters.

Table 5 shows the translations of these clusters. These code translations are provided at http://icd9cm.chrisendres.com/.

We want to examine the relationship between lung cancer and other diseases. Hence, we use concept links for the ICD9 code of 1620; the links for 1622, 1623,1624,1625,1628 and 1629 are similar (Figure 8).

Note that most of the links are to code 1618 (shown with the widest line), malignant neoplasm of other specified sites of larynx. The other large links are to 5303 (Stricture and stenosis of esophagus), v1011 (Personal history of malignant neoplasm of Bronchus and lung), and 49390(Asthma). It shows that patients with lung cancer often have other problems that are also related to smoking.

Again, kernel density estimation was use to make a comparison of age, length of stay and cost by clusters. The code was the following:

```
data emws1.clusternis (keep=_cluster_ _
freq_ _rmsstd_
clus_desc);
set emws1.text_cluster;
run;
```

Table 4. Cluster table for diagnosis strings

Cluster #	Descriptive Terms	Frequency	Percentage	RMS Std.
1	5990, 486, 2859, 25000, 42731	1236	0.1504	0.1260
2	25000, 41401, 4280, 412, 41400	938	0.1142	0.1187
3	1629, 486, 4280, 42731, 2765	1666	0.2028	0.1284
4	3051, 1623, 5121, 496, v1582	399	0.0486	0.1100
5	311, 1972, 1622, 53081, 3051	1387	0.1688	0.1286
6	1985, 2768, 1628, 2765, 1983	1641	0.1997	0.1243
7	3051, v1582, 1961, 1625, 49121	949	0.1155	0.1241

Table 5. Translation for the clusters

Cluster #	Description	Label
1	Unspecified Urinary tract infection, Pneumonia, Unspecified Anemia, Diabetes mellitus without mention of complication, Atrial fibrillation	Diabetes and Heart Problems
2	Diabetes mellitus without mention of complication, Coronary atherosclerosis, Unspecified Congestive heart failure, Old myocardial infarction	Diabetes and Heart Problems (CHF)
3	Unspecified Bronchus and lung, Pneumonia, Unspecified Congestive heart failure, Atrial fibrillation, Volume depletion	COPD and Heart problems
4	Tobacco use disorder, Upper lobe, bronchus or lung, Iatrogenic pneumothorax, Chronic airway obstruction, History of tobacco use	COPD and smoking
5	Depressive disorder, Pleura, Main bronchus, Esophageal reflux, Tobacco use disorder	Depression
6	Secondary malignant neoplasm of Bone, bone marrow, Brain and spinal cord, Hypopotassemia, Malignant neoplasm of Other parts of bronchus or lung,	Metastasizing Cancer
7	Tobacco use disorder, History of tobacco use, Secondary and unspecified malignant neoplasm of Intrathoracic lymph nodes, Malignant neoplasm of Lower lobe, bronchus or lung, Chronic bronchitis With (acute) exacerbation	COPD and cancer in the lymph nodes

```
data emws1.desccopynis (drop=_svd_1-_
svd_500
_roll_1-_roll_1000 prob1-prob500);
set emws1.text_documents;
run;
proc sort data=emws1.clusternis;
by _cluster_;
proc sort data=emws1.desccopynis;
by _cluster_;
data emws1.nistextranks;
merge emws1.clusternis emws1.desccopynis;
by _CLUSTER_;
run;
proc kde data=emws1.nistextranks;
univar totchg/gridl=0 gridu=100000
out=emws1.kdecostbycluster;
by _cluster_;
run;
proc kde data=emws1.nistextranks;
univar age/gridl=0 gridu=100
out=emws1.kdeagebycluster;
by _cluster_;
run;
proc kde data=emws1.nistextranks;
univar los/gridl=0 gridu=35
out=emws1.kdelosbycluster;
by _cluster_;
run;
```

The average cost for cluster 6 is greater compared to other clusters. There is no big difference between clusters 1, 2, 3 and 7, which mean that they have similar severity conditions. Cluster 5 has a slightly higher probability of a higher cost than cluster 4 (Figure 9).

For the average age of each cluster (Figure 10), note that cluster 5 has the youngest average age, around 61, compared to other clusters. Clusters 1, 4 and 6 have a similar average age of 70. Similarly, clusters 2, 3 and 7 have an average age of 75.

Note that cluster 6 has a higher probability of a longer stay compared to the others (Figure 11). It would seem reasonable that patients at higher risk will stay longer and have higher cost.

Time Series and Forecasting

Next, we want to investigate and forecast the total costs of treatment for lung cancer to determine the future costs based on the inflation rate, with consideration of the patient outcomes and conditions of the patients undergoing different treatments.

Consider Figure 12, for example, which shows the trend of the total cost for lung cancer over the period January, 2000 to December, 2004 with 60 monthly average charges. For the 4-year period,

Figure 8. Concept links for 1620, malignant neoplasm of trachea

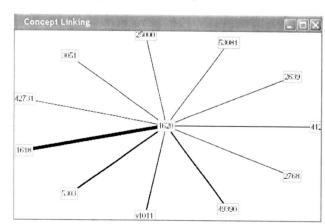

Figure 9. Kernel density estimate for total charges by clusters

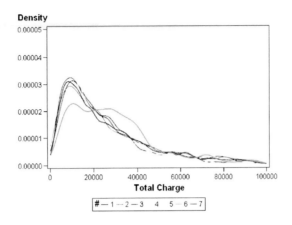

Figure 10. Kernel density estimate for age by clusters

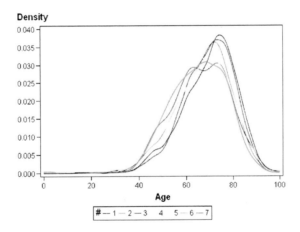

Figure 11. Kernel density estimate for length of stay by clusters

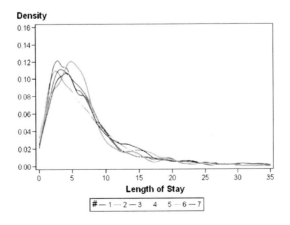

Figure 12. The trend of total charge from Jan 2000 to Dec 2004

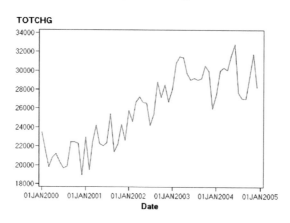

Figure 13. The means plots of total charges by LOS and Age

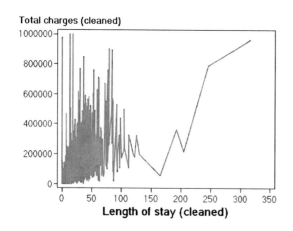

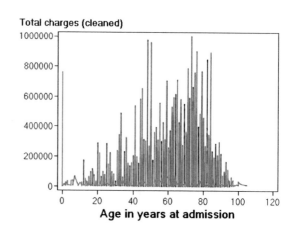

the price increases from 20,000 in 2000 to 32,000 in 2004.

Time series models were also used to analyze the total cost, Age, Length of Stay (LOS) and Inflation Rate. We used some time series features in SAS Enterprise Guide to create time series data. Here, we accumulated using the average. After accumulating, the number of records decreased to 60 with the time interval of month. The inflation rate data over the same period were collected from the website, inflationrate.com, and added to those monthly average data. Different models

were considered with or without an inflation rate. Enterprise Guide was used to create a SAS dataset. Then, Time Series models were used to examine the data. It made the information of price more visible with respect to date.

Note that the relationship between total charges and length of stay is approximately increasing (Figure 13). The amount of total charges increases as the number of days of stay is increasing. The plot of total charge and age shows that the amount of charges of patients with age from 50 to 80 is much higher than those of patients with age less than 45. There exists some relationship between them, which is not clear just by the information from these graphs.

The inflation rate was selected as a dynamic regressor. We specify a denominator factor with a simple order of 1, which represents a shifting of the inflation rate by one time unit, implying that the inflation rate leads the total cost by one month. Then, Age and Length of Stay were selected as regressors to predict the total cost. Since the actual data are increasing as shown in Figure 6, we added the linear trend as a trend model.

ARIMA (3, 1, 0) and ARMA (2, 1) were selected as a seasonal model and error model, respectively.

We applied all possible models on the data by switching values for p and d (for ARIMA(p,d,q). Also, other models were applied in order to choose the best fit model for the data. We compared all models by looking at the Root Mean Square Error and R Square. All these diagnostic measures show that INFLATION[/D(1)]+LOS+LINEAR TREAD +AGE+ARIMA(2,0,1)(3,1,0)s is the

best model for our data. Figure 14 shows the list of models used. The smallest Root Mean Square Error is 1330.8.

Note that the ACF, PACF, and IACF all suggest white noise residuals (Figure 15). The white noise tests fail to reject a null hypothesis of white noise. Thus, we conclude that this model is an adequate model based on the white noise check, autocorrelation plot and the smallest Root Mean Square Error.

Note that this model (Figure 16) fits the data well. The predicted total charges values for the next 12 months will still keep increasing, averaged at $31,500. There was a large drop at the end of 2004, and the predicted charge after 2004 is predicted to increase to the highest level, and then decrease a little.

Logistic Model for Mortality

It is the purpose of this part of the study to examine the relationship between the death and conditions of the patients undergoing different treatments.

Figure 14. Root Mean Square Error for different model used

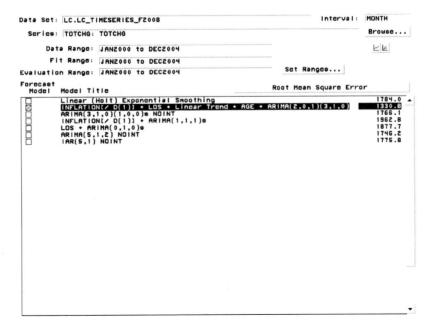

Results show that Death was highly related to Age, Length of Stay, and Total Charges, and we also found the Logistic model for mortality.

We filtered the patients who have lung diseases using the DRG codes. We used SAS Enterprise Guide and CATX and RXMATCH along with other functions in several lines of code to get a summary of the codes defining Lung cancer.

After preprocessing the data, we had 5457 patient records involving Lung cancer.

Regression analysis can characterize the relationship between a response variable and one or more predictor variables. In linear regression, the response variable is continuous. In logistic regression, the response variable is categorical. The logistic regression model uses the predictor

Figure 15. Prediction error autocorrelation plots and white noise

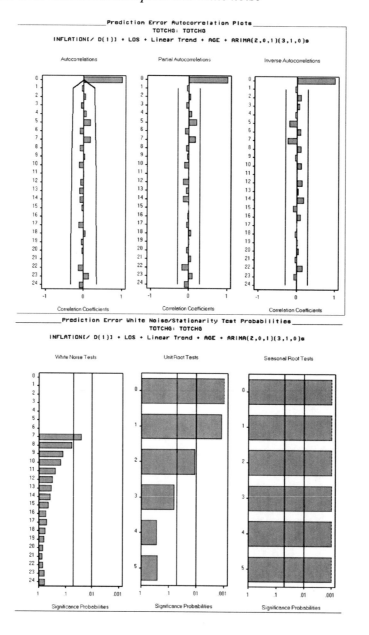

Figure 16. The forecast of total cost based on an ARIMA model with regressors

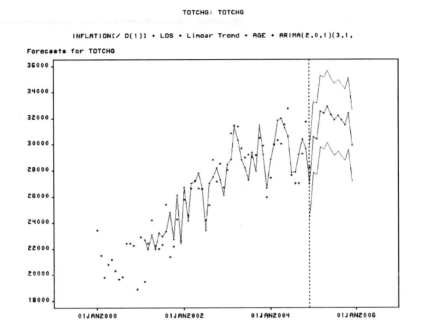

TOTCHG: TOTCHG

INFLATION[/ D(1)] + LOS + Linear Trend + AGE + ARIMA(2,0,1)(3,1,

Forecasts for TOTCHG

variables, which can be categorical or continuous, to predict the probability of specific outcomes.

The Logistic Regression Model is defined by

$$Logit(p_i) = \beta 0 + \beta 1 x_i,$$

where *Logit (p_i)* logit transformation of the probability of the event

β0 intercept of the regression line
β1 slope of the regression line

Unlike linear regression, the categorical response is not normally distributed and the variances are not the same. Also, logistic regression usually requires a more complex iterative estimation method to estimate the parameters than linear regression.

Here, we focus on the relationship between Died (death) and other conditions of the patients, such as Age (Age in years at admission), Atype (Admission type), Elective (Elective versus non-

elective admission), LOS (Length of stay), Totchg (Total charges), Zipinc_qrtl (Median household income for patient). Here, the variable, Died, was selected as the Dependent variable, and Age, Los, Totchg and Zipinc_qrtl were continuous variables. The Atype and Elective were chosen as classification variables.

Note that there were total 5457 observations, and 766 observations were deleted due to missing values for the response or explanatory variables (Table 6).

We evaluated the significance of all variables in the model by using the backward elimination method. The criterion to stay in the model was set at 0.05. Note that ELECTIVE was removed because of its redundancy.

Note that Zipinc_qrtl effect, Atype effect and the interaction effect were removed because they had large p-values in the model, which were 0.777, 0.496 and 0.6102, respectively (Table 7).

Table 8 shows that the Age and Totchg are significant at the 0.05 level in the model when LOS is slightly significant and the p-value of

Table 6. Basic information about the data set

Model Information		
Data Set	WORK.SORTTEMPTABLESORTED	
Response Variable	DIED	Died during hospitalization
Number of Response Levels	2	
Model	Binary logit	
Optimization Technique		
Number of Observations Read		5457
Number of Observations Used		4691

Table 7. The variables removed from the model

	Summary of Backward Elimination					
Step	Effect Removed	DF	Number In	Wald Chi-Square	Pr>ChiSq	Variable Label
1	AG*LO*TO*ZIP*ATY*ELE	5	6	3.5876	0.6102	
2	ZipInc_Qrtl	1	4	0.0802	0.7770	Median household income quartile by zip code
4	ATYPE	5	3	4.3809	0.4960	Admission Type

Table 8. Type III analysis of effects table

Effect	DF	Wald Chi-Square	Pr>ChiSq
Age	1	41.5927	<0.0001
LOS	1	8.8093	0.0030
TOTCHG	1	20.4203	<0.0001

interaction effect of Age and LOS is not statistically significant.

Note that all the effects are highly significant. From this table, we obtained the estimates of intercept, Age, LOS, and Totchg, 9.84, -0.08, 0.11, and -0.00002, respectively (Table 9). Hence, the model is:

Logit(p)=9.84-0.08*Age+0.11*Los-0.00002*Totchg

Note that the odds ratio estimate for Age is 0.924, which is an estimate of the relative risk for

the death adjusted for the effects of lung disease (Table 10). A 95% confidence interval for this adjusted relative risk is (0.902, 0.946). The 95% confidence interval for the odds ratio for LOS is (1.037, 1.195), which is slightly significant in the model.

Analysis of MarketScan Data

We next examine the lung cancer data from the Medstat MarketScan database, and we had two years of data, 2000 and 2001. Each year of data included medical and surgical claims, aggregated populations and enrollment information. Here, we consider inpatient cases first. There are a total of 4,718 observations for two years related to lung disease out of 800,000 records. Note that approximately 1.05% of the inpatient population has a diagnosis of lung disease.

First, we use PROC KDE to examine the variables in relationship to the data using kernel

Table 9. The analysis of maximum likelihood estimates

Parameter	DF	Estimate	Standard Error	Wald Chi-Square	Pr>ChiSq
Intercept	1	9.8407	0.9565	105.8488	<0.0001
AGE	1	-0.0795	0.0123	41.5927	<0.0001
LOS	1	0.1072	0.0361	8.8093	0.0030
TOTCHG	1	-0.00002	4.673E-6	20.4203	<0.0001

Table 10. The confidence interval for adjusted odds ratios

Effect	Point Estimate	95% Wald Confidence Limits	
AGE	0.924	0.902	0.946
LOS	1.113	1.037	1.195
TOTCHG	1.000	1.000	1.000

density estimation. The main advantage of using kernel density estimation is that the graphs can be overlayed for more direct comparisons. For example, we consider the relationship of lung cancer to Age, Length of Stay and Costs (Figures 17, 18, and 19, respectively).

Note that the patients without lung diseases have a relatively constant likelihood of an inpatient event regardless of age (except for the interval of 0 to 20 and 60 to 80, where there is a slight change. However, patients with lung diseases increase

inpatient events starting at age 38, accelerating at age 45, and decreasing at age 64.

Those with lung diseases have a higher probability of a stay of 4 or more days, and a lower probability of staying 3 or fewer days compared to patients without lung diseases.

Note that there is an intersection point of costs for patients at around 7,000, indicating that there is a higher probability of higher cost if the patient has lung disease.

Next, we considered the procedure codes and examined more in-depth the types of treatments that patients have in relation to lung cancer. Recall that there are 4,718 patients with a diagnosis of lung cancer. The procedures of treatment can be represented in multiple categories. Here, Text Miner in Enterprise Miner was used to examine the data according to text strings of treatment procedure. Cluster analysis was used to find the

Figure 17. The kernel density of lung cancer by age using kernel density estimation

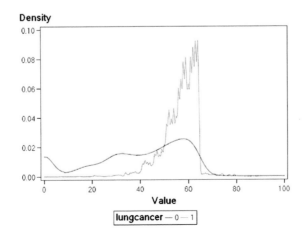

categories of documents. For example, the text analysis defined four different clusters in the data that are given in Table 11.

Table 12 shows the translations of these clusters by using the CPT codes.

According to the results of the NIS data analysis, cluster 6, Secondary malignant neoplasm of Bone, bone marrow, and Brain, is related to Biopsy Examination with an average cost that is higher. Cluster 4, COPD and smoking, is related to Screening by Scan (X-Ray or Other).

Again, kernel density estimation was use to make a comparison of age, length of stay and cost by clusters. The average cost for cluster 2 is greater compared to other clusters. There is no big difference between clusters 3 and 4, which means that they have similar severity conditions. Cluster 1 has a slightly higher probability of a lower cost than other clusters (Figure 20).

For the average age of each cluster, note that all four clusters have similar shapes, which indicates that the average ages for each cluster is 60 (Figure 21).

Note that clusters 2 and 4 have a higher probability of a longer stay compared to the others (Figure 22). It would seem reasonable that

Figure 18. The density of lung cancer by days (length of stay) using kernel density estimation

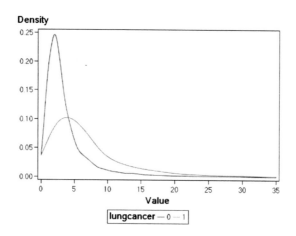

Figure 19. The density of lung cancer by total charge using kernel density estimation

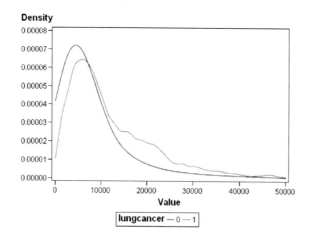

Table 11. Cluster table for procedure strings

Cluster #	Descriptive Terms	Frequency	Percentage	RMS Std.
1	99238, 99232, 99222, 71020	538	0.1140	0.0937
2	88305, 36620, 88331, 32480, 88309	1263	0.2677	0.1315
3	71260, 99238, 99223, 99231, 99233	2431	0.5153	0.1325
4	93320, 93325, 93307, 93010, 99254	486	0.1030	0.1186

Table 12. Translation for the clusters

Cluster #	Description	Label
1	Initial and subsequent hospital care, Radiologic examination, chest, two views, frontal and lateral	Screening by Scan (X-Ray or Other)
2	Level IV and VI- Surgical pathology, gross and microscopic examination, Pathology consultation during surgery; first tissue block, with frozen section(s), single specimen	Biopsy Examination
3	Initial and subsequent hospital care, Computed tomography, thorax; with contrast material(s)	MRI
4	Doppler echocardiography, Inpatient consultation for a new or established patient	Doppler

Figure 20. Kernel density estimate for total charges by clusters

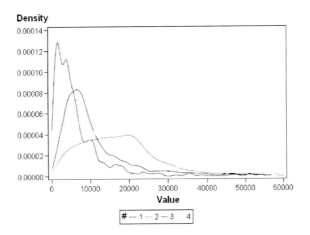

patients at higher risk will stay longer and have higher cost.

Next, we want to predict the occurrence of lung cancer according to patient age, gender, days of stay and total charges. Since lung cancer remains a rare occurrence, we use stratification as the sampling method and the sample proportion is 50/50. Figure 23 shows the predictive modeling in Enterprise Miner.

Here, the model comparison node is used to compare the results of all the models to determine which model gives the most accurate or least costly results. Figure 24 shows the model choice using the 50/50 proportion, stratified sampling and the misclassification rate.

Note that the Decision Tree is optimal with a 22.9% misclassification rate in the testing set. Figure 25 gives us the details of the Decision Tree.

Figure 21. Kernel density estimate for age by clusters

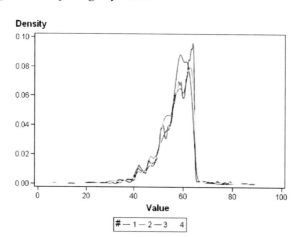

Figure 22. Kernel density estimate for length of stay by clusters

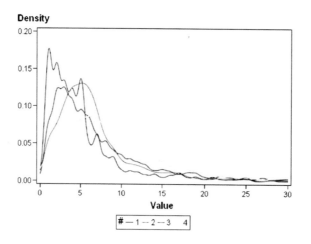

Note that the age of the patient is the first major predictor based on age with patients older than 40.5 years. The next split is based on length of stay with patients staying more than 4.5 days at higher risk compared to patients staying less than 4.5 days. The decision tree clearly shows that age and length of stay are the leading predictors of lung cancer diagnosis.

CURRENT AND FUTURE CHALLENGES FACING THE ORGANIZATION

Kernel Density Estimation was used to compare graphs that can be overlayed to give us more information. Here, we might conclude that older patients are more likely to have lung cancers that would lead to a higher probability of longer stay and higher costs for the treatment procedure. With text analysis on the diagnosis codes and KDE, it shows that malignant neoplasm of the lobe, bronchus or lung is of higher risk and has a higher cost

Figure 23. Predictive modeling process

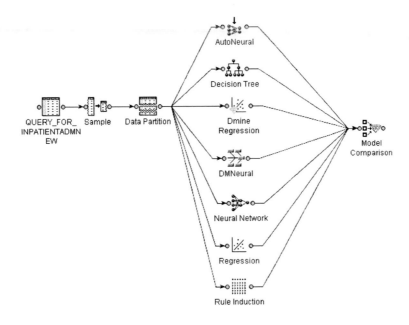

Figure 24. Model choice with profit/loss criterion

Fit Statistics
Model selection based on _APROF_

Selected Model	Model Node	Train: Average Profit for lungcancer	Train: Average Squared Error.	Valid: Average Squared Error.	Test: Average Squared Error.	Train: Akaike's Information Criterion.	Train: Misclassification Rate.	Valid: Misclassification Rate.	Test: Misclassification Rate.
	AutoNeural	0.72893	0.19296	0.20344	0.18606	4564.37	0.27107	0.28763	0.26589
	DMNeural	0.24430	0.16501	0.17096	0.15919	-4141.89	0.24430	0.25406	0.22887
	DmineReg	0.24351	0.15969	0.16898	0.15534	.	0.24351	0.25654	0.22669
	Neural	0.76603	0.15748	0.16664	0.15500	3590.64	0.23397	0.24311	0.22987
	Reg	0.75172	0.16681	0.17313	0.16018	3787.99	0.24828	0.25654	0.23164
	Rule	0.22390	.	.	.	.	0.22390	0.26078	0.22881
Y	Tree	0.77107	0.15929	0.17003	0.15811	.	0.22893	0.25053	0.22881

compared to other lung cancers. It also shows that Levels IV and VI of Surgical pathology, gross and microscopic examination are used for patients of higher risk and have a higher cost compared to other procedures to diagnose lung cancer.

The ARIMA model with ordinary and dynamic regressors was used to analyze the hospital's financial data. It provides the hospital with the ability to predict total charges of lung cancer based on previous costs. The ordinary and dynamic regressors modeled showed the effect of

the length of stay and age on the predicted values of total charges.

Then, the Logistic model was used to examine the relationship between death and conditions of patients with lung diseases. Here, we just focused on Age in years at admission, Admission type, Elective versus non-elective admission, Length of stay, Total charges, and Median household income for patient. By using the backward elimination method with level 0.15, we removed Admission type, Elective versus non-elective admission and

Figure 25. Decision tree results

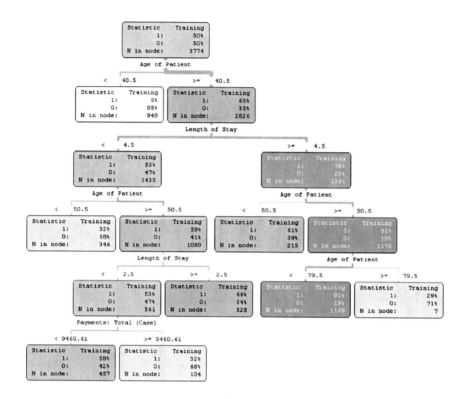

Median household income for the patient, which are not statistically significant. Then we refit the data with Age, Los and Totchg effects, which are all highly statistically significant. Finally, we obtained the model:

Logit(p)=9.84-0.08*Age+0.11*Los -0.00002*Totchg.

Last, predictive modeling is used to define patients at high risk for lung cancer. The model comparison node identified the decision tree as the optimal model to predict lung cancer. We might conclude that age and length of stay are the leading predictors of lung cancer based on the decision tree. However, this is still not enough to predict the mortality of lung cancer.

There has been an increasing interest in developing methods of assessing individual risk for lung cancer, and the National Cancer Institute has identified risk modeling as an area of extraordinary opportunity (Institute NC, 2006). Risk modeling has been successfully developed for coronary heart disease and was first published in 1976 (W. B, Kannel, 1976). The 1980s heralded the initial breast cancer risk modeling, which calculated the probability that an individual would develop breast cancer over a defined period of time (M. H, Gail, 1989). Very few models have been developed to estimate lung cancer risk, in contrast with more prevalent modeling in the breast and certain other sites. Lung cancer risk modeling has come of age in this decade. The direction of new model development is to combine clinical and epidemiologic risk factors with new biological and genetic data to more accurately assess cancer risk (A. N, Freedman, 2005).

REFERENCES

Alberg, A. J. (2003). Epidemiology of Lung Cancer. *Chest, 123,* 21–49. doi:10.1378/chest.123.1_suppl.21S

Anonymous-Medstat. (2007). *Thomson Healthcare.* Retrieved from http://home.thomsonhealthcare.com/

Anonymous-NIS. (2007). *Overview of the National Inpatient Sample.* Retrieved from http://www.hcup-us.ahrq.gov/nisoverview.jsp

Earle, C. C., & Earle, C. C. (2004). Outcomes research in lung cancer. [Review]. *Journal of the National Cancer Institute. Monographs, 33,* 56–77. doi:10.1093/jncimonographs/lgh001

Freedman, N. (2005). Cancer risk prediction models: a workshop on development, evaluation, and application. *Journal of the National Cancer Institute, 97,* 715–723.

Gail, M. H. (1989). Projecting individualized probabilities of developing breast cancer for white females who are being examined annually. *Journal of the National Cancer Institute, 81,* 1879–1886. doi:10.1093/jnci/81.24.1879

Hopenhayn-Rich, C. (2001). Lung cancer in the commonwealth: A closer look at the data. *Lung Cancer Policy Brief 2001, 1*(2).

Institute, N. C. (2006). *The nation's investment in cancer research. A plan and budget proposal for the year 2006.* Retrieved from http://plan.cancer.gov/

Kannel, W. B. (1976). A general cardiovascular risk profile: the Framingham Study. *The American Journal of Cardiology, 38,* 46–51. doi:10.1016/0002-9149(76)90061-8

Parkin, D. (2005). Max Global Cancer Statistics, 2002. *CA: a Cancer Journal for Clinicians, 55,* 74–108. doi:10.3322/canjclin.55.2.74

Thompson Cancer Survival Center. (2008). *Lung Cancer Diagnosis and Staging.* Retrieved from Thompson Cancer Survival Center web site http://www.thompsoncancer.com/tcsc-lungcancer-diagnosis.cfm

Travis, W. D. (1995). Lung cancer. *Cancer, 75*(Suppl. 1), 191–202. doi:10.1002/1097-0142(19950101)75:1+<191::AID-CNCR2820751307>3.0.CO;2-Y

Wingo, P. A. (2003). Long-Term Trends in Cancer Mortality in the United States, 1930–1998. *Cancer, 97*(11Suppl), 3133–3275. doi:10.1002/cncr.11380

ADDITIONAL READING

Bach, P. B., & Kattan, M. W. (2003). Variations in Lung Cancer Risk among Smokers. *Journal of the National Cancer Institute, 95,* 470–478.

Beane, J., & Sebastiani, P. (2008, June). A Prediction Model for Lung Cancer Diagnosis that Integrates Genomic and Clinical Features. *Cancer Prevention Research (Philadelphia, Pa.), 1*(1), 56–64. doi:10.1158/1940-6207.CAPR-08-0011

Cerrito, P. *Data mining healthcare and clinical databases.*

Heinavaara, S., & Hakulinen, T. (2006). Predicting the lung cancer burden: Accounting for selection of the patients with respect to general population mortality. *Statistics in Medicine, 25,* 2967–2980. doi:10.1002/sim.2443

Spitz, M. R., & Etzel, C. J. (2008, September). An Expanded Risk Prediction Model for Lung Cancer. *Cancer Prevention Research (Philadelphia, Pa.), 1*(4), 250–254. doi:10.1158/1940-6207.CAPR-08-0060

Spitz, M. R., & Hong, W. K. (2007). A Risk Model for Prediction of Lung Cancer. *Journal of the National Cancer Institute, 99,* 715–726. doi:10.1093/jnci/djk153

Tang, G. (n.d.). Text and Data Mining to Investigate Expenditures on Prescribed Medicines. *SAS Global Forum Proceedings2008.* Retrieved from http://www2.sas.com/proceedings/forum2008/244-2008.pdf

Chapter 7
Outcomes Research in Physical Therapy

Jennifer Ferrell Pleiman
University of Louisville, USA

ABSTRACT

This research investigates the outcomes of physical therapy by using data fusion methodology to develop a process for sequential episode grouping data in medicine. By using data fusion, data from different sources will be combined to review the use of physical therapy in orthopedic surgical procedures. The data that were used to develop sequential episode grouping consisted of insurance claims data from the Thomson Medstat MarketScan database. The data will be reviewed as a continuous time lapse for surgery date; that is, the utilization of physical therapy for a defined time period both before and after surgery will be used and studied. The methodology of this research will follow a series of preprocessing cleaning and sequential episode grouping, culminating in text mining and clustering the results to review. Through this research, it was found that the use of physical therapy for orthopedic issues is not common and was utilized in under 1% of the data sampled. Text mining was further utilized to examine the outcomes of physical rehabilitation in cardiopulmonary research. The functional independence measures score at discharge can be predicted to identify the potential benefits of physical rehabilitation on a patient by patient basis. By text mining and clustering comorbidity codes, the severity of those clusters were used in a prediction model to determine rehabilitation benefits. Other information such as preliminary functional independence scores and age (in relation to independence scores) were used in the prediction model to provide the prescribing physician a way to determine if a patient will benefit from rehabilitation after a cardiopulmonary event.

INTRODUCTION

The purpose of this study is to use claims data to investigate the use of physical therapy as a way to avoid surgery in the treatment of orthopedic problems. In order to investigate this problem, the period from the start of treatment through surgery (if surgery happens) needs to be defined and identified.

Currently, episode groupers are used in medicine to examine specific conditions that occur within a

DOI: 10.4018/978-1-61520-723-7.ch007

Copyright © 2010, IGI Global. Copying or distributing in print or electronic forms without written permission of IGI Global is prohibited.

set time period. Therefore, any medical condition, usually gathered from insurance claims data, that occurs outside of that time period is not defined in that episode, regardless of its pertinence to the prior conditions. Hence, the time limits place unnecessary restrictions on prior events. This can cause concern when trying to make medical decisions based on defined episodes. A data mining process that is similar in nature to episode groupers is data fusion. Data fusion is defined as gathering data from different sources and combining them in a way that gives a different view of the situation. Data fusion is used in image processing to combine images taken at different times and overlapped to increase relevant information. This method requires taking parts from different sources and making them whole. Once the data are gathered from the different sources, data mining techniques can then be used to determine outcomes such as classification or predictions.

This research will use data fusion methodology to develop processes for sequential episode grouping data in medicine. By using data fusion methodology, data from different sources can then be combined to give more information about the totality of patient treatment. The combination of these two ideas will be used to develop processes for sequential episode grouping. This technique will be used to identify the outcomes of certain conditions and include a more complete review of the patient's experience from beginning to end. This technique will allow a review of the data that occurs both before and after the outcome in question takes place. Additionally, these processes will assist researchers with the preprocessing of multidimensional data from different sources.

Specifically, this study will be focused on patients with orthopedic conditions. It is expected that doctors advise patients with orthopedic problems, such as knee injuries, to participate in months of physical therapy, only to have surgery as the outcome. By using the developed process for episode grouping, the data will be reviewed to define episodes for patients with orthopedic

conditions. By defining these episodes, classification and prediction models will be developed to determine outcomes based on these episodes.

Developing this process will be no easy task. A common issue in data fusion is weeding out the data that are not pertinent to the needed information. With medical claims data, this will undoubtedly occur. Therefore, the process must take into account that not every medical claim will define an episode.

The benefits of the newfound processes will be to allow researchers to combine multiple datasets into one. Applications in the healthcare field would be greatly enhanced by allowing doctors to make more informed decisions based on previous outcomes of patients with similar conditions. Also, insurance companies will be able to anticipate more accurately the next steps in patient care and can be prepared for future claims. Other fields, such as finance, will be able to apply this process to more accurately value organizational worth and to predict future cash flows and investment opportunities by looking at multiple datasets. The development of this process can provide multiple benefits in different areas of study.

BACKGROUND

Preprocessing

When working with real world data, certain revisions will need to be made to the raw data to turn the information into usable inputs for processing within a statistical software system. Unless working with a manufactured data set, it will be necessary to review the data for data integrity as well. Preprocessing is the series of steps to clean and refine the data into a useful set. Not only will preprocessing put the data into a usable format, it assists the researcher to become more familiar with the complete data. In preprocessing, familiarization with how the data appear in a raw state will allow the researcher to make early connections. Preprocessing is not an easy task and is typically the most time-consuming part of a research project. In fact, "the data extraction and preparation steps could occupy up to 80% of the project time" according to Mamdouh Refeaat (Refeaat, 2007).

Preprocessing is important to ensure the usability of data. Since real world data are rarely provided to a researcher in a clean and consistent manner, it is necessary to make certain revisions to ensure quality. In careful preparation of the data for use, errors that may cause problems later in analysis can be identified and fixed or removed from the data set entirely.

When preprocessing, a few parameters that need to be examined in the data are

- **Consistency.** Review the formatting of each column of data to ensure that the data remain consistent. For example, if a column of data is used to represent gender, ensure that all of the records include the same format. In this case, all of the records of the column would hold an "F" or "M;" a record with "Female" would not be in an appropriate format.
- **Usability.** Ensure that the format supplied is usable in the system. Dates should be entered in a format that is useful for each system needed. For example, Microsoft Excel often uses dates in a 5-digit number format, but this may not be a good method for entering into SAS.
- **Accuracy.** Reviewing for the accuracy of data can assist by highlighting issues within the data set. If the researcher was not involved directly in the data collection, it may be useful to look for certain cases that are not possible. For example, in medical data, a woman should not be reported as having a vasectomy. In reviewing for accuracy, it will help provide a first impression of the data for the researcher to begin

noticing trends and recognizing areas for further exploration.

- **Size Reduction.** Dealing with a large dimension data set can be overwhelming and result in unnecessary time and complexity in processing. By removing variables that are unnecessary to the review, it will assist in providing timely and accurate analyses. While retaining a master data set with the complete information, creating subsets for specific review can help in providing more manageable sizes.
- **Missing/Null Values.** Invariably, data sets will include records where some information may be missing. By recognizing this situation early, it may help the researcher to decide which tools and techniques would be appropriate (or inappropriate) for data sets with a number of records with missing values.

This list is a beginning point to consider in preprocessing a data set. This list is not all-inclusive as each different data set may require different steps. After initial preprocessing, the data should be in a form where it can be combined with other sources to supplement and expand the data set. This process is data fusion.

Data Fusion

Data fusion is the process of gathering data from different sources and combining the information in a way that provides a more complete view of the situation.

Developed in the late 1980's and early 1990's, multisensor data fusion is primarily used by the military for intelligence gathering, target recognition, and threat detection. Data fusion can be used to combine a series of photographs to provide a more complete view of a geographic area. As the specialty of data fusion has grown, additional fields such as law enforcement and medicine have begun to utilize the potential of data fusion (Hall, et al., 2004).

Consistent time measurement is an important factor in data fusion. If the order of images (or in this research case, medical events) is inaccurate, it will result in a skewed view of the real image. In this way, cleanliness and accuracy in preprocessing is essential. Preprocessing must ensure that the time stamp or other key factors on which the data are fused are consistent. If the elements that are used in the fusion are not consistent, then the overall image may be inaccurate and could misrepresent what is really happening.

Data fusion systems aim to perform several tasks. The system must "identify when data represents *[sic]* different views of the same object, when data is *[sic]* redundant, and when mismatch occurs between data items" (McKerrow, et al., 1996). Data fusion is a form of preprocessing data. In fusion systems, data fusion is considered to be at the low level. There are three different levels of fusion systems: low, intermediate and high. The different levels represent the level at which the fusion takes place (Royal Military Academy, nd). A low level would be the combination of the raw data sources to produce a new source. An intermediate level is also referred to as feature level fusion and is the level at which "various features extracted from several sources of raw data are combined into a composite feature that may then be used by further processing stages" (Yuhang, et al., 2006). High-level fusion is the stage at which decisions are made or fused. This level of fusion incorporates fuzzy logic and statistical methods (2006).

Since the first development, data fusion is now being expanded to other fields of interest. The field of information retrieval has been studying the concept of data fusion. In fact, some statistical methods have been developed by Wu, Bi and Mclean to be used as guidelines for fusion in information retrieval (Wu, et al., 2007). Other areas using data fusion are meteorology and intelligence data. Meteorology has used data fusion in efforts to fight forest fires. Meteorological data, winds, humidity, temperature and precipitation data are fused with tracks of tankers so that command centers can accurately direct the fire fighters to the fire's path (Akita, et al., 2002). Medical research is also starting to use elements of data fusion.

Data fusion is useful in medical research, and particularly for insurance companies, where software packages are being created with aspects of data fusion. This data fusion is important to assist in episode grouping.

Episode Grouping

Episode grouping is becoming more widely used in medical insurance because it combines data from different claims sources, such as inpatient and outpatient claims, to examine specific medical conditions. Episodes are defined by a specific time frame and insurance companies use this information to predict costs for their members. Episode grouping can also be used by healthcare providers to make better decisions on care through better information. Episode grouping tends to focus on a single condition. Currently, most software available for episode grouping is used mostly to make decisions about financial matters and is not as concerned with patient outcomes. Insurance companies heavily utilize episode groupers for economic profiling. Claims are lumped into an episode based on diagnostics (usually DRG or diagnosis related groups) and by the time stamp of the claim. Software developed for episode grouping helps assign costs by calculating the episode as "the sum of costs associated with included claims, and episode expected costs are determined, typically as the mean cost of all episodes of the same type (e.g., ETG) in the database" (Thomas, 2006). However, this software does not take into account the past episodes of a patient.

Episode grouping is typically focused on the current conditions and often provides less weight to historical information. Also, current episode grouping software sets predefined buckets for the episode groups. While there are only so many diseases commonly found in claims data, this does not factor in any previous cases or causal episodes. The software systems that offer episode grouping are often used as a product for insurance companies and are not greatly noted in research work. By using episode grouping with greater historical information, it may become a more powerful tool for predictive modeling.

Sequential Episode Grouping

By using the data fusion processes with episode grouping, a new technique can be considered in sequential episode grouping. This takes the two ideas above and utilizes the time factor needed in data fusion and provides a basis for the episode grouping to review the totality of patient treatment. By using the time element from data fusion, one issue that may occur in the episode grouping is that certain conditions and claims may be included in the data set that are not pertinent to another condition for an individual.

Sequential episode grouping is built upon combining all of the data for an individual regardless of apparent pertinence to a condition at hand. In this way, it may happen that an individual who has been hospitalized with three separate conditions within the defined time period may find that the first and third conditions are linked, but the second is unrelated. The sequential episode grouping must recognize the relevance of each record and must take into account that each claim may not be germane to an episode.

Sequential episode grouping is a daunting task to complete by hand. Currently, episode grouping has dedicated software for this processing; however, the software is expensive and often does not allow for customization by the end user. To allow for more flexibility (and cost savings), this research will show how existing statistical software can be used to complete the tasks of the off-the-shelf products.

Sequential episode grouping is a way of preprocessing the data into defined groups. It is important to note that once the data are defined, statistical methods and data mining techniques can be used to further analyze the data for data-driven insights and decisions.

Statistical Methodologies

Statistics is the science of characterizing a population based on known information, or data, collected about that population. By collecting information about the population, statistics allows for previously unknown relationships and information to be discovered.

Statistics can be used to describe the data. This information is most commonly used in data analysis to making inferences about the data. Information such as means, distributions and correlations give basic insights into the data. This information is usually the basis of more advanced statistical methodologies, such as predictive modeling.

Statistics can also be inferential, such as in predictive modeling. Predictive models such as general linear models and mixed models are commonly used to model potential outcomes of known data and to help describe the relationship between the input and output variables. These models use linearly independent and normally distributed data as inputs to predict a dependent output variable using information already collected. These models may have many fixed variables, such as the general linear models, or may include random variables, such as those found in mixed models. These models will also help describe the similarities and differences between the variables.

To visualize the differences in the data, kernel density estimation can be applied. Kernel density approximates a hypothesized probability density function from the observed data. It is a nonparametric technique in which a known density function is averaged across the observed data points to create a smooth approximation. By graphing the output from kernel density estimations, the data can be visually represented to show peaks in distributions. For example, kernel density estimation can be used to show differences between two groups of patients to see the distribution of changes in patient outcomes. Kernel density can also be used to show geographic distances to providers. In this research, kernel density estimation will be used to show the difference in time between different procedures.

Data Mining Techniques

Data mining is defined as "the search for new, valuable, and nontrivial information in large volumes of data" (Kantardzic, 2003). Data mining techniques are concerned with identifying differences occurring within the data. There are two main goals of data mining: prediction and description (2003). Predictive data mining is used to develop models that describe the known data, whereas descriptive data mining is used to find new insights in the data. Data mining is a part of a larger process called knowledge discovery (Tan, et al., 2006). This process gives the start to finish of how to turn raw data into useful information. This process starts with preprocessing, which leads into the use of data mining techniques; then the outcomes can be used for post-processing, which validates and incorporates the data into decision making.

Data mining includes a multitude of techniques. One such technique is association rules. This technique looks for patterns within data to provide information that may not have been seen by using common statistical methods. The outputs or rules can then be used to build decision models. One such method in association rules is Market Basket Analysis.

Market basket analysis is used to discover patterns in a customer's market basket. This refers to the collection of items purchased by a customer in a single transaction (Kantardzic, 2003). This information can be combined to see which items are commonly purchased together among multiple customers, or which items are routinely purchased together in a single purchase, called itemsets. This information is then mined for patterns and used to build rules showing the frequency of the patterns. One common example is the Kroger Card (http://www.kroger.com/mykroger/Pages/default.aspx). Kroger, Inc. allows customers to sign up for a free rewards card for special sale prices. However, Kroger uses this card as a tracking mechanism to see which items are purchased together in a single transaction. Kroger then uses this information to place certain items near each other and determines which items to put on sale prices to move that item. The rules built from these transactional data are then turned into information that can be used in decision making.

Another data mining technique is clustering. Clustering is a technique used to find similarities between observations and groups the observations together. The purpose of cluster analysis is to organize previously unclassified data into meaningful and useful information (SAS Text Miner Manual, 2004). Cluster analysis is an exploratory data analysis tool that aims to classify information without any explanation or interpretation (Statsoft.com, nd).

While text mining is not technically a data mining technique, it is used to process textual information so that it can be used in other data mining techniques. The main difference between data mining and text mining is the nature of the data that are used. Data mining uses ordinal and interval structured data, whereas text mining uses unstructured data. The process of text mining involves a largely automated system of complex mathematical algorithms. To achieve the desired outcomes of text mining, a series of procedures must be conducted on the data. These procedures are preprocessing, parsing, stemming, tagging, and transforming. Text mining helps to combine similar responses into meaningful clusters. For example, text mining can be used to examine the difference in procedures performed on patients in claims data. This information can then be clustered to see any trends in patients who are prescribed similar procedures and used in predictive models to show potential outcomes based on the known information.

SAS

The Statistical Analysis Software (SAS®) is a software package that was developed in the late 1960's for statisticians. The system was built for programming statistical methodologies such as analysis of variance (ANOVA) and multiple regression models on larger data sets. The SAS® Institute was incorporated in 1976 and is located in Cary, North Carolina.

Over the years, SAS® has developed from a simple system with relatively few capabilities into a more user-friendly, comprehensive tool. Until recent developments, much of the SAS system was based upon direct programming and required expert users who were proficient in the programming language to accomplish calculations. SAS® is now a market leader in data mining with the Enterprise Miner® Package. Enterprise Miner® allows advanced techniques such as neural networks, decisions trees, clustering, etc. SAS® also has a Text Miner® available to integrate with the Enterprise Miner to perform text mining applications. SAS® provides certain functions for preprocessing. The functions used in this research will include query functionality, filtering, random sampling, transposition and other functions. To aid in sequential episode grouping, SAS® will be used to fuse the different claims data sources together, preprocess the data, and run predictive models on the data.

Physical Therapy

Physical Therapy is used to "improve your mobility (such as walking, going up stairs, or getting in and out of bed), to relieve your pain, and to restore your physical function and overall fitness"

according to WebMD (webmd.com). There were two major events that resulted in the evolution of physical therapy in the US: the spread of polio in the 1800's and World War I. During the wars, physical therapists were used to aid soldiers who suffered injuries affecting their mobility. As medicine advanced, physical therapists were utilized to help patients recover from the new surgical techniques. In the 1960's and 1970's, heart surgeons started recommending physical therapy to patients before and after surgery to help with their recovery (Moffat, 2003). In the present time, physical therapy is prescribed for patients with varying types of afflictions. For this study, orthopedic issues will be the focus.

Orthopedics refers to any disorder of the musculoskeletal system. This can be anything such as a knee injury, carpal tunnel syndrome or a broken hip. Many physicians prescribe orthopedic physical therapy for these types of injuries before and after surgery (if needed). One common treatment for orthopedic problems is arthroscopic surgery. Arthroscopic surgeries involve inserting a small camera into a joint to view and aid the surgeon in making repairs. Other incisions are made to insert the tools and correct the problem at hand. Arthroscopic surgeries are usually performed on larger joints, such as knees and shoulders, but can be performed on smaller areas such as wrists, hips and ankles. Arthroscopic surgeries may be followed up (or preceded) by physical therapy (Cluett, 2006). If this is the case, episode grouping may be needed.

It is unknown how often physical therapy is prescribed as a way to avoid surgery in the treatment of orthopedic problems. Sequential episode grouping may answer this. By fusing outpatient data (where most physical therapy occurs) with inpatient data (where surgeries can occur either as inpatient or outpatient), episode grouping may shed light on how physical therapy is prescribed. The next section shows how to investigate this issue.

Physical therapy is also often prescribed for patients who have had strokes or severe heart at-

Table 1. FIM score indications

Score	Indication	Classification
1	Total Assistance	Complete Dependence
2	Maximal Assistance	Complete Dependence
3	Moderate Assistance	Modified Dependence
4	Minimal Contact Assistance	Modified Dependence
5	Needs some supervision Or will ask for help	Modified Dependence
6	Modified Independence independent but may use a wheelchair or other assistive devices	Independent
7	Total Independence	Independent

tacks. For these patients, functional independence measure scores (FIM) are measurements used to assess how well a patient is mentally and physically performing on their own. These scores range from 1 to 7 on each item in an 18-item questionnaire. The lowest, 1, means that a person is totally dependent and the highest, 7, means that the person is completely independent. These scores are used to measure the ability of the rehab patient in everyday tasks. These include physical tasks such as bathing, dressing, walking, and eating. The scores also measure social and cognitive tasks such as problem solving, social interaction, and comprehension of task. Each score has an individual meaning. Table 1 shows what each score means and the classification given to a patient with that score. (Medfriendly.com, n.d.).

SETTING THE STAGE

Rehabilitation after Stroke or Heart Attack

The first data analyzed in this study was collected at a Rehabilitation facility Louisville, Kentucky. The data consist of 555 patients who were all receiving inpatient care at this facility for either cardiac or pulmonary disorders. There were 254 (45.8%) patients with cardiac disorders and 301 (54.2%) patients with pulmonary disorders. There were 247 (44.5%) males and 308 (55.5%) females ranging in age from 2 to 96 with a mean age of 70.93 (std dev=14.38). The patients were predominately Caucasian (476 out of 555 patients (85.8%)). There were also 78 (14%) African-Americans and 1 (0.2%) Pacific Islander enrolled in the study. The majority of patients were admitted from an acute care unit. The average length of stay for Rehabilitation was 13.29 days (std dev=6.81).

Each patient who was in this study had a main diagnosis code, which represents the primary reason for receiving care. The diagnosis codes allowed us to define a patient as cardiac or pulmonary in condition. No other conditions were included in the study. Each patient had a string of comorbidity codes, which were secondary to the diagnosis code. These strings range from 1 code to 10 codes, depending on the patient (Table 2). These codes were used in the text mining stage of the analysis.

Thomson Medstat MarketScan Data

The second data set that was used in this study to develop sequential episode grouping algorithms consists of insurance claims data from the Thomson Medstat MarketScan® database (Thomson Medstat, 2002). This database contains aggregate information from approximately 100 different insurance companies from 2000 and 2001. The database contains information from inpatient admission, inpatient and outpatient services, outpatient pharmaceutical claims, population, enrollment summary and enrollment detail. The data include more than 40 million insurance members belonging to Commercial medical insurance plans from one of 45 large employers, health plans and government organizations. The database contains more than 500 million claims records (2002). This study will focus on the datasets containing commercial claims for inpatient and outpatient services

Table 2. Primary conditions for patients in rehabilitation

ICD-9 codes	Descriptions
244.9	Unspecified Hypothyroidism
250	Diabetes mellitus
276.8	Hypopotassemia (potassium deficiency)
278.01	Morbid obesity
285.9	Unspecified anemia
300	Neurotic disorders
305.1	Tobacco use disorder
357.2	Polyneuropathy in diabetes
401.9	Essential hypertension (unspecified)
428	Heart failure
496	Chronic airway obstruction
518.83	Chronic respiratory failure
530.81	Esophageal reflux
593.9	Unspecified disorder of the kidney or ureter
715.9	Osteoarthrosis, unspecified where
787.2	Dysphagia
799.3	Debility
v44.0	Tracheostomy
v45.01	Cardiac pacemaker

as well as ICD9 codes and how the two systems need to be integrated for your analysis.

Preprocessing

Sequential episode grouping is a multi-step process. Without designated episode grouping software, data are not usually in the correct format for grouping. Therefore, some data preprocessing must occur. To accomplish sequential episode grouping, several steps must be taken to begin the analysis. Among the steps that must occur are variable selection, sorting, transposing, concatenating, parsing, filtering, and data fusing. Each step should be completed in order as the order, can make a difference in the data set's composition.

The first step for preprocessing the data is variable selection. When working with large datasets, there are sometimes more variables than are needed for an analysis. Reducing the size of the data set will make preprocessing more manageable, and can make procedures run faster. Just be sure to keep all variables that may be needed. For this research, there are only three variables of concern: patient id, date of service and procedure code. The patient id will serve as the unique claim identifier. The service date will be used for sequencing and grouping. The procedure code will be the variable of interest; in particular, we want to extract arthroscopic surgeries and physical therapy. Other information such as demographics can be added later, if needed. However, as mentioned in the introduction, there are 14 outpatient files and 2 inpatient files. Each file is very large, so it is not recommended to append the tables before starting preprocessing. Instead, it is recommended that for each set of procedures, the researcher runs 16 iterations in one swipe to process all 16 tables. Just change the input and output data to account for all of the tables. Another tip is that unless the computer used has a large hard drive, it is recommended to utilize an external hard drive to save the tables being created. To assist with this process, SAS® Enterprise Guide will be used. It is recommended that a program that can handle large data sets, such as SAS®, be used for these steps.

With claims data, each claim is considered an individual data observation. Therefore, one patient can have many observations. In the MarketScan® data, this is the case and it can be daunting to try to analyze and group the data of this type. Also, this increases the size of the data set. Now that the necessary variables have been identified, the data can be sorted. In sorting, the data will be ordered based on the variable that the user defines. Sorting will allow for ordering the data sequentially by patient identifier so that information by patient identifier can be grouped.

The next step is to use transposing to reduce dimensionality and make the data more manageable. Since the procedure codes are the target for grouping, the procedure variable will be transposed. By defining the procedure to transpose by patient identifier and service date, the procedure codes will be placed on the same row for each service date. The SAS code below shows how to sort and transpose the data.

```
Libname pre 'J:\medstat sas files';
proc sort data=pre.ccae001h
out=work.ccae01hsorted;
by patid svcdate;
proc transpose data=work.ccae001hsorted
out = work.01htrans (drop=_name_ _label_)
prefix=proc_;
var proc1;
by patid svcdate;
run;
```

The code above will produce an output table that is sorted by patient id and date, and has many columns of procedure codes for each date of service per patient. This shows that most patients have multiple procedures conducted in one visit. While this has reduced the size of the table, the data are still not in a very usable format. This is where concatenation occurs.

Concatenation is the joining of two character strings into one cell. This will allow for grouping all of the procedures from one date into one column/variable. However, each patient has a varying number of procedure codes per visit. Therefore, the code must take this into account. The code below shows how to concatenate the procedure codes for each row of data, regardless of how many columns.

```
Libname pre 'J:\medstat sas files';
data pre.01hconcat(keep= patid svcdate
proc1) ;
length proc1 $2000 ; /*# of characters in
cell*/
set work.01htrans ;
array chconcat {*} proc_: ;
proc1 = left(trim(proc_1)) ;
```

```
do i = 2 to dim(chconcat) ;
proc1 = left(trim(proc1)) || ' ' ||
left(trim(chconcat[i]));
/* ' ' inputs space between CPT codes*/
end ;
run ;
```

After the concatenation step, there should only be 3 columns again: patient id, date of service and procedure. However, the procedure column will be much larger since all of the procedures for a given date will be included in this field.

The next few steps are defined based on the problem at hand. To define the episode, it is recommended that you know what procedure codes are tied to the problem (or ICD codes if looking for specific ailments). In this research, we are trying to investigate the use of physical therapy as a way to avoid surgery in the treatment of orthopedic problems. In order to investigate this problem, the period from the start of treatment through surgery (if surgery happens) needs to be defined and identified. Therefore, we will need the CPT codes related to physical therapy, as well as arthroscopic surgery. All together, there are 63 CPT codes related to arthroscopic surgery and 5 related to physical therapy. To help identify these codes, prxparse with the call function prxchange will be used. These functions will find the codes defined, then substitute in with surgery or pt (physical therapy) based on the code. Now if the hypothesis was to see if or how physical therapy was related to specific arthroscopic surgeries, this step would not be recommended. The code below shows the prxparse and prxchange functions.

```
Libname pre 'J:\medstat sas files';
data pre.01hconcat (keep = patid svcdate
proc1);
set pre.01hrecoded;
IF _N_=1 THEN Recode = prxparse('s/29892|
29898|29897|29895|29899|29894|29891|29827
|29999|29830|29838|29837|29836|29835|2983
4|29860|29862|29861|29863|29800|29804|298
```

```
70|29871|29888|29889|29851|29850|29879|29
877|29886|29887|29885|29874|29875|29876|2
9873|29884|29880|29881|29883|29882|29900|
29901|29902|29805|29806|29823|29822|29826
|29824|29807|29821|29820|29825|29819|2985
6|29855|29840|29846|29843|29847|29845|298
44/surgery/');
Call Prxchange (Recode, -1, proc1);
IF _N_=1 THEN Recode2 = prxparse('s/4018F
|97799|97039|97530|97110/pt/');
run;
```

Since the data have now been recoded to better identify surgery or physical therapy codes, it will be beneficial to create two new columns to flag when these codes are present. To do this, a procedure called rxmatch will be utilized. This procedure just uses basic pattern matching to see if any of the codes in the procedure strings match the arthroscopic surgery or physical therapy codes we are looking for. The code is given below.

```
/* arthroscopic codes*/
/* if any of the codes are found, a 1
will appear in new column surg*/
Libname pre 'J:\medstat sas files';
data pre.01hsurg (keep = patid svcdate
proc1 surg pt);
set pre.01hrecoded;
surg = rxmatch('surgery',proc1)>0;
if surg >0 then put 'surgery';
retain surg;
/* Physical Therapy codes*/
/* if any of the codes are found, a 1
will appear in new column pt*/
pt = rxmatch('4pt',proc1)>;
if pt >0 then put 'pt';
retain pt;
run;
```

Now, the dataset has 2 columns that help identify whether arthroscopic or physical therapy were conducted. Since this particular problem is only concerned with those patients with surgery or physical therapy, the data can be filtered to only show those patients. The code below filters out the patients if a 1 is present in the POS (surgery) column or the PT (physical therapy) column.

```
Libname pre 'J:\medstat sas files';
data pre.01hfilter (keep = patid svcdate
proc1 surg pt);
set pre.01hsurg;
By patid svcdate;
If (surg or pt=1);
run;
```

For this research problem, the only concern is for those patients who have had physical therapy or arthroscopic orthopedic surgery. For a more general review of the data where the researcher wants to discover all possible outcomes in relation to episodes, filtering is not necessary. Filtering is helpful if the researcher is trying to identify the frequency of specific outcomes and/or treatments.

The datasets should be reduced in size quite a bit. At this point, it is safe to fuse the data sets together. This problem is not concerned with when or where the procedure took place (inpatient or outpatient), so it suffices to append all of the tables. To do this, proc append is recommended.

Now that all of the data are contained in one large dataset, another iteration of proc sort, proc transpose and concatenation should occur. This will ensure that the episodes get defined correctly should a patient exist in multiple tables, such as inpatient and outpatient.

Before coding the episodes, there is one last step that will be beneficial for this research. The data can be further filtered out into three groups: Patients with surgery and no physical therapy, patients with surgery and physical therapy, and patients with surgery only. By filtering out the data by these groups, then the group(s) that are not of interest (in this case, the patients with pt or surgery only) can be filtered out so as not to distort the group of interest. To do this, the filter and query builder in Enterprise Guide may be used.

Create two new columns of sum (distinct) for the physical therapy and the surgery indicators. Group the data by patient id, and run. This query will show for each patient those who have physical therapy only, who have surgery only and who have both. Furthermore, place a filter on this query where physical therapy = 1 and surgery =1 to show the patient ids that should be included in the episode grouping. This list can be used to query the appended dataset where patient id = the patient id in the filtered list. The following screen shots show this process (Figures 1, 2, and 3).

At this point, the episodes can be defined on the patients who were identified as having both physical therapy and surgery. To do this, the time between service dates must be examined. Since the data are sorted, the date differences will be sequential. To define the episode, we want to see which records fall within 30 days (before and after) the surgery. This will allow us to see how many patients were prescribed physical therapy. We are assuming that if physical therapy is conducted 30

days before surgery, then the physical therapy is related to the injury that required the arthroscopic surgery. Therefore, to test how physical therapy is prescribed with patients who received arthroscopic surgery, the episodes will be defined as the start of an episode minus 30 days from the presence of surgery and the end of the episode will be plus 30 days from the presence of surgery.

To do this, the code will first sort the data by patient and the surgery indicator (descending). Then, a new column will be created to copy down the date of the surgery for each observation for that patient by utilizing the retain function. Last, the code will take the difference between the surgery date and the row's service date. This code is given below.

```
proc sort data=pre.appended1
out=work.appendedsorted;
by patid descending surg;
run;
Libname pre 'J:\medstat';
data pre.surgdate (keep = patid svcdate
proc1 pt surg Surgdate diffsurg);
```

Figure 1. Screenshot of query to create 2 new columns

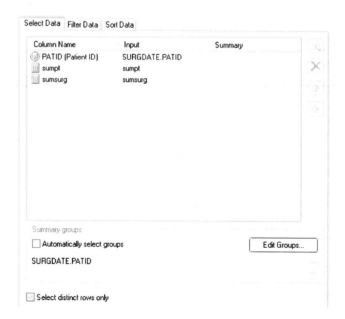

```
set work.appendedsorted;
by Patid descending Surg;
retain Surgdate;
format Surgdate mmddyy10.;
if first.patid then Surgdate=svcdate;
/*Calculate Difference between Surgery
Date and Service Date*/
diffsurg = surgdate - svcdate;
format episode $char10.;
/*Code for Pt Before or After Surgery*/
if diffsurg = 0 then episode = 'surgery';
if -30=< diffsurg <0 then episode = 'pt
after';
if 0 < diffsurg =< 30 then episode = 'pt
before';
run;
```

Now the data are coded as an episode, and researchers can now identify how the physical therapy relates to the surgery. The case description will show how many episodes by patient, as well as the frequency of physical therapy before surgery.

By defining the episode sequentially, researchers will see how often physical therapy is prescribed as a first course treatment to surgery. This method also allows for deeper investigations into the groups of patients. Researchers can then fuse the episode groups with other information, such as demographics, to see if there are any trends with the groups. Also, the patients who received physical therapy before surgery can then be compared to those who did not receive surgery at all or those who only received surgery to try to identify if there are any key differences into why a patient may or may not receive physical therapy before surgery (such as gender, age, other conditions, etc.)

Figure 2. Screenshot of query to create list of patients with surgery & physical therapy

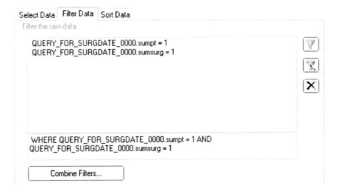

Figure 3. Screenshot of query to filter out patients with surgery & physical therapy observations

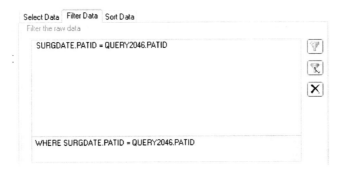

In completing the preprocessing noted above, the work for sequential episode grouping has been completed. Through preprocessing, the data are now in a suitable format for further analysis.

Validation

To see if the definition of the episodes is on the right track, text mining can be used. This technique will show linkages between the procedures. The terms can then be filtered by physical therapy and surgery to see if there is a strong linkage between the two procedures. A strong link would suggest that we should see many episodes of patients with both procedures.

Text mining is a useful technique to identify patterns within textual data. Using a largely automated system of complex mathematical algorithms, text mining can not only show basic statistics of terms, but also show linkages between the terms. To achieve the desired outcomes of text mining, a series of procedures must be conducted on the data. These procedures are preprocessing, parsing, stemming, tagging, and transforming. SAS Text Miner will be used for this analysis.

The data from the sequential episode grouping needs to be reorganized for text mining. First, it helps to pare down the data to only the variables that will be used in the text mining. For this project, only the patient id and procedure strings will be needed. Therefore, another iteration of sorting, transposing and concatenation will be needed to ensure that each patient only has one row of data.

Next, the variable must be marked for parsing. Parsing is the selection of a variable that will be used to discover trends among the documents. This variable will be used in the text mining to find meaningful similarities among the observations. Since the data set only contains 2 variables, patient id and procedure strings, it is apparent that the procedure string will be the variable parsed. However, it is important to select the roles as such when bringing the data source into Text Miner. The variable to be parsed, proc1, needs to be set to text as shown in the screen shot of Figure 4.

Stemming refers to the process of taking similar terms and combining into one umbrella term. For example, if the word is "small", then small, smaller and smallest would all fall under "small". Also, synonyms can be input to combine terms, such as little for "small". For this process, a list of synonyms usually needs to be specified. This can be done by the user and input to the text mining program. This is optional and is used to help reduce the number of words.

Tagging is utilized to exclude certain words, such as articles of speech. For instance, if the phrase was "milking the cow", tagging can be used to exclude the word, "the". If the word has no importance to the phrase, then it can be excluded. In the Text Miner node in Enterprise Miner 5.3, tagging properties are listed out under the Parse section as shown in Figure 5. For instance, punctuation and terms in a single document can be specified. For this project, and any project that would be mining codes, it is important to set Numbers to yes. Also, noun groups would allow

Figure 4. Screenshot of data source input into text miner

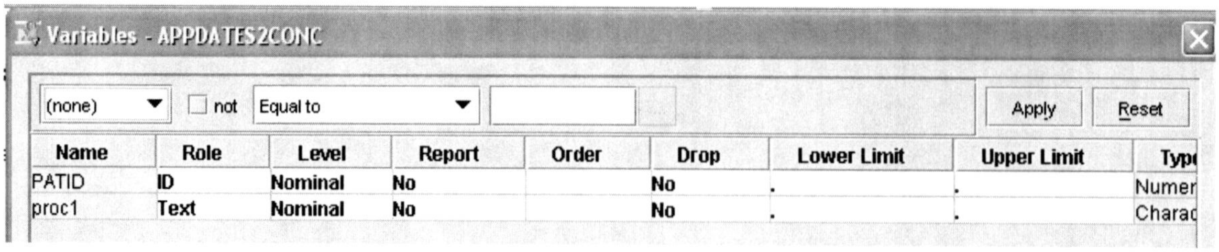

Name	Role	Level	Report	Order	Drop	Lower Limit	Upper Limit	Type
PATID	ID	Nominal	No		No	.	.	Numer
proc1	Text	Nominal	No		No	.	.	Charac

multiple instances of a code found in one string to be its own term. For instance, "pt" would be a term as well as "pt pt pt" (for three instances of pt for a patient). In this case, the noun groups will be set to no since we are only concerned with one instance of physical therapy or surgery (or any other procedure).

Last, transforming involves the actual creation of the matrices to convert the words into numerical indices. This includes creating a term by document frequency matrix, weighting the frequencies and transforming the frequencies.

A term by document frequency matrix gives the frequencies of the unstructured text by transposing the matrix as variables by observations or terms by documents. Frequency weights can then be applied to the matrix to account for the distribution of terms in a document. There are two types of frequency weights: binary and log. The user can also specify not to weight the terms. The binary weighting system assigns a "1" if the term is in the document or a "0" if otherwise. The log weights even the distribution since certain words occur more often than other words. This basically means that the term with a higher frequency in the dataset receives a smaller weight and a term with a lower frequency receives a larger weight. Term weights can also be used to adjust the local weights to even the distribution of terms among the documents. There are also two types of term weights: entropy and normal. Entropy weighting

is used when terms appearing exactly once in each document do not provide any new information about the data, and therefore give a weight of 0. Otherwise, if a term appears only one time in one document, then the weight is 1. Normal term weighting is used when the frequency of terms within documents is more informative rather than the rarity of those terms. As the frequency of term i across documents increases, the normal weight tends towards zero. These options are listed under the Transform section of Text Miner as shown in Figure 6.

Transforming the matrix can help reduce dimensionality, and help correct for empty cells. Singular Value Decomposition can be used to further transform the term by document matrix. This method reduces dimensionality while preserving information.

Singular Value Decomposition takes the term document frequency matrix, A, and expresses it in equivalent form as $A=U\Sigma V$, where Σ is the diagonal matrix of singular values, σ, and U and V are orthogonal with right- and left-singular vectors. Left- and right-singular vectors means that for the singular value σ of A, $AV= \sigma U$ and $A^T U=V$ where U is left-singular and V is right-singular. The transpose of the U matrix by A produces SVD document vectors and A by the transpose of the matrix; V is the SVD term vectors.

To attempt the maximum dimension reduction of the SVD matrix that can be used without losing

Figure 5. Screenshot of parse properties in text miner

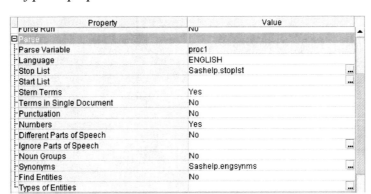

Property	Value	
Force Run	No	▲
Parse		
Parse Variable	proc1	
Language	ENGLISH	
Stop List	Sashelp.stoplst	...
Start List		...
Stem Terms	Yes	
Terms in Single Document	No	
Punctuation	No	
Numbers	Yes	
Different Parts of Speech	No	
Ignore Parts of Speech		...
Noun Groups	No	
Synonyms	Sashelp.engsynms	...
Find Entities	No	
Types of Entities		...

too much information, there are some guidelines to follow if using SAS Text Miner. First, if the document collection is larger, say in the thousands, the SVD dimension should be between 10 and 200. Otherwise, a dimension from 2 to 50 is more appropriate. If the goal is prediction, then a larger dimension, from 30-200, is appropriate. If the goal is clustering or exploration, then 2-50 is appropriate. If a high resolution is specified, then the Heuristic SVD cutoff rule uses the maximum dimension specified by the user. A higher resolu-

tion should summarize the data better, but requires more computing resources. If low or medium resolution is selected, then the Heuristic cutoff rule is applied (SAS Text Miner Manual, 2004). There must be a minimum of six documents, but at least 100 documents are recommended to get meaningful results. It is not clear as to whether these guidelines are general and would work with other text mining programs. The values generated by the Singular Value Decomposition can then be used for clustering the data (Ferrell, 2006). These

Figure 6. Screenshot of transform properties in text miner

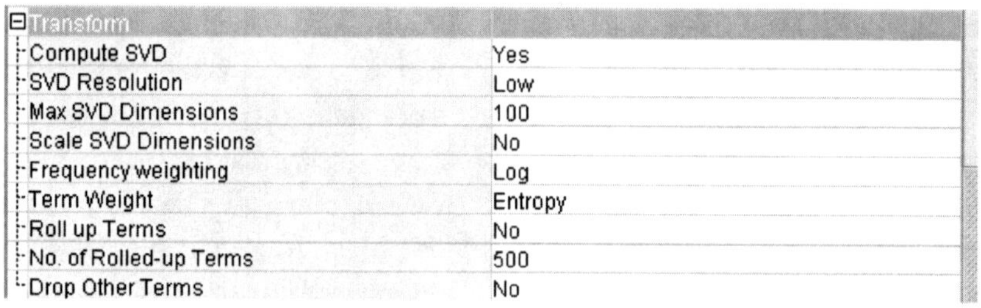

Transform	
Compute SVD	Yes
SVD Resolution	Low
Max SVD Dimensions	100
Scale SVD Dimensions	No
Frequency weighting	Log
Term Weight	Entropy
Roll up Terms	No
No. of Rolled-up Terms	500
Drop Other Terms	No

Figure 7. Screenshot of terms list in text miner

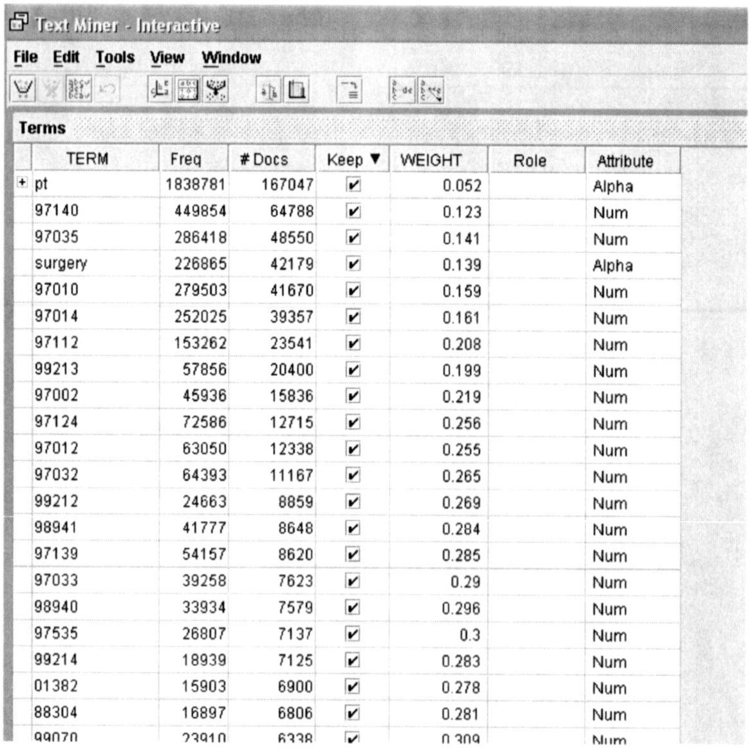

Text Miner - Interactive

File   Edit   Tools   View   Window

Terms

TERM	Freq	# Docs	Keep ▼	WEIGHT	Role	Attribute
+ pt	1838781	167047	✔	0.052		Alpha
97140	449854	64788	✔	0.123		Num
97035	286418	48550	✔	0.141		Num
surgery	226865	42179	✔	0.139		Alpha
97010	279503	41670	✔	0.159		Num
97014	252025	39357	✔	0.161		Num
97112	153262	23541	✔	0.208		Num
99213	57856	20400	✔	0.199		Num
97002	45936	15836	✔	0.219		Num
97124	72586	12715	✔	0.256		Num
97012	63050	12338	✔	0.255		Num
97032	64393	11167	✔	0.265		Num
99212	24663	8859	✔	0.269		Num
98941	41777	8648	✔	0.284		Num
97139	54157	8620	✔	0.285		Num
97033	39258	7623	✔	0.29		Num
98940	33934	7579	✔	0.296		Num
97535	26807	7137	✔	0.3		Num
99214	18939	7125	✔	0.283		Num
01382	15903	6900	✔	0.278		Num
88304	16897	6806	✔	0.281		Num
99070	23910	6338	✔	0.309		Num

options are also listed under the transform section of Text Miner.

The information just given is more of the theory behind text mining. Most of the functions listed previously occur behind the scenes. After the node has run, results will be given by clicking on the ... box after interactive (under the Training section); the user can see the terms (with frequencies and weights) as shown in Figure 7.

Here, the user can right click on a term to filter the data based on a specific term, treat terms as equivalent (which can then be used in synonym lists), and view concept links (Figure 8).

A concept link is useful when trying to identify which terms are highly identified with a specific term. In the case description section, concept maps of physical therapy and surgery will be shown to see if they are highly associated with each other.

Another useful technique that can be used in conjunction with text mining is clustering. Clus-

tering is used to give an assigned numeric index to observations that share similar information. When used with text mining, clustering is used to group observations that have similar terms with each other. This information can then be used to identify further areas of exploration or in statistical methods such as predictive modeling.

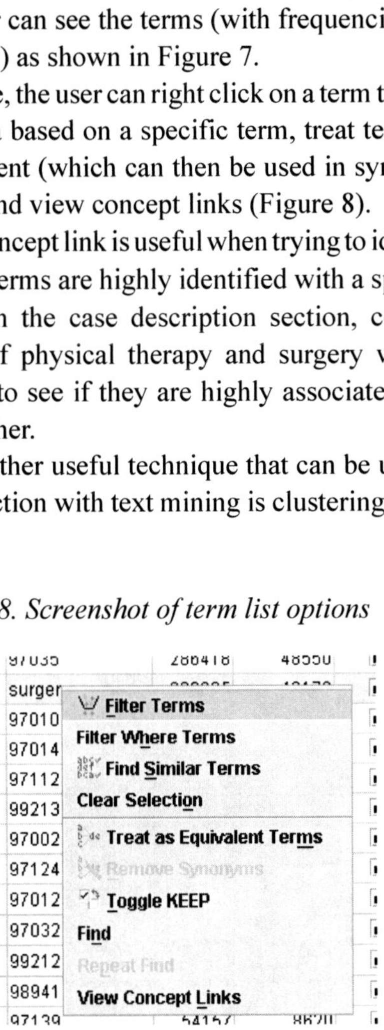

Clustering is an option within the Text Miner node (Figure 9). The user can input a specific number of clusters to identify, the clustering algorithm, and what to cluster (among other options).

SAS offers two algorithms for clustering: Expectation Maximization and Hierarchical. Expectation Maximization can apply to categorical or continuous variables to create a best-fit probability distribution. This algorithm is very similar to K-means in that it tried to determine the best distribution of k clusters given a mixture of k multivariate normal distributions of all the clusters. Hierarchical clustering is an agglomerative process in which each cluster contains a single observation at first. This process works from the bottom-up, starting with each observation as its own cluster. The algorithm continues by iteratively merging the two least dissimilar clusters until only one cluster is left.

A maximum number of clusters may be specified, or an exact number. If left at maximum, SAS will calculate the optimal number of clusters based on the user inputs. The clustering may be run at the same time as the text mining, so results will appear with the text mining output. The assigned cluster index will appear in the data so that this information can be used in other techniques.

Figure 8. Screenshot of term list options

Figure 9. Screenshot of cluster property in text miner

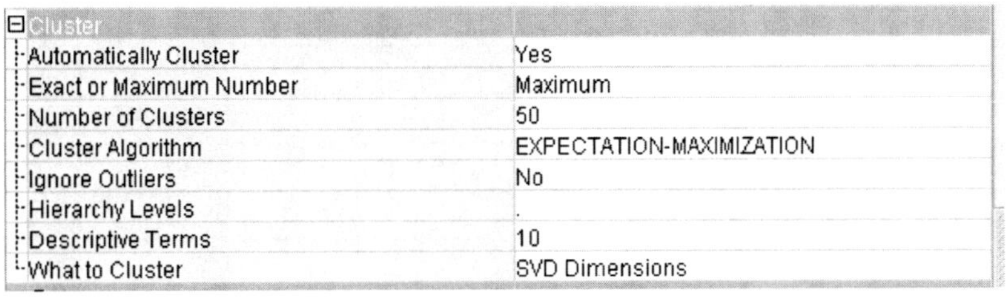

Cluster	
Automatically Cluster	Yes
Exact or Maximum Number	Maximum
Number of Clusters	50
Cluster Algorithm	EXPECTATION-MAXIMIZATION
Ignore Outliers	No
Hierarchy Levels	.
Descriptive Terms	10
What to Cluster	SVD Dimensions

CASE DESCRIPTION

Rehabilitation Related to Arthroscopic Surgery

Through sequential episode grouping, the data will show how many times physical therapy is prescribed before a surgery occurs. The sequential episode grouping will also show how often surgery occurs without physical therapy or with physical therapy only after the surgery takes place.

From the data reduction due to preprocessing, only 0.06% of the original sample falls into an episode. The episode is defined as 30 days minus surgery and 30 days plus surgery. Figure 10 shows the results.

As shown in Figure 10, only 1,845 patients had physical therapy prescribed before surgery. This frequency is lower than all of the other possibilities. It appears that most patients receive surgery without any physical therapy (from a provider) prescribed. It is very possible that patients are given exercises at home to aid with pre- or post surgical treatment.

Even though physical therapy only is shown as a group, this cannot really be used for comparison, because the physical therapy could be related to something besides arthroscopic surgery.

Figure 10. Episode groups

Groups	Count	% of Original Sample (Concatenated)
Physical Therapy Only	152,224	0.30%
Surgery Only	27,454	0.05%
Physical Therapy Only Before Surgery	534	0.00%
Surgery with Physical Therapy both Before and After	1,311	0.00%
Surgery with Physical Therapy at least before	1,845	0.00%
Physical Therapy Only After Surgery	8,631	0.02%
Surgery with physical therapy NOT in an episode	4,162	0.01%
Total Patients	196,161	

Table 3. Text mining terms

Term	Translation	Frequency	Documents
Pt		1838781	167047
97140	Manual therapy	449854	64788
97035	Ultrasound therapy	286418	48550
Surgery		226865	42179
97010	Hot or cold packs therapy	279503	41670
97014	Electronic stimulation therapy	252025	39357
97112	Neuromuscular reeducation	153262	23541
99213	Office or outpatient visit, est.	57856	20400
97002	Patient reevaluation	45936	15836
97124	Massage therapy	72586	12715
97012	Mechanical traction therapy	63050	12338
97032	Electrical stimulation	64393	11167
99212	Office or outpatient visit, est.	24663	8859
98941	Chiropractic manipulation	41777	8648

In fact, those patients should be matched up to the ICD-9 codes to see what the physical therapy was related to.

Therefore, it can be concluded that physical therapy is not prescribed much as a first course treatment for orthopedic problems. In fact, it appears that physical therapy is very seldom prescribed (or used) in conjunction with surgery. To validate that this conclusion is correct, text mining was performed to see how often physical therapy and surgery were linked in the procedure text strings. First, a term list was generated to show the frequency of terms in the dataset. Table 3 shows the top terms.

As the term list shows, physical therapy is the term or procedure that appears most throughout the data. Surgery is the fourth highest term. Therefore, we know that the terms have some significance in the data. Next, by looking at the concept maps of physical therapy (Figure 11) and surgery (Figure 12), we will be able to see if there are strong linkages between the two terms.

As the concept maps show, surgery does not even appear on the physical therapy map and vice versa. This indicates that the two terms do not show a strong linkage together in the text strings. This helps validate what the sequential episode groupers show, since physical therapy was rarely seen in a group with surgery.

The concept maps also point out a couple of other things. First, there are terms in the surgery map that are not in the researchers listing of CPT codes. This may indicate coding errors, or that there may be company-specific codes. Another interesting thing with the text mining is that there are procedure codes that could possibly be treated as equivalent with physical therapy. It is recommended that further investigations include a domain knowledge expert (such as a physician or physical therapist) to see if any of the codes can be rolled up together. If so, linkages could change. However, it is not expected that any changes such as those would change the outcome of the physical therapy link (or lack thereof).

Clustering was also defined to see if any clusters found physical therapy and surgery together. There were 23 clusters formed from the text mining. Table 4 shows the clusters.

As shown in the tables, there are no clusters that contain physical therapy and surgery, even

Figure 11. Physical therapy text concept map

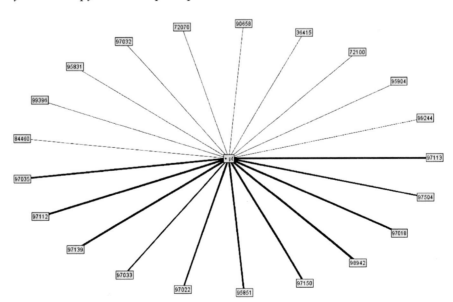

163

Figure 12. Surgery text concept map

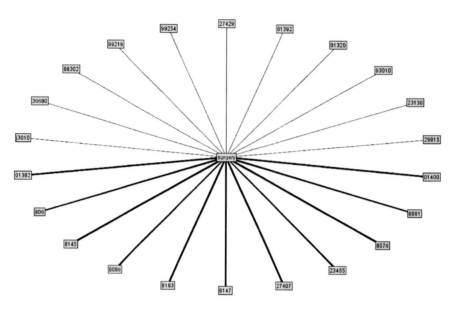

Table 4. Clusters

Cluster #	Terms	Translation	Frequency	Percent
1	97035, 97140, a4556, 97001, 97010, 97003, 97033, j1100, pt, 97002	Ultrasound therapy, manual therapy, electrodes (eg, apnea monitor), per pair, pt evaluation, hot or cold packs therapy, ot evaluation, electric current therapy, injection, dexamethasone sodium phosphate, 1 mg, pt, pt re-evaluation	4033	0.0207
2	98942, 98940, 72100, 99203, 99212, 98941, 99214, 99204, 97012, 98943	Chiropractic manipulation, chiropractic manipulation, x-ray exam of lower spine, office/outpatient visit new, office/outpatient visit est, chiropractic manipulation, mechanical traction therapy, chiropractic manipulation	6368	0.0327
3	97010, 97124, 97035, 97001, pt, a9300, 97250, 95117, 76092, 90471	Hot or cold packs therapy, massage therapy, ultrasound therapy, pt evaluation, electrical stimulation, manual therapy, electric stimulation therapy, pt re-evaluation, diathermy eg, microwave, pt	9961	0.1381
4	97140, 97001, 97010, 97035, pt, a9300, 97250, 95117, 76092, 90471	Manual therapy, pt evaluation, hot or cold packs therapy, ultrasound therapy, pt, exercise equipment, immunotherapy injections, mammogram, screening, immunization administration	8791	0.0452
5	88305, 27425, e0114, surgery, 88311, 806,88304, e0135, 37202, 93010	Lat retinacular release open, crutches, underarm, surgery, decalcify tissue, tissue exam by pathologist, walker, folding, transcatheter therapy infuse, electrocardiogram report	3462	0.0178
6	99243, 73610, pt, 99212, 99213, 20610, 99211, 73030, 99203, 99204	x-ray exam of ankle, pt, office/outpatient visit, est, drain/inject joint/bursa, x-ray exam of shoulder, office/outpatient visit, new	5529	0.0284
7	97012, 99203, 98940, 97014, 72070, 72040, 99204, 97032, pt, 97124	Mechanical traction therapy, office/outpatient visit new, chiropractic manipulation, electric stimulation therapy, x-ray exam of thoracic spine, x-ray exam of neck spine, office/outpatient visit new, pt, massage therapy	9959	0.0512

continued on the following page

Table 4. continued

Cluster #	Terms	Translation	Frequency	Percent
8	Pt, 98940, 97140, 97010, 97001, 99202, 99203, 72040, 72100, a9300	Pt, chiropractic manipulation, manual therapy, not or cold packs therapy, pt evaluation, office/outpatient visit, new, x-ray exam of neck spine, x-ray exam of lower spine, exercise equipment	6350	0.1275
9	97010, a9300, 97112, 97140, 97001, pt, 97014, 97250, 86092, a4556	Hot or cold packs therapy, exercise equipment, neuromuscular reeducation, manual therapy, pt evaluation, pt, electric stimulation therapy, mammogram, screening,, electrodes (eg, apnea monitor), per pair	7981	0.0410
10	97124, 97002, 97112, 99211, 97012, 97140, 97750, 99213, 97035, 99212	Massage therapy, pt re-evaluation, neuromuscular reeducation, office/outpatient visit est, mechanical traction therapy, manual therapy, physical performance test, ultrasound therapy	14861	0.0764
11	97036, 97139, 99199, pt, 97001, 90658, 97002, 97150, 97144, 99212	Hydrotherapy, physical medicine procedure, special service/proc/report, pt, pt evaluation, flu vaccine 3 years & >, im, pt re-evaluation, group therapeutic procedures, manual therapy, office/outpatient visit, est	5334	0.0274
12	97116, 97112, 97002, 36415, 97750, 97001, 97535, 99214, 99213, 01382	Gait training therapy, neuromuscular reeducation, pt reevaluation, routine venipuncture, physical performance test, pt evaluation, self care management training, office/outpatient visit est	3077	0.0158
13	97116, 99392, 97535, 92526, 97532, 92506, 92507, 97004, 90471, 97533	Gait training therapy, previous visit est, age 1-4, self care management training, oral function therapy, cognitive skills development, speech/hearing evaluation, ot re-evaluation, immunization administration, sensory integration	838	0.0043
14	27428, 01382, e0114, e0188, i1832, 01320, 64450, e0218, 8145, 88304	Reconstruction, knee, crutches, underarm, synthetic sheepskin pad, knee orthosis, n block, other peripheral, water circulating cold pad with pump	724	0.0037
15	97001, a4556, pt, 97010, 97140, 97014, 97035, 97016, a9300, 99202	Pt evaluation, electrodes (eg, apnea monitor), per pair, pt, hot or cold packs therapy, manual therapy, electric stimulation therapy, ultrasound therapy, vasopneumatic device therapy, exercise equipment, office/outpatient visit, new	12087	0.0622
16	97033, 97033, 99070, 97004, 97010, 97014, 97002, 99203, 99212, 97112	Electric current therapy, ot evaluation, special supplies, ot re-evaluation, hot or cold packs therapy, electric stimulation therapy, pt re-evaluation, office/outpatient visit, new	4457	0.0229
17	97002, 97001, 99078, 97750, 97139, 97535, 97112, 97116, 010, 97003	Pt re-evaluation, pt evaluation, group health education, physical performance test, physical medicine procedure, self care management training, neuromuscular reeducation, gait training	4855	0.0250
18	Pt, 97001, i1800, e1130, i3002, e0601, i1906, 92542, i1815, i0500	Pt, pt evaluation, knee orthosis, standard wheelchair, continuous airway pressure device, ankle foot orthosis, positional nystagmus test, lumbar-sacral orthosis	22136	0.1139
19	01382, 99214, 36415, 80061, 80053, 97002, 85025, 97150, 97022, 97113	Office/outpatient visit, est, routine venipuncture, lipid panel, comprehensive metabolic panel, pt re-evaluation, complete cbc w/auto differ wbc, group therapeutic procedures	23694	0.1219
20	97001, pt, 97140, 99205, a9300, 76075, 97265, 76092, 95117, 95115	Pt evaluation, pt, manual therapy, office/outpatient visit, new, exercise equipment, dxa bone density, axial, mammogram screening, immunotherapy injections, immunotherapy, one injection	6396	0.0329
21	23420, 29815, 23120, 23410, 03010, 01382, 29909, 73560, 8363, 23412	Repair of shoulder, partial removal, collar bone, repair rotator cuff, acute electrocardiogram report, x-ray exam of knee, 1 or 2, repair rotate cuff	5988	0.0308

continued on the following page

Table 4. continued

Cluster #	Terms	Translation	Frequency	Percent
22	97124, 99070, 95831, 99214, 97504, 97018, 95851, 97003, 97750, 97535	Massage therapy, special supplies, limb muscle testing manual, office/outpatient visit, est, paraffin bath therapy, range of motion measurements, ot evaluation, physical	9048	23
23	88311, 8076, 27425, 8086, 20680, 29908, 88300, 64450, 8046, 93010	Decalcify tissue, lat retinacular release open, removal of support implant, surgical path, gross, n block, other peripheral, electrocardiogram report	18474	0.0950

though both are highly present in the strings. The text mining and clustering outcomes have helped validate what was seen with the initial sequential episode grouping. While these two techniques do not incorporate a sequential element, they demonstrate the presence of the two procedures together. Had the text mining shown strong linkages between physical therapy and surgery, it would be an indicator that the episodes were poorly defined. However, the results of the cluster analysis indicate that the codes used in the prxparse code may not have been inclusive. After further evaluation of the cpt codes, there are more procedures that can be coded as surgery and physical therapy.

The text mining and clustering outcomes have helped validate what was seen with the first iteration of sequential episode grouping. While these two techniques do not incorporate a sequential element, they demonstrate the presence of the two procedures together. Had the text mining shown strong linkages between physical therapy and surgery, it would be an indicator that the episodes were poorly defined.

At this point, another iteration of the sequential episode grouping will be conducted adding the additional codes. Since the data was saved throughout the preprocessing steps, the iteration can start at the prxparse functions. As with many preprocessing methods as well as data mining techniques, multiple iterations are common. Since these techniques are very exploratory in nature, patterns and additional knowledge are gained with

each run. In this case, it was discovered that some codes that could be included were missing from the code. This could indeed produce different results depending on how common the additional codes are in the claims data.

The results of the investigation have led to conclusions, which may not have been foreseeable at the outset of this research. Based on information reported, physical therapy is not being used prior to or after surgery. The episode grouping has led to a rounded 0% of the records having physical therapy in conjunction with a surgical procedure. This information may be somewhat misleading, though, as there are possible reasons why this is occurring. Three different scenarios are most likely. First, the doctor may have chosen not to prescribe physical therapy. Given the medical history of the patient, the doctor may have found it expedient to forego this process. Second, the doctor may have prescribed physical therapy, but the patient may not have gone. This is possible as physical therapy is a voluntary exercise that the patient must actively participate in. The final explanation may be that the doctor is prescribing physical therapy exercises as part of the post-operative instructions. If doctors are giving instruction for exercises that would help in rehabilitation, this information would not be contained in this dataset and would not be available for review.

The processes of this research have demonstrated the use of several techniques in data preprocessing. Primarily, the use of sequential episode

Table 5. Table of clusters

Cluster #	Descriptive Terms	Frequency	Percentage
1	518.83, 733, 278.01, 250.6, 357.2	37	7%
2	799.3, 715.9, 530.81, 428, 250	122	22%
3	285.9, 276.8, 593.9, 787.2, 414	88	16%
4	357.2, 250.6, v45.81, v43.3, 496	94	17%
5	v68.61, 244.9, 250, 45.01, 401.9	113	20%
6	305.1, 787.91, 300, 799, 599	52	9%
7	v44.0, 44.1, 780.57, 787.2, 278.01	49	9%

grouping has helped to produce many of the results used in this research. This method demonstrates an ability to find previously unrecognized trends and series within large datasets. This method, though, is best used where a previous notion of the data is held. In using episode grouping, a defined outcome is necessary to set the first baseline of the group. In the research presented above, the use of physical therapy was the issue that was under question. By relating physical therapy to surgery, the episode grouping was allowed to present information about how the prescription of physical therapy was utilized. Thus, episode grouping is most useful when looking at outcome measures, but would be less appropriate if a particular outcome of interest is not defined.

Rehabilitation after Stroke or Heart Attack

Even though text mining showed that physical therapy was not linked to surgery, it can be used in investigating rehabilitation for cardiopulmonary patients. To start, for each patient, text strings of the comorbidity codes were created. These strings were then used for text mining and clustering to create severity rankings. Using Text Miner, the variable selected to be parsed was the text strings. Since the strings contained numbers, the numbers option, as well as stemmed words as root form, was selected for identifying the terms. A singular value decomposition was selected for the transformation, with a low resolution and a maximum of 100 dimensions. A log weighting scale was used as well as entropy term weighting. Clustering was also performed using Text Miner. The clusters were based on the SVD dimensions using an expectation maximization approach. Initially, the number of clusters was arbitrarily selected to be seven. Table 5 shows the first five terms of each cluster as well as the frequency of the clusters.

The clusters are translated in Table 6.

In the data, it appeared that there were several outliers, and the handling of these data is useful to discuss. In particular, there were several cases where the age, FIM score sums or length of stay appeared to be irregular. For this study, the average age was 70.93 years (Std. Dev=14.38). However, the minimum age was almost 2 years old. In fact, there were 10 patients under the age of eighteen. Since the majority of the patients were elderly, and Medicare was involved with this study, it was not clear whether to include children or not. After looking through the literature, there was nothing stating whether children should or should not be included in cardiopulmonary rehabilitation studies. Therefore, to maintain the possible maximum number of observations, patients under the age of eighteen were excluded. Also, there were outliers in regards to length of stay. The average length of stay for a cardiopulmonary rehabilitation program is supposed to be two weeks. For this study, the average was 13.29 days, fairly close to the stan-

Table 6. Translations of cluster codes

Cluster 7	**Definition of Codes**
v44.0	Tracheostomy
v44.1	Gastrostomy
780.57	other & unspecified sleep apnea
787.2	Dysphagia
278.01	Morbid obesity
Cluster 6	
305.1	tobacco use disorder
787.91	Diarrhea
300	neurotic disorders
799	ill-defined and unknown cause of morbidity and mortality (or asphyxia)
599	other disorders of urethra and urinary tract
Cluster 5	
v58.61	long term (current) use of anticoagulants
244.9	Unspecified Hypothyroidism
250	Diabetes mellitus
v45.01	cardiac pacemaker
401.9	essential hypertension (unspecified)
Cluster 4	
357.2	polyneuropathy in diabetes
250.6	Diabetes with neurological manifestations
v45.81	aortocoronary bypass status
v43.3	heart valve
496	chronic airway obstruction
Cluster 3	
285.9	unspecified anemia
276.8	Hypopotassemia (potassium deficiency)
593.9	unspecified disorder of the kidney or ureter
787.2	Dysphagia
414	other forms of chronic ischemic heart disease
Cluster 2	
799.3	Debility
715.9	osteoarthrosis, unspecified where
530.81	esophageal reflux
428	heart failure
250	Diabetes mellitus
Cluster 1	
518.83	chronic respiratory failure
733	other disorders of bone and cartilage

continued on the following page

Table 6. continued

278.01	Morbid obesity
250.6	Diabetes with neurological manifestations
357.2	polyneuropathy in diabetes

dard. However, the minimum was one day and the maximum was 46 days. Looking at these patients, there was no noticeable trend, such as patients with longer length of stays coming in with the highest or lowest FIM sum score at admission, nor were they of a certain age group. The outliers for length of stay did not appear to be related to age or condition. Again, since there was nothing that stated that these patients should be discarded, the patients remained in the study. In the future, it would be beneficial to consult with a physician to try to identify causes for these outliers.

We attempted to determine whether patients are receiving benefits from cardiopulmonary rehabilitation. We are hypothesizing that the sum of FIM scores at discharge can be predicted by the sum of admission FIM scores and the age of the patient, the severity of comorbidities and the interaction between the sum of admission FIM scores and age. Common sense tells us that if a patient enters the hospital with low FIM score sums and leaves with high FIM score sums, then the rehabilitation helped. The model also allowed for an interaction between age and admission FIM score sum. Lastly, the severity of the patients' illnesses will most likely affect the FIM

Table 7. Ranking of clusters

Cluster #	Rank
7	1
1	2
2	3
3	4
4	5
5	6
6	7

scores. A severity ranking was assigned to each of the clusters obtained through text mining, as described below.

Assigning severity rankings based on the code definitions in Table 7 was out of the domain knowledge of the author. Therefore, an expert having knowledge of medical illnesses and terms (a pharmacist through personal communication) was contacted to rank these clusters in order of severity. The pharmacist has years of experience in ranking conditions and was a good resource for this issue. Using only the table of the clusters and codes/definitions, the consulted pharmacist was asked to rank the clusters on the basis of severity.

The higher the rank, the more severe the associated comorbidities, so a cluster with Rank=1 is most severe and a cluster with Rank=7 is least severe. Eventually, the ranking will be used for insurance reasons. For this study however, the actual ranking was not used in the model. The variable, "rank," is just severity assigned to the clusters, which was still used as a nominal class variable. Therefore, the order assumed by the severity ranking was not used. Results for the general linear model described above are shown in Table 8.

It is clear that the rank is marginally statistically significant, and needs to be taken into consideration for the patient outcomes.

CURRENT AND FUTURE CHALLENGES FACING THE ORGANIZATION

More and more, treatment units such as physical therapy will need to demonstrate patient benefit,

Table 8. Results of the general linear model

GLM with Rank Source	DF	SS	Mean Square	F value	Pr>F
Model	9	148948.0549	16549.7839	97.03	<.0001
Error		545	92961.5378		170.5716
Corrected Total		554			241909.5928
R-Square					0.615718

Source	DF	Type III SS	Mean Square	F value	Pr>F
ADFIMSUMS	1	26472.13645	26472.13645	155.2	<.0001
AGE	1	1342.0686	1342.0686	7.87	0.0052
RANK	6	2113.80454	352.300076	2.07	0.0556
ADFIMSUMS*AGE	1	1570.95921	1570.95921	9.21	0.0025

or the treatments will be discontinued. This model does not fully demonstrate that patients are benefiting from cardiopulmonary rehabilitation. However, this model does suggest that age has an impact on the sum of the FIM scores at discharge after adjusting for the sum of the FIM scores at admission. We can see from the parameter estimates that as FIM sum scores at admission and age increase, the discharge sum of FIM scores also increases. However, if both age and admission FIM sum score are higher, there will be a relatively lower increase. Also, the interaction term implies that the relationship between age and the discharge FIM scores depends on the admission FIM scores. Therefore, age does influence the benefits of the rehabilitation program, but is dependent on the FIM score sum with which the patients enter the program.

From this model, we can predict the discharge FIM scores sum. This could aid physicians who are deciding whether a person should enter rehabilitation. By assessing the patient's age, severity, and preliminary FIM scores, the physician could use this model to predict the possible benefits of the rehabilitation.

It is also important to understand how and why physicians are prescribing physical rehabilitation. The results of the investigation of the Thomson Medstat data have led to the conclusion that physi-

cal therapy is not being used in advance of or after arthroscopic surgery. The episode grouping has led to a rounded 0% of the records having physical therapy in conjunction with a surgical procedure. This information may be somewhat misleading, though, as there are possible reasons why this is occurring. Three different scenarios are most likely. First, the doctor may have chosen not to prescribe physical therapy. Given the medical history of the patient, the doctor may have found it expedient to forego this process. Second, the doctor may have prescribed physical therapy, but the patient may not have gone. This is possible as physical therapy is a voluntary exercise that the patient must actively participate in. The final explanation may be that the doctor is prescribing physical therapy exercises as part of the post-operative instructions. If doctors are giving instruction for exercises which would help in rehab, this information would not be contained in this dataset and would not be available for review.

Further research may be required to investigate the benefits of physical therapy. It is important that providers have an understanding of factors, such as age and FIM scores, that may influence the benefit of physical therapy. Reviewing the usefulness of physical therapy with respect to actual usage by prescribing physicians may reveal additional insights into potential benefits.

REFERENCES

Akita, R. M. (2002). Silver Bullet Solutions Inc., San Diego, CA. "User Based Data Fusion Approaches". Information Fusion. In *Proceedings of the Fifth International Conference*. (Volume: 2, pp 1457- 1462).

Cluett, J. (2006) *"What is arthroscopic surgery?"* Retrieved from http://orthopedics.about.com/cs/arthroscopy/a/arthroscopy.htm

Hall, D. L., & McMullen, S. A. H. (2004). *Mathematical Techniques in Multisensor Data Fusion*. Norwood, MA: Artech House, Inc.

Kantardzic, M. (2003). *Data Mining: Concepts, Models, Methods, and Algorithms*. Hoboken, NJ: IEEE.

McKerrow, P. J., & Volk, S. J. (1996, November). "A Systems Approach to Data Fusion". In *Proceedings of ADFS-96, IEEE* (pp 217-222).

Medfriendly, Inc. (n.d.). *Functional Independence Scores*. Retrieved 2004, from http://www.medfriendly.com/functionalindependencemeasure.html

Moffat, M. (2003). History of Physical Therapy Practice in the United States, The. *Journal of Physical Therapy Education*. Retrieved from FindArticles.com

Refaat, M. (2007). *Data Preparation for Data Mining Using SAS*. San Francisco: Morgan Kaufmann Publications.

Royal Military Academy. (n.d.). *Introduction to Data Fusion*. Retrieved from http://www.sic.rma.ac.be/Research/Fusion/Intro/content.html

SAS® (2004). *Text Miner Manual*. Cary, NC: SAS Institute.

Tan, P. -N., Steinbach, M., & Kumar, Vi. (2006). *Introduction to Data Mining*. . Boston: Pearson Education

The Statistics Homepage. (1984-2005). *Statsoft, Inc.* Retrieved from http://www.statsoft.com/textbook/stathome.html=

Thomas, J. W. (2006). Should Episode-Based Economic Profiles Be Risk Adjusted to Account for Differences in Patients' Health Risks? *Health Services Research, 41*(2), 581–598. doi:10.1111/j.1475-6773.2005.00499.x

Thomson Medstat. (2002). *MarketScan® Research Databases User Guide and Database Dictionary*. Ann Arbor, MI: Michigan University Press.

Wang, Y., Dunham, M. H., Waddle, J. A., & McGee, M. (2006). *Classifier Fusion for Poorly-Differentiated Tumor Classification using Both Messenger RNA and MicroRNA Expression Profiles*. Accepted by the 2006 Computational Systems Bioinformatics Conference (CSB 2006). Stanford, California.

ADDITIONAL READING

Cerrito, P. (2010). Clinical Data Mining for Physician Decision Making and Investigating Health Outcomes. Hershey, PA: IGI Publishing. Cerrito, P. B. (2009). Data Mining Healthcare and Clinical Databases. Cary, NC: SAS Press, Inc.

Ferrell, J. (n.d.). *Text Mining Comorbidity Codes in the Analysis of Cardiopulmonary Rehabilitation Data* (MA Thesis). Retrieved from http://etd.louisville.edu.echo.louisville.edu/data/UofL0161t2006.pdf

Groll, D., Heyland, D., Caeser, M., & Wright, J. (2006). Assessment of long-term physical function in acute respiratory distress syndrome (ARDS) patients. *American Journal of Physical Medicine & Rehabilitation, 85*(7), 574–581. doi:10.1097/01.phm.0000223220.91914.61

Horn, S. D., Gassaway, J., Horn, S. D., & Gassaway, J. (2007). Practice-based evidence study design for comparative effectiveness research. *Medical Care, 45*(10 Supl 2), 50-57.

Iezzoni, L. I., Ngo, L. H., Li, D., Roetzheim, R. G., Drews, R. E., & McCarthy, E. P. (2008). Treatment disparities for disabled Medicare beneficiaries with stage I non-small cell lung cancer. Review]. *Archives of Physical Medicine and Rehabilitation, 89*(4), 595–601. doi:10.1016/j.apmr.2007.09.042

Kennedy, J., Tuleu, I. B., Kennedy, J., & Tuleu, I. B. (2007). Working age Medicare beneficiaries with disabilities: population characteristics and policy considerations. [Review]. *Journal of Health and Human Services Administration, 30*(3), 268–291.

Meyers, A. R., Andresen, E. M., & Hagglund, K. J. (2000). A model of outcomes research: spinal cord injury. [Research Support, Non-U.S. Gov't. *Archives of Physical Medicine and Rehabilitation, 81*(12Suppl 2), 81–90.

Ottenbacher, K. J., Hsu, Y., Granger, C. V., & Fiedler, R. C. (1996). The reliability of the functional independence measure: a quantitative review. *Archives of Physical Medicine and Rehabilitation, 77*, 1226–1232. doi:10.1016/S0003-9993(96)90184-7

Chapter 8

Analyzing the Relationship between Diagnosis and the Cost of Diabetic Patients

Xiao Wang
University of Louisville, USA

ABSTRACT

The purpose of this study is to examine the relationship between the diagnosis and the cost of patient care for those with diabetes in Medicare. In this analysis, the author used data sets about outpatient claim, inpatient claim as well as beneficiary demography information for the year 2004, all of which were taken from the Chronic Condition Data Warehouse provided by the Centers for Medicare and Medicaid. The author analyzed the cases for diabetic inpatients and outpatients by different methods. For outpatient analysis, exploratory data analysis and linear models were used .The results show that the total charges for diagnoses are reduced considerably for payment. The distribution of the total charges follows a Gamma distribution. The output of the generalized linear model demonstrates that only 15 out of the top 20 primary treatments for charges are statistically significant to the expenditures on outpatients.

BACKGROUND

Information about Diabetes and its Co-Morbid Diseases

Diabetes is a devastating disease that greatly impacts long-term care. In recent years, diabetes has become a serious problem. According to the Centers for Disease Control and Prevention (CDC) (2007), 23.6 million children and adults had diabetes in the US in 2007, and 12.2 million are over 60 years old. Diabetes can lead to many complications such as heart disease, renal failure, high blood pressure and anemia. Statistics carried out by the American Diabetes Association showed that heart disease strikes people with diabetes twice as often as people without diabetes. Diabetes is the leading cause of new cases of blindness in people ages 20-74 and the primary cause of end-stage renal disease. The CDC also states that about 60% to 70% of people with diabetes have mild to severe forms of nervous system damage, and severe forms of diabetic

DOI: 10.4018/978-1-61520-723-7.ch008

Copyright © 2010, IGI Global. Copying or distributing in print or electronic forms without written permission of IGI Global is prohibited.

Table 1. Health care expenditures attributed to diabetes (in millions of dollars) (Anonymous-ADA, 2008)

Setting	Diabetes	Chronic Complications					General medical conditions	Total
		Neurological	Peripheral vascular	Cardio-vascular	Renal	Ophthalmic		
Hospital inpatient	1,535	3,115	2,719	20,790	3,285	36	23,473	58,344
Physician's office	2,899	382	382 279	1,004	323	899	3,830	9,897
Emergency department	234	138	43	403	132	11	2,717	3,870
Hospital out-patient	842	75	135	317	87	130	1,321	2,985

nerve disease are a major contributing cause of lower-extremity amputations. In addition, the co-morbidities often suffered by patients with diabetes can affect each other. For example, diabetes is the leading cause of renal failure. The National Institute of Diabetes and Digestive and Kidney Diseases study (2008) showed that nearly 24 million people in the United States have diabetes; the Annual Data Report supported by United States Renal Data System (2007) illustrated that nearly 180,000 people are living with kidney failure as a result of diabetes. Diabetic nephropathy likely contributes to the development of anemia in patients with diabetes. Anemia often develops early in the course of chronic kidney disease in patients with diabetes and also contributes to the high incidence of cardiovascular disease observed in diabetic patients.

Each year, it takes a large amount of resources to treat diabetes and its complications including organ dysfunctions and neurological disorders. (See Table 1). According to the American Diabetes Association (2007), the total annual economic cost of diabetes in 2007 was estimated to be $174 billion; medical expenditures totaled $116 billion, including $27 billion for diabetes care and $58 billion for chronic diabetes-related complications. Therefore, it is very essential to control diabetes. Among all the measures to control diabetes, blood

glucose monitoring is the best. The Diabetes Control and Complications Trial funded by the National Institutes of Health reported in 1993 that intensive glucose control prevents or delays the eye, nerve and kidney complications of type I diabetes (as cited in the Glucose Control Cuts Risk of Heart Disease in Type 1 Diabetes, 2005); and the DCCT/EDIC study (2005), which illustrated that intensive glucose control lowers the risk of heart disease and stroke by about 50 percent in people with type I diabetes. However, renal failure treatment is expensive since the treatment includes dialysis, an artificial blood-cleaning process, or transplantation to receive a healthy kidney from a donor. Since the expenditures for the treatment of renal failure account for 30 per cent of the costs of the treatment of diabetes, it is essential to find and examine the factors that impact on renal failure in order to reduce the total charges of diabetes treatment.

Information about the Data

Two data sets about claim information were used in this analysis: the outpatient_base_claims with 2,030,078 records and the inpatients_base_claims recorded 244,299 items. Since both of them do not cover demography information, the beneficiary_summary_file was needed. They were all

Table 2. Variables and explanations

CLM_PMT_AMT	Claim Payment Amount
NCH_BENE_PTB_COINSRNC_AMT	NCH Beneficiary Part B Coinsurance Amount
NCH_BENE_PTB_DDCTBL_AMT	NCH Beneficiary Part B Deductible Amount
CLM_OP_PRVDR_PMT_AMT	Claim Outpatient Provider Payment Amount
CLM_TOT_CHRG_AMT	Claim Total Charge Amount
ICD9_DGNS_CDn	Claim Diagnosis Code n
ICD9_PRCDR_CDn	Claim Procedure Code n
REN	Renal failure
HEA	Heart disease
ANE	Anemia
UCTRL	Uncontrolled diabetes
BENE_ID:	Encrypted 723 Beneficiary ID
BENE_SEX_IDENT_CD	Sex
BENE_RACE_CD	Beneficiary Race Code
ICD9	AN abbreviation for the 9th edition of the International Classification of Diabetes and Related Health Problems.
NCH	A nonprofit, multi-facility healthcare system located in Naples, Florida, U.S.

from CMC Chronic Condition Data Warehouse, which provides researchers with Medicare beneficiary, claims, and assessment data linked by beneficiary across the continuum of care.

SETTING THE STAGE

We first discuss the details of the data sets. Table 2 gives a list of the variables that will be used in the paper.

Outpatient Analysis

Since the study was concerned with the cost and the diagnosis, the author used Filter and Query procedures to select the columns related to these variables and to generate the Query data set; then, the author used Data->Random Sample to choose a sample of size 10,000. Next, the author used Describe->Summary Statistics to Summarize Claim Total Charges, Coinsurance Amount, Deductible Amount, Claim Payment and Provider Payment.

Usually, a general linear model is used to analyze cost data. However, the author used the generalized linear model, which extends the general linear model by allowing a non-normal distribution while the generalized mixed linear model extends the generalized linear model by incorporating normally distributed random effects. The GLIMMIX procedure is a production download from the SAS website (SAS Institute, Inc; Cary, NC). Like the generalized linear model, the GLIMMIX model assumes normal random effects, and conditional on these random effects, data can have any distribution in the exponential family (The GlMMIX Procedure, 2006). The reason why the author used the generalized linear model is that the variable, total charges, follows a Gamma distribution; the reason for using GLIM-MIX is that the response variable, renal failure, follows a binary distribution and the author also had random effects in the model since the author chose the diagnoses to examine in the model. The logistic regression was also utilized since the author wanted to examine the binary target variable, renal failure, as a function of 14 diagnoses vital to total charges. Since the event has a low probability of happening, Enterprise Miner was used rather than SAS Enterprise Guide because only the former can analyze data on a rarest event level.

After the study, the author concluded that there are 15 diseases, particularly chronic kidney diseases, that have important effects on the total charges. Anemia and heart disease have vital relationships to renal failure; hence, anemia and heart disease should be considered for diabetic outpatients with renal failure in order to reduce the total charges.

Inpatient Analysis

Information in the model shows that both heart disease and anemia have important relationships to renal failure. For inpatient analysis, the Text Miner node in SAS Enterprise Miner and Kernel Density Estimation were used. The CATX function was used to put all possible diagnosis codes into one text string. To find those patients with organ diseases or neurological disorders, the RXMATCH function was used. It is discovered that below 34,350 dollars, the North American Natives' expenditures are greater than any other races while after that, the Asian costs are the highest. Another discovery is that before the expenditures arrive at 40,000 dollars, kidney disease does not affect the costs as much as the other organ diseases do; after that amount, kidney disease has important effects on the cost.

Before the analysis, the author also needed to preprocess the data. Random Sampling in SAS Enterprise Guide was used to reduce the size of the data to 10,000; then, the sample data were added to the beneficiary data set by beneficiary ID. Next, kernel density estimation (KDE) was utilized to see how the total charges were distributed among different races. The CATX statement was used to put all possible diagnosis codes into one column.

Now, the Text Miner node can be used. This node in SAS Enterprise Miner can process volumes of textual data; hence, its data source must contain at least one variable assigned the text role; in this analysis, the variable diagnosis was assigned as the text variable. After running this node, document clustering and concept linkage can be performed. Cluster analysis (first used by Tryon, 1939) encompasses a number of different algorithms and methods for grouping objects of similar kind into respective categories. In most cases, it is only a useful starting point for other purposes. In this paper, it was used for Kernel density estimation of the costs. Concept linkage connects related documents by identifying shared concepts between two unrelated data sets (Lavengood & Kiser, 2007).

The results demonstrate that under a threshold amount of costs, kidney disease does not impact the expenditures of the inpatients as much as the other organ diseases do; however, as the costs increase, the effects of kidney disease become more and more important.

CASE DESCRIPTION

Outpatient Case

Table 3 shows the summary results.

The output in table 3 shows that the average claim for total charges is around 1168.88 dollars, while the average claim payment is only 254 dollars; the differences are in the other payments such as coinsurance and the deductible amount. Therefore, the total charges are reduced considerably for payment. The author used kernel density estimation for total charges. The method is SNR (SAS/STAT User's Guide, 1999) and the upper bound is at 9000 dollars; the lower bound is at 0 dollars for the total charges. The SAS code (Cerrito, 2007) is as follows:

Table 3. Summary of claim charges

Variable	Mean	Std Dev	Minimum	Maximum	N	Median
CLM_PMT_AMT	254.9002600	628.7453260	-64.6900000	19401.07	10000	58.4400000
NCH_BENE_PTB_COINSRNC_AMT	84.1978490	188.6815001	0	2550.97	10000	13.29000000
NCH_BENE_PTB_DDCTBL_AMT	1.3519630	9.5368202	0	100.0000000	10000	58.4400000
CLM_OP_PRVDR_PMT_AMT	254.9002600	628.7453260	-64.6900000	19401.07	10000	212.0000000
CLM_TOT_CHRG_AMT	1168.88	3261.83	1.0000000	70903.60	10000	

```
proc kde data=sasuser.sampledata;
univar CLM_TOT_CHRG_AMT / gridl=0
gridu=6000
method=SNR out=KDEtotalcharges;
run;
```

Graph->Line Plot->Spline Plot in Enterprise Guide was used to get Figure 1.

Figure 1 visualizes the distribution of the total charges. It illustrates that the distribution of the total charges is a gamma distribution. The density increases before the total charges reach almost 500 dollars and decreases sharply after that. Most of the total charges are under 3500 dollars.

Since the raw data cannot be utilized directly in the generalized linear model, preprocessing is needed. The author followed the methods used in the book, *A Casebook of Pediatric Diseases*

(Cerrito, 2009). First, the author used Filter and Query to select Claim ID and ICD9_DGNS_CD1 to generate a new data set that contains two columns, and changed the name of ICD9_DGNS_CD1 to ICD9. It was the same for the left nine ICD9_DGNS_CDn and six ICD9_PRCDR_CDn to generate 16 tables. Then, the author opened one table, and used Data->Append Table; after that, the ICD9 table (Figure 2) was generated. This was followed by Describe->One-way Frequencies to count the frequencies of ICD9 Codes to find the top 20 ICD9 codes as displayed in Table 4.

Next, the author used Filter and Query->Compute Column to recode the ICD9 codes in Figure 2 to generate the Recode_ICD9 table (Figure 3) and performed One- way frequency, choosing Recode as the analysis variable and Group analysis by Claim ID to generate the

Figure 1. KDE of total charges

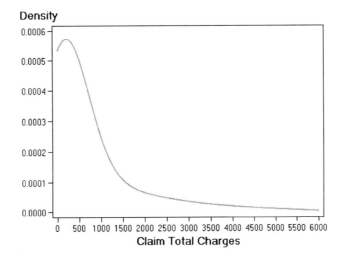

One-way frequency table. The following step is to use 0-1 indicator functions to generate 20 new variables and get a new dataset (Figure 4).The SAS code is as follows:

Figure 2. ICD9 table

	CLM_ID	ICD9
1	VVVVVVvRRRVE	V5883
2	VVVVVVvRRRVE	V5883
3	VVVVVVvRRRVE	7038
4	VVVVVVvRRRVt	71947
5	VVVVVVvRRRVtp	5130
6	VVVVVVvRRRVB	4010
7	VVVVVVvRRRVB	25000
8	VVVVVVvRRRVB	25000
9	VVVVVVvRRRVB	7859
10	VVVVVVvRRRV7	25000
11	VVVVVVvRRRVp	29620
12	VVVVVVvRRRVp	V825
13	VVVVVVvRRRVp	25000
14	VVVVVVvRRRVp	25001
15	VVVVVVvRRRvV	V5861

```
data sasuser.Recodedata; set sasuser.
freqofrcode;
IF(Recode_ICD9 EQ:'25000')
THEN R25000=1;
ELSE R25000=0;
IF(Recode_ICD9 EQ:'4019')
THEN R4019=1;ELSE R4019=0;...
```

Next, the author performed Summary Statistics->Maximum for the 20 newly-generated variables, with Claim ID as the Classification variable; then, the Max variable data set was generated as shown in Figure 5. Finally, the author added the Max Variable table to the original sample data to get Figure 7 for the generalized linear model and the process is shown in Figure 6.

Now, the Generalized Linear Model could be used. First, the author chose the Claim Total

Table 4. Top 20 ICD9 diagnosis codes

ICD9	Diagnosis	Frequency	Percent
25000	Diabetes mellitus without complication type ii or unspecified type not stated uncontrolled	2264	8.90
4019	Unspecified essential hypertension	1351	5.31
585	Chronic kidney disease (ckd)	629	2.47
V5861	Long-term (current) use of anticoagulants	509	2.00
2724	Other and unspecified hyperlipidemia	508	2.00
42731	Atrial fibrillation	469	1.84
2859	Anemia unspecified	452	1.78
4280	Congestive heart failure unspecified	429	1.69
V5869	Long-term (current) use of other medications	402	1.58
28521	Anemia in chronic kidney disease	357	1.40
4011	Benign essential hypertension	339	1.33
2720	Pure hypercholesterolemia	314	1.23
41400	Coronary atherosclerosis of unspecified type of vessel native or graft	296	1.16
25001	Diabetes mellitus without complication type i not stated as uncontrolled	244	0.96
5990	Urinary tract infection site not specified	232	0.91
2809	Iron deficiency anemia unspecified	230	0.90
2449	Unspecified acquired hypothyroidism	225	0.88
496	Chronic airway obstruction not elsewhere classified	210	0.83
25002	Diabetes mellitus without complication type ii or unspecified type uncontrolled	203	0.80
78079	Other malaise and fatigue	194	0.76

Charges as the dependent variable and the newly-generated variables as the classification variables. Then, the author chose the Gamma function and used the Log link function as well as Type I analysis. The results are given in the following tables. The output displayed in Table 6 shows that the dependent variable follows a Gamma distribution; the link function is a Log function.

In Table 7, the value of deviance divided by degree is 2.32, and the scaled deviance divided by degree is 1.26. These two variables demonstrate the adequacy of this model, which means that the generalized linear model fits the data reasonably well. Type I analysis shows that the following factors (shown in Table 8) are statistically significant to the model since their

Figure 3. Recode_ICD9 table

	CLM_ID	ICD9	Recode_ICD9
1	WWWWvRRRVE	V5883	other
2	WWWWvRRRVE	V5883	other
3	WWWWvRRRVE	7038	other
4	WWWWvRRRVt	71947	other
5	WWWWvRRRVtp	5130	other
6	WWWWvRRRVB	4010	other
7	WWWWvRRRVB	25000	25000
8	WWWWvRRRVB	25000	25000
9	WWWWvRRRVB	7859	other
10	WWWWvRRRV7	25000	25000
11	WWWWvRRRVp	29620	other
12	WWWWvRRRVp	V825	other
13	WWWWvRRRVp	25000	25000
14	WWWWvRRRVp	25001	25001
15	WWWWvRRRvV	V5861	V5861

Figure 4. New 20 variables (part of columns and rows)

CLM_ID	Recode_ICD9	COUNT	PERCENT	R25000	R4019	R585	RV5861	R2724	R42731
WWWWvE	other	16	100	0	0	0	0	0	
WWWWvE	42731	1	6.25	0	0	0	0	0	
WWWWvE	V5861	1	6.25	0	0	0	1	0	
WWWWvE	other	14	87.5	0	0	0	0	0	
WWWWvE	42731	1	6.25	0	0	0	0	0	
WWWWvE	V5861	1	6.25	0	0	0	1	0	
WWWWvE	other	14	87.5	0	0	0	0	0	
WWWWvE	other	16	100	0	0	0	0	0	
WWWWvE	2859	1	6.25	0	0	0	0	0	
WWWWvE	5990	1	6.25	0	0	0	0	0	
WWWWvE	other	14	87.5	0	0	0	0	0	

Figure 5. Max variable

CLM_ID	_WAY_	_TYPE_	_FREQ_	R25000_Max	R4019_Max	R585_Max	RV5861_Max	R2724_Max	R427:
WWWWvEEVO7	1 1		1	0	0	0	0	0	
WWWWvEEVOE	1 1		3	0	0	0	1	0	
WWWWvEEVOE	1 1		3	0	0	0	1	0	
WWWWvEEVOO	1 1		1	0	0	0	0	0	
WWWWvEEVOR	1 1		3	0	0	0	0	0	
WWWWvEEVOb	1 1		1	0	0	0	0	0	
WWWWvEEVOb	1 1		1	0	0	0	0	0	
WWWWvEEVOp	1 1		1	0	0	0	0	0	
WWWWvEEVOp	1 1		3	0	0	0	0	0	
WWWWvEEVOp	1 1		3	1	0	0	0	0	

Figure 6. Add tables

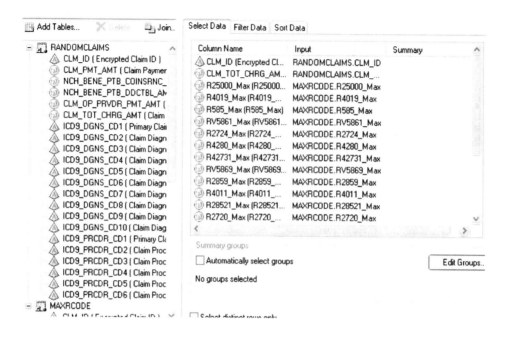

Figure 7. Table for GLM

CLM_ID	CLM_TOT_CHRG_AMT	R25000_Max	R4019_Max	R585_Max	RV5861_Max	R2724_Max	R4280_Max	R4273
WWWvEWvv	262.00	0	0	1	0	0	0	
WWWvEWvb	327.42	0	1	0	0	0	0	
WWWvEWv	2055.00	0	0	0	0	0	0	
WWWvEWb	288.94	0	0	0	0	0	0	
WWWvEWb	163.00	0	0	0	0	0	0	
WWWvEWb	384.50	0	0	0	0	0	0	
WWWvEW0	200.00	0	0	0	0	0	0	
WWWvEW0	140.00	0	0	0	0	0	0	
WWWvEWR	410.00	0	0	0	0	0	0	
WWWvEWE	2446.00	0	0	0	0	0	0	

Table 6. Overall mode information

Model Information		
Data Set	WORK.SORTTEMPTABLESORTED	
Distribution	Gamma	
Link Function	Log	
Dependent Variable	CLM_TOT_CHRG_AMT	Claim Total Charge Amount

p-values are smaller than 0.05. The chi-square value of 23.68 for type II Diabetes mellitus without complication represents twice the difference in the log likelihoods between fitting a model with only an intercept and a model with an intercept and type II diabetes mellitus without complications. Similarly, every chi-square value for each variable represents the differences in log likelihoods between successive models. Since the value of the chi-square for a variable represents the importance of that value, and the chi-square value for chronic kidney disease ranks the first

Table 7. Criteria for assessing goodness of fit

Criteria For Assessing Goodness Of Fit			
Criterion	**DF**	**Value**	**Value/DF**
Deviance	9980	23196.7333	2.3243
Scaled Deviance	9980	12550.5608	1.2576
Pearson Chi-Square	9980	79786.4792	7.9946
Scaled Pearson X2	9980	43168.3655	4.3255
Log Likelihood		-75829.4983	

Table 8. Type I analysis

LR Statistics For Type 1 Analysis		2*Log Likelihood	DF	Chi-Square	Pr
Source					
Intercept		-154184.45			
R25000_Max	Diabetes mellitus without complication type II or unspecified type uncontrolled	-154160.76	1	23.68	<.0001
R4019_Max	Unspecified essential hypertension	-154078.23	1	82.53	<.0001
R585_Max	Chronic kidney disease (ckd)	-152265.81	1	1812.42	<.0001
RV5861_Max	Long-term (current) use of anticoagulants	-152018.52	1	247.29	<.0001
R2724_Max	Other and unspecified hyperlipidemia	-151969.30	1	49.21	<.0001
R4280_Max	Congestive heart failure unspecified	-151953.57	1	15.74	<.0001
R42731_Max	Atrial fibrillation	-151889.81	1	63.76	<.0001
RV5869_Max	Long-term (current) use of other medications	-151886.98	1	2.82	0.0929
R2859_Max	Anemia unspecified	-151880.30	1	6.69	0.0097
R4011_Max	Benign essential hypertension	-151782.39	1	97.91	<.0001
R28521_Max	Anemia in chronic kidney disease	-151737.71	1	44.68	<.0001
R2720_Max	Pure hypercholesterolemia	-151736.64	1	1.07	0.3014
R41400_Max	Coronary atherosclerosis of unspecified type of vessel native or graft	-151731.99	1	4.65	0.0311
R5990_Max	Urinary tract infection site not specified	-151731.98	1	0.01	0.9287
R25001_Max	Diabetes mellitus without complication type i not stated as uncontrolled	-151729.57	1	2.41	0.1203
R78079_Max	Other malaise and fatigue	-151729.57	0	0.00	.
R2809_Max	Iron deficiency anemia unspecified	-151708.85	1	20.72	<.0001
R2449_Max	Unspecified acquired hypothyroidism	-151707.74	1	1.11	0.2922
R496_Max	Chronic airway obstruction not elsewhere classified	-151698.50	1	9.24	0.0024
R25002_Max	Diabetes mellitus without complication type ii or unspecified type uncontrolled	-151659.00	1	39.50	<.0001

among all the values (shown in Table 9); kidney disease is the most important variable related to the total charges.

Since chronic kidney disease has the most important effect on the costs and since chronic kidney disease counts for a large per cent of renal failure, the logistic regression in Enterprise Miner would be used to analyze the relationship between renal failure and the other diseases vital to the total charges. Before using it, some preprocessing was still needed. The 0-1 indicator functions were used in the ICD9 table (Figure 3) to get a new table shown in Figure 8. The SAS code is as follows:

```
data sasuser.renal; set sasuser.appcal-
imtable;
IF(ICD9 EQ:'586') or (ICD9 EQ:'5849')
THEN R=1;ELSE R=0;Run
```

Next, the author used Summary Statistics to analyze the maximum of the variable R (for renal failure) and chose claim ID as the classification variable. After getting another new table, the author added the new table to the Max variable table (Figure 5) to get the following Figure 9.

After preprocessing the data, the following steps were utilized in Enterprise Miner. First, the author chose Renal Table as the data source, set R (Renal Failure) as the Target and set the variables on binary level. Then, the author added a Sample node and connected it from the data and the author used Stratify Method, chose Level Based as the stratified criterion and Rarest Level in the Level Based options. The results of the logistic regression are as follows in Tables 11, 12, and 13.

The output in Table 11 shows the overall information of the Logistic Regression Model. Fourteen variables are used to analyze their relationships to Renal Failure. Table 12 indicates that the error of the model is MBernoulli and the link function is logit. The misclassification rate in Table 13 is 0.386, which is accepted.

The results in Table 14 indicate that only unspecified anemia is significant to renal failure since only its p-value in the Type 3 analysis is less than 0.05 out of the 15 diseases that are considered for renal failure. The odds ratio (Table 15) for Anemia shows that if the diagnosis is not Anemia, then the chance that it is related to renal failure is only 9 per cent of the probability that it is Anemia. Hence, Anemia has the most important relationship to renal failure.

Table 16 shows that the false negative rate is 32 per cent, which means it is 32 per cent likely for the model to predict that renal failure is not

Table 9. Variables significant to the model

R25000_Max	Diabetes mellitus without complication type II or unspecified type uncontrolled
R4019_Max	Unspecified essential hypertension
R585_Max	Chronic kidney disease (ckd)
RV5861_Max	Long-term (current) use of anticoagulants
R2724_Max	Other and unspecified hyperlipidemia
R4280_Max	Congestive heart failure unspecified
R42731_Max	Atrial fibrillation
R2859_Max	Anemia unspecified
R4011_Max	Benign essential hypertension
R28521_Max	Anemia in chronic kidney disease
R41400_Max	Coronary atherosclerosis of unspecified type of vessel native or graft
R78079_Max	Other malaise and fatigue
R2809_Max	Iron deficiency anemia unspecified
R496_Max	Chronic airway obstruction not elsewhere classified
R25002_Max	Diabetes mellitus without complication type ii or unspecified type uncontrolled

Figure 8. R table

⚠ CLM_ID	⚠ ICD9	R
VVVVVvRRRVE	78650	0
VVVVVvRRRVE	7038	0
VVVVVvRRRVt	43310	0
VVVVVvRRRVB	78900	0
VVVVVvRRRV7	2252	0
VVVVVvRRRVp	585	0
VVVVVvRRRvV	37489	0
VVVVVvRRRvv	25000	0
VVVVVvRRRvb	5738	0
VVVVVvRRRvOt	07819	0
VVVVVvRRRvR	585	0
VVVVVvRRRvR	79380	0
VVVVVvRRRvR	9961	0
VVVVVvRRRvE	55090	0
VVVVVvRRRvE	25000	0

Figure 9. Renal table

	⚠ CLM_ID	R_Max	R25000_Max	R4019_Max	R585_Max	RV5861_Max	R2724_Max	R42731_Max	R2859_Max
1	VVVVVvEEVO7	0	0	0	0	0	0	0	0
2	VVVVVvEEVOE	0	1	0	0	0	0	1	0
3	VVVVVvEEVOE	0	0	0	0	0	0	0	0
4	VVVVVvEEVO0	0	0	0	0	0	0	0	0
5	VVVVVvEEVO0	0	0	0	0	0	0	0	0
6	VVVVVvEEVO0	0	0	0	0	0	0	0	1
7	VVVVVvEEVO0	0	1	1	0	0	0	0	0
8	VVVVVvEEVO0	0	0	0	0	0	0	0	0
9	VVVVVvEEVOR	0	0	0	0	0	0	0	0
10	VVVVVvEEVOR	0	0	0	1	0	0	0	0

Table 11. Variable summary

ROLE	LEVEL	COUNT
INPUT	BINARY	14
REJECTED	BINARY	6
REJECTED	NOMINAL	1
TARGET	BINARY	1

Table 12. Model information

Training Data Set	EMWS1.SMPL_DATA.DATA
DMDB Catalog	WORK.REG2_DMDB
Target Variable	R_Max (R_Max)
Target Measurement Level	Ordinal
Number of Target Categories	2
Error	MBernoulli
Link Function	Logit
Number of Model Parameters	15
Number of Observations	114

Table 13. Misclassification rate

TARGET	Fit statistics	Statistic Label	Train	Validation	Test
R_Max		Misclassification Rate	0.38596491	NaN	NaN

Table 14. Type 3 analysis of effects

Effect	Diagnosis	DF	Wald ChiSquare	Pr > ChiSq
R2449_Max	Unspecified acquired hypothyroidism	1	0.028	0.866
R25000_Max	Diabetes mellitus without complication type ii or unspecified type not stated as uncontrolled	1	1.131	0.288
R25001_Max	Diabetes mellitus without complication type i not stated as uncontrolled	1	0.360	0.548
R25002_Max	Diabetes mellitus without complication type ii or unspecified type uncontrolled	1	0.027	0.868
R2859_Max	Anemia unspecified	1	4.708	0.030
R4011_Max	Benign essential hypertension	1	0.264	0.607
R41400_Max	Coronary atherosclerosis of unspecified type of vessel native or graft	1	0.012	0.910
R42731_Max	Atrial fibrillation	1	0.151	0.697
R4280_Max	Congestive heart failure unspecified	1	0.226	0.634
R496_Max	Chronic airway obstruction not elsewhere classified	1	0.562	0.453
R585_Max	Chronic kidney disease (ckd)	1	0.428	0.513
R5990_Max	Urinary tract infection site not specified	1	2.596	0.107
RV5861_Max	Long-term (current) use of anticoagulants	1	0.00	0.929
RV5869_Max	Long-term (current) use of other medications	1	0.015	0.902

occurring when it in fact is; the false positive rate is 12, which means that it is only 12 percent likely to predict the diagnosis of renal failure when it actually does not occur. Since a false negative is more critical than a false positive, the model is fairly good.

Just as the results of the logistic regression show, the model probably needs improving; hence, it is necessary to utilize another model to analyze the relationship. Next, the author utilized the generalized linear mixed model. Again, preprocessing the data was needed first. The author used the following SAS code in the ICD9 table to get the renal failure table (Figure 10). Then, the author performed Summary Statistics->Max for the analysis variables: Renal failure, Heart

Table 15. Odds ratio estimates

Effect	Diagnosis	Point Estimate
R2449_Max 0 vs 1	Unspecified acquired hypothyroidism	0.745
R25000_Max 0 vs 1	Diabetes mellitus without complication type ii or unspecified type not stated as uncontrolled	2.057
R25001_Max 0 vs 1	Diabetes mellitus without complication type i not stated as un-controlled	0.602
R25002_Max 0 vs 1	Diabetes mellitus without complication type ii or unspecified type uncontrolled	0.840
R2859_Max 0 vs 1	Anemia unspecified	0.093
R4011_Max 0 vs 1	Benign essential hypertension	0.562
R41400_Max 0 vs 1	Coronary atherosclerosis of unspecified type of vessel native or graft	1.145
R42731_Max 0 vs 1	Atrial fibrillation	1.551
R4280_Max 0 vs 1	Congestive heart failure unspecified	0.704
R496_Max 0 vs 1	Chronic airway obstruction not elsewhere classified	0.402
R585_Max 0 vs 1	Chronic kidney disease (ckd)	0.626
R5990_Max 0 vs 1	Urinary tract infection site not specified	0.121
RV5861_Max 0 vs 1	Long-term (current) use of anticoagulants	1.139
RV5869_Max 0 vs 1	Long-term (current) use of other medications	0.794

Table 16. Event classification table

Data Role	Target	False Negative	True Negative	False Positive	True Positive
Train	R_Max	32	45	12	25

disease, Anemia and Uncontrolled diabetes, and chose Claim ID as the classification variable to get the renal failure_max (Figure 11).

```
data sasuser.mixmodel; set sasuser.ap-
pcalimtable
IF(ICD9 EQ:'586') or (ICD9 EQ:'5849')
THEN Ren=1; ELSE Ren=0;
IF(ICD9 EQ:'4280') or(ICD9 EQ:'4281')
or(ICD9 EQ:'4289')THEN Hea=1; ELSE Hea=0;
IF(ICD9 EQ:'2811') or (ICD9 EQ:'2819')
or (ICD9 EQ:'2849')or(ICD9 EQ:'2851')
or(ICD9 EQ:'2858') or(ICD9 EQ:'2859')
or (ICD9 EQ:'28521')or(ICD9 EQ:'28529')
THEN Ane=1; ELSE Ane=0;
```

```
IF(ICD9 EQ:'25003')or(ICD9 EQ:'28042')
or (ICD9 EQ:'28052')or(ICD9 EQ:'28062')
or (ICD9 EQ:'28092')or(ICD9 EQ:'28093')
THEN Unctrl=1; ELSE Unctrl=0; run;
```

Now, the GLIMMIX procedure in SAS can be used to perform the generalized linear model analysis: selecting Ren_max as the response variable, which is a binary variable; selecting Ane_max, Hea_max and Unctrl_max as the classification variables; analyzing Ane_max and Hea_max in the fixed effects while analyzing Unctrl_max in the random effects. The author also analyzed the least-squares means for Ane_max and Hea_max; and set the link function to logit. The following

Figure 10. Renal failure tables

CLM_ID	ICD9	Ren	Hea	Ane	Unctrl
VVVVVVvRRRVE	78650	0	0	0	0
VVVVVVvRRRVE	7038	0	0	0	0
VVVVVVvRRRVt	43310	0	0	0	0
VVVVVVvRRRVB	78900	0	0	0	0
VVVVVVvRRRV7	2252	0	0	0	0
VVVVVVvRRRVp	585	0	0	0	0
VVVVVVvRRRvV	37489	0	0	0	0
VVVVVVvRRRvv	25000	0	0	0	0
VVVVVVvRRRvb	5738	0	0	0	0
VVVVVVvRRRvOt	07819	0	0	0	0

Figure 11. Renal failure_max table

CLM_ID	_WAY_	_TYPE_	_FREQ_	Ren_Max	Hea_Max	Ane_Max	Unctrl_Max
VVVVVvEEV07	1 1		16	0	0	0	0
VVVVVvEEV0E	1 1		16	0	1	0	0
VVVVVvEEV0E	1 1		16	0	0	0	0
VVVVVvEEV00	1 1		16	0	0	0	0
VVVVVvEEV00	1 1		16	0	0	0	0
VVVVVvEEV00	1 1		16	0	1	1	0
VVVVVvEEV00	1 1		16	0	1	0	0
VVVVVvEEV00	1 1		16	0	0	0	0
VVVVVvEEV0R	1 1		16	0	0	0	0
VVVVVvEEV0R	1 1		16	0	0	1	0

SAS code (The GLIMMIX Procedure, p.17) is used:

```
proc glimmix data=sasuser.Rmixwctrl;
class Hea_Max Ane_Max Unctrl_max;
model Ren_max=Ane_Max Hea_Max/
DIST=Binary link=logit; LSMEANS Ane_Ma
Hea_Max / ; Random Unctrl_max; run;
```

The model results of this analysis are shown in Table 18. Table 19 provides information about the methods and size of the optimization problems. Iteration history is shown in Table 19. The output in Table 20 shows that after the initial optimization, the GLIMMIX procedure performed 7 times before the convergence criterion was met.

In Table 21, the first two measures indicate that the model is statistically significant; and the third measure demonstrates that the model fits the dataset very well.

Table 22 lists the covariance parameter estimates for a random variable. The variance for Unctrl_max is rather small and hence the variable is significant to the model. The output in Type 3 analysis (Table 23) shows that both Anemia and Heart disease are significant to the model since their p-values are less than or almost equal to 0.05. Table 24 lists the information about the least-squares means. The output in Table 23 shows that the estimate mean for anemia is 4.0978 and the standard error is 0.3677 while the value for heart disease is 3.9192 and its standard error is 0.4. Therefore, the two diseases are almost equally important to renal failure.

Inpatient Case

After the author combined the claim data set and beneficiary data set together, Kernel Density Estimation could be used. The SAS code and KDE are shown below:

```
proc sort data=sasuser.
ipclaimdemoout=sasuser.sortipclaim; by
bene_race_cd; run;
proc kde data=sasuser.sortipclaim;
```

Table 18. Overall information

Model Information	
Data Set	SASUSER.RMIXWCTRL
Response Variable	Ren_Max
Response Distribution	Binary
Link Function	Logit
Variance Function	Default
Variance Matrix	Not blocked
Estimation Technique	Residual PL
Degrees of Freedom Method	Containment

Table 19. Optimization information

Optimization Information	
Optimization Technique	Dual Quasi-Newton
Parameters in Optimization	1
Lower Boundaries	1
Upper Boundaries	0
Fixed Effects	Profiled
Starting From	Data

Table 20. Iteration history

Iteration History					
Iteration	Re-starts	Sub-iterations	Objective Function	Change	Gradient Max Gradient
0	0	4	44901.333748	2.00000000	2.258999
1	0	0	55044.975544	0.88254455	0.899126
2	0	0	65383.492191	0.66480678	0.386994
3	0	0	74538.584524	0.33901645	0.204332
4	0	0	79678.668813	0.06599228	0.150173
5	0	0	80708.172067	0.00198498	0.141884
6	0	0	80738.777631	0.00000168	0.141649
7	0	0	80738.803026	0.00000000	0.141649

```
univar clm_tot_chrg_amt/gridl=0
gridu=60000 method=snrout=sasuser.kdesor-
tipclaim;
by bene_race_cd;run;
```

Figure 12 gives the estimates of the total charges. Before the value of 40,000 dollars occurs, the North American natives > the Whites>the Blacks>the Hispanics, and all of them are far greater than the Asians in terms of costs; while

Table 21. Fit statistics

Fit Statistics	
-2 Res Log Pseudo-Likelihood	80738.80
Generalized Chi-Square	10055.61
Gener. Chi-Square / DF	1.01

Table 22. Covariance parameter estimates

Covariance Parameter Estimates		
Cov Parm	Estimate	Standard Error
Unctrl_Max	8.21E-22	.

Table 23. Type 3 analysis for fixed effects

Type III Tests of Fixed Effects				
Effect	Num DF	Den DF	F Value	Pr > F
Ane_Max	1	9996	3.68	0.0551
Hea_Max	1	9996	6.77	0.0093

Table 24. Least –square means analysis

Ane_Max Least Squares Means					
Ane_Max	Estimate	Standard Error	DF	t Value	Pr > |t|
0	4.7986	0.2116	9996	22.67	<.0001
1	4.0978	0.3677	9996	11.14	<.0001
Hea_Max Least Squares Means					
Hea_Max	Estimate	Standard Error	DF	t Value	Pr > |t|
0	4.9771	0.1895	9996	26.26	<.0001
1	3.9192	0.4000	9996	9.80	<.0001

after that point, the Asians cost more than the other races.

Next, we needed to preprocess the data before using Enterprise Miner. We defined a string containing all possible diagnosis codes using the CATX statement, which concatenates character strings, removes leading and trailing blanks, and inserts separators. We used the following code:

```
data sasuser.ipclaim(keep=bene_id bene_
sex_ident_cd bene_race_cd
clm_tot_chrg_amt diagnoses);
set sasuser.ipclaimdemo;
diagnoses=catx('',ICD9_DGNS_CD1,ICD9_
DGNS_CD2,ICD9_DGNS_CD3,ICD9_DGNS_
CD4,ICD9_DGNS_CD5,ICD9_DGNS_CD6,ICD9_
DGNS_CD7,ICD9_DGNS_CD8,ICD9_DGNS_
CD9,ICD9_DGNS_CD10,ICD9_DGNS_CD11,ICD9_
```

Figure 12. KDE of total charges among different races

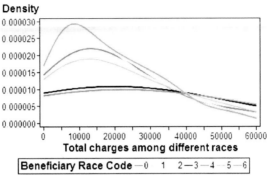

0:unkown ;1: white; 2: black; 3: other; 4: Asian; 5: Hispanic;
6: north American native

Table 25. Clusters of diagnoses

Cluster #	Descriptive Terms	Frequency	Percentage	RMS Std.
1	27800, 29570, 25000, 3051, 2724	327	0.0327	0.0994
2	412, 41401, v4581, 41400, v4582	1414	0.1414	0.1202
3	4139, 42789, 2948, 41401, 2720	539	0.0539	0.1213
4	4019, 25000, 2449, 71590, 311	1949	0.1949	0.1284
5	25060, 36201, 25050, 3572, 2724	362	0.0362	0.0988
6	5849, 4280, 49121, 40391, 486	1826	0.1828	0.1267
7	4240, 25001, 4280, 4254, 42731	1276	0.1276	0.1260
8	3310, 5990, 2859, 2765, 486	1515	0.1515	0.1238
9	25000, 53081, 2724, 4019, 2720	790	0.079	0.1177

```
DGNS_CD12,ICD9_DGNS_CD13,ICD9_DGNS_
CD14,ICD9_DGNS_CD15,ICD9_DGNS_CD16);run;
```

Now, we use Enterprise Miner. We used the data set named ipclaim as the data source, and used the Text Miner node, setting the default of number to Yes and Different parts of speech and Noun groups to No. Then we used Interactive-> Cluster documents to group the diagnoses. The results are displayed in Table 25 and the clusters are translated in Table 26. In order to view how the clusters of diagnoses affect the total charges, we still used kernel density estimation. Before that, we needed to preprocess the data sets using the following SAS code:

```
libname emst "C:\Documents and Settings \
Administrator\My Documents\ My SAS Files\
```

Table 26. Translations for the clusters

Cluster #	Diagnoses	Cluster label
1	Unspecified Obesity, Schizoaffective disorder, Diabetes mellitus without mention of complication, Tobacco use disorder, Other and unspecified hyperlipidemia	Diabetes
2	Old myocardial infarction, Of native coronary artery, Aortocoronary bypass status, Of unspecified type of vessel or native or graft, Percutaneous transluminal coronary angioplasty status	Heart disease
3	Other and unspecified angina pectoris, Other specified cardiac dysrhythmias, Other persistent mental disorders due to conditions classified elsewhere, Of native coronary artery, Pure hypercholesterolemia	Heart disease vascular disease
4	Unspecified Essential hypertension, Diabetes mellitus without mention of complication, Unspecified hypothyroidism, Osteoarthrosis which unspecified whether generalized or localized, Depressive disorder	vascular disease Diabetes
5	Diabetes with neurological manifestations, Background diabetic retinopathy, Diabetes with ophthalmic manifestations, Diabetes with ophthalmic manifestations, Other and unspecified hyperlipidemia	Ophthalmic disease Neurological disorder
6	Unspecified Acute renal failure, unspecified Congestive heart failure, Obstructive chronic bronchitis with exacerbation, Unspecified Hypertensive chronic kidney disease, Pneumonia	Heart disease Kidneydisease
7	Mitral valve disorders, Diabetes mellitus without mention of complication, unspecified Congestive heart failure, Other primary cardiomyopathies, Atrial fibrillation,	Diabetes Heart disease
8	Alzheimer's disease, Urinary tract infection, unspecified Anemia, Volume depletion, Pneumonia	Others
9	Diabetes mellitus without mention of complication, Esophageal reflux, Other and unspecified hyperlipidemia, Unspecified Essential hypertension, Pure hypercholesterolemia	Diabetes vascular disease

```
9.1\EM_Projects\IPorganfailure\Workspac-
es\EMWS1";
data sasuser.ipclus(keep= _cluster_ _
freq_ _rmsstd_ clus_desc);
set emst.text_cluster; run;
data sasuser.iptchdem (keep= bene_sex_
ident_cd bene_race_cd clm_tot_chrg_amt
diagnoses _cluster_);
set emst.text_documents; run;
proc sort data=sasuser.ipclus; by _clus-
ter_;
proc sort data=sasuser.iptchdem; by _
cluster_;
data sasuser.ipkdetchdem;
merge sasuser.ipclus sasuser.iptchdem;
by _cluster_ ; run;
proc sort data=sasuser.ipkdetchdem
out=sasuser.sortipkdetchdem;
by _cluster_ bene_sex_ident_cd ; run;
proc kde data=sasuser.sortipkdetchdem;
```

```
univar clm_tot_chrg_amt/ gridl=0
gridu=60000
method=snr out=sasuser.cluster;
by _cluster_ bene_sex_ident_cd ; run;
```

After running the SAS code, we got the KDE of total charges between the males and the females shown in Figure 13. The distributions of the costs for the male inpatients are different from the ones for the females. The first link graph in Figure 13 gives the relationships of the text cluster to male inpatient costs. From the shape of the graph, the clusters yield the relationships in terms of ordering; before the first cutpoint occurs at 19,200 dollars, cluster #5 is much greater than the other clusters; #1, #4 and #9 are almost the same and they are all greater than #2, 3; #6, 7, 8 are also almost the same, but they are all much smaller than the other clusters. Between the cutpoints of 19,200 dollars and 33,000 dollars, the ordering is

Figure 13. KDE of Total charges for diabetic inpatients by clusters

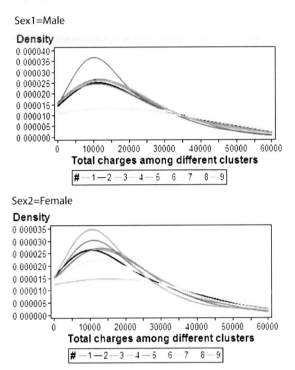

1, 4, 5, 9>2, 3>6, 7, 8. After 33,000 dollars, there are no differences among all clusters. The graph for the female inpatients shows the relationships of the text cluster to the costs in terms of ordering is 9>5>2>1,3>7.8>4,6 before the first cutpoint 10,650 occurs; between 10,650 and 16,800 dollars, 9>5>1>3>2>7,8>4,6; between 16,800 and 19500 dollars, # 1,3>2,5,7,8,9>4,6; and when the costs are above 34,650 dollars, cluster#6 is the greatest, and the cluster # 1,2,3,4,5,7,8 are almost the same; but all of them is greater than cluster # 9.

The cluster analysis just shows the costs by grouping the diagnoses; we needed to see how organ diseases are related to diabetes. We used the concept link in Text Miner to show the relationships with the results displayed in Figure 14. The ICD9 codes not analyzed below are translated in Table 27.

Output 1 shows the links to 25000 (diabetes mellitus without mention of complication). It indicates that the most prominent connections to

diabetes are cardiovascular diseases such as 4019 (Unspecified Essential hypertension), 2720 (Pure hypercholesterolemia), 2724 (Other and unspecified hyperlipidemia). It also demonstrates that 41041 (Of the native coronary artery, one kind of heart disease) has a strong connection to diabetes. Output 2 shows the links to 25040 (Diabetes with renal manifestations). It indicates that the larger links are to kidney diseases such as 58381 (Nephritis and nephropathy), 40391 (Unspecified Hypertensive chronic kidney disease) and 585 (Chronic kidney disease). The Display in Output 3 shows that 36201 (Background diabetic retinopathy, one kind of eye disease) has the highest association with 25050 (Diabetes with ophthalmic manifestations). The other, larger links to 25050 are 25040, 25060, 3572 (Polyneuropathy in diabetes) as well as 4039 (Unspecified Hypertensive chronic kidney disease).

Output 4 shows that the most prominent connection to 25060 (Diabetes with neurologi-

Figure 14. Linkages of organ diseases to diabetes

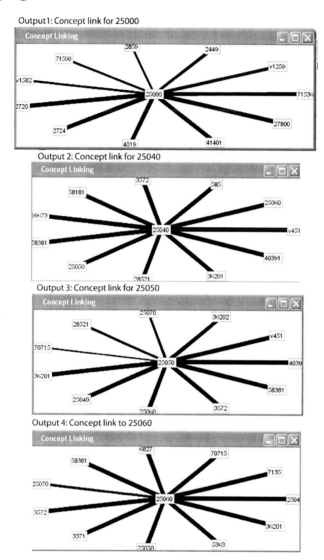

cal manifestations) is 3572. The other diseases closely related to 25060 are 3371 (Peripheral autonomic neuropathy in disorders classified elsewhere), 36201 (Background diabetic retinopathy), 25040 and 7135 (Arthropathy associated with neurological disorders). Translations are given in Table 27.

All the results in Figure 14 indicate that diabetes is related to many diseases such as Hypertension, blood diseases, Obesity and so on. Since we wanted to discuss organ diseases, we mainly focused on heart disease, kidney disease (including renal failure), ophthalmic disease and neurological disorders. We still needed to preprocess the data. We again used the CATX function to concentrate different diagnosis codes into one column; we used the RXMATCH statement to look for the initial code of '4280' that finds all inpatients with a diagnosis code related to heart disease. We used the same method for the other organ diseases. After that, we used IF, THEN statements to generate a new column.

Table 27. Translations for ICD9 diagnosis codes

2449	Unspecified hypothyroidism
27800	Unspecified Obesity
28521	Anemia in chronic kidney disease
2859	unspecified Anemia
36202	Proliferative diabetic retinopathy
5363	Gastroparesis
58181	Nephrotic syndrome in diseases classified elsewhere
6827	Other cellulitis and abscess:Foot(except toes)
70715	Ulcer of other part of foot
71536	Osteoarthrosis which not specified whether primary or secondary
71590	Osteoarthrosis which unspecified whether generalized or localized
99673	Due to renal dialysis device, implant, and graft
V1259	Other Diseases of circulatory system
V1582	History of tobacco use
V451	Renal dialysis status

Then, we used the kernel density estimation to show the costs by organ diseases. The results are displayed in Figure 15.

```
data sasuser.iporgan(keep=CLM_ID CLM_TOT_
CHRG_AMT CLM_DRG_CD diagnoses Hea Kid
Oculo Neu);
set sasuser.ipclaimdemo;
Hea=0;Kid=0;Oculo=0;Neu=0;
diagnoses=catx('',ICD9_DGNS_CD1,ICD9_
DGNS_CD2,ICD9_DGNS_CD3,ICD9_DGNS_
CD4,ICD9_DGNS_CD5,ICD9_DGNS_CD6,ICD9_
DGNS_CD7,ICD9_DGNS_CD8,ICD9_DGNS_CD9,
ICD9_DGNS_CD10,ICD9_DGNS_CD11,ICD9_DGNS_
CD12,ICD9_DGNS_CD13,ICD9_DGNS_CD14,ICD9_
DGNS_CD15,ICD9_DGNS_CD16);
if(rxmatch('4280',diagnoses)>0)then
Hea=1;
if(rxmatch('4254',diagnoses)>0)then
Hea=1;
if(rxmatch('42731',diagnoses)>0)then
Hea=1;
if(rxmatch('4240',diagnoses)>0)then
Hea=1;
if(rxmatch('4281',diagnoses)>0)then
```

```
Hea=1;
if(rxmatch('4282',diagnoses)>0)then
Hea=1;
if(rxmatch('4283',diagnoses)>0)then
Hea=1;
if(rxmatch('4284',diagnoses)>0)then
Hea=1;
if(rxmatch('4289',diagnoses)>0)then
Hea=1;
…

data sasuser.organfailure;set sasuser.
iporgan;if Hea=1 then Organ=1;if Kid=1
then Organ=2;if Oculo=1 then Organ=3;if
Neu=1 then Organ=4;run;
proc sort data=sasuser.ror-
gan out=sasuser.sortrorgan; by
rorgan;run;proc kde data=sasuser.
sortrorgan;univarclm_tot_chrg_amt/
gridl=0 gridu=60000 method=snr
out=sasuser.kdesrorgan;by rorgan; run;
```

The graphs in Figure 15 indicate that before the costs reach the value of 9,900 dollars, the cost with heart disease, the cost with ophthalmic diseases and the cost with neurological disorders

Figure 15. Total charges by different organ diseases

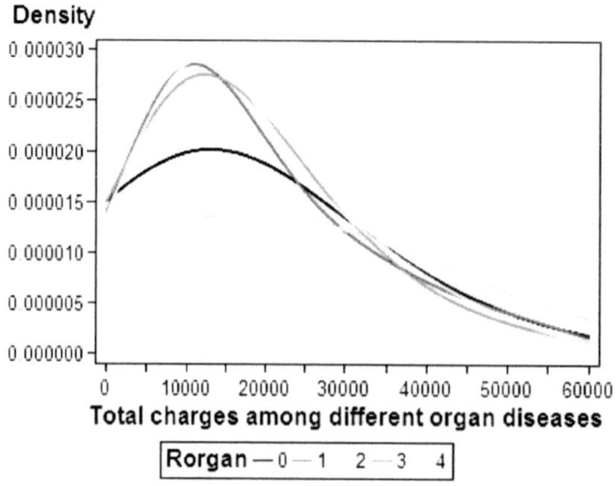

0: None of the organ diseases; 1:Heart diseases; 2:Kidney diseases; 3: ophthalmic diseases, 4: Neurological disorders

have almost the same probability, which is much higher than the cost without any of the organ diseases; and the probability for the cost with kidney disease is the smallest. However, after the cutpoint at 34,350 dollars, the density of the cost with kidney disease is higher than any other densities.

CURRENT AND FUTURE CHALLENGES FACING THE ORGANIZATION

After the study, the author can draw conclusions about the 15 diseases that have important relationships to the costs for the diabetic outpatients; among them, chronic kidney disease affects the charges most. Both heart disease and anemia are important to renal failure. The outcome of inpatients shows that many organ diseases and neurological disorders indeed have important effects on the costs of inpatients with diabetes: heart diseases, eye diseases and nervous system diseases all raise the inpatient costs. The results demonstrate that under a threshold amount of costs, kidney disease does not impact the expenditures of the inpatients as much as the other organ diseases do; however, as the costs increase, the effects of kidney disease

become more and more important. The results also show that that the expenditures of the Asians are much smaller than those on the other races when the costs are below 40,000 dollars; but after that, the Asians spend more than the others. Hence, to reduce the expenditures, the diabetic outpatients with renal failure should frequently monitor their heart disease and anemia; the Asians should take more care of their organ dysfunctions before the disease gets worse; all inpatients with diabetes should pay more attention to their kidney disease, and to avoid kidney disease. However, in the future, the following information is still needed for further study: to find the relationship between total charges and the deductibles, to see how the treatments of diabetes affect the costs, to see how the procedures impact the expenditures. and to see how such factors as the visit time, hospice care day and nursing facility day affect the costs.

REFERENCES

American Diabetes Association. (2008, March). Economic Costs of Diabetes in the U.S. in 2007. *DIABETES CARE, 31*(3).Retrieved Dec.10th, 2008, from http://care.diabetesjournals.org/misc/econcosts.pdf

American Diabetes Association. (n.d.). *Diabetes and Cardiovascular (Heart) Disease*.Retrieved Feb.5th, 2009, fromhttp://wwww.diabetes.org/ diabetes-statistics/heart-disease.jsp

Anonymous. (2006, June). *The GLIMMIX Procedure*. RetrievedNov.10th, 2008, from http://support. sas.com/rnd/app/papers/glimmix.pdf

Anonymous. (n.d.). *Cluster Analysis*. Retrieved Feb.20th, 2009, from http://www.statsoft.com/ textbook/stcluan.html

Centers for Disease Control and Prevention.(2007). *National Diabetes Fact Sheet, 2007.* Retrieved Nov.3rd, 2008, from http://www.cdc.gov/diabetes/ pubs/pdf/ndfs_2007.pdf

Cerrito, P. (2007) *Exploratory Data Analysis: An Introduction to Data Analysis Using SAS.* Retrieved from Lulu.com

Cerrito, P. (2008). *Student Papers in Introductory Statistics for Mathematics Majors*. Retrieved from Lulu.com

Cerrito, P. (2008). *Data Mining Healthcare and Clinical Database.* Hershey, PA: IGI Global.

Lavengood, K. A., & Kiser, P. (2007)Information Professionals in the Text Mine. *ONLINE, 31*(3)Retrieved Mar.3rd, 2009, from http://www.infotoday. com/online/may07/Lavengood_Kiser.shtml

National Institute of Diabetes and Digestive and Kidney Diseases. (2008). *National Diabetes Statistics, 2007.* Retrieved November 3rd, 2008, from http://diabetes.niddk.nih.gov/dm/pubs/statistics/

SAS Institute. (1999). *SAS/STAT User's Guide.* Cary, NC: SAS Publishing.

The Diabetes Control and Complications Trial/ Epidemiology of Diabetes Interventions and Complications (DCCT/EDIC) Study Research Group. (2005,December). Intensive Diabetes Treatment and Cardiovascular Disease in Patients with Type 1 Diabetes. *The New England Journal of Medicine, 353,* 2643-2653. Retrieved Dec.12th, 2008, from http://content.nejm.org/cgi/content/ full/353/25/2643

United States Renal Data System. (2007). *USRDS 2007 Annual Data Report.* Retrieved Dec.10th, 2008, from http://www.usrds.org/atlas_2007. htm

University of Iowa Health Science Relations. (2005, December). *Glucose Control Cuts Risk Of Heart Disease In Type 1 Diabetes.* Retrievedfrom http://www.news-releases.uiowa.edu/2005/ december/122205glucose_control.html

ADDITIONAL READING

American Diabetes Association. (2008, March) Economic Costs of Diabetes in the U.S. in 2007. *DIABETES CARE, 31*(3).Retrieved Dec.10th, 2008, from http://care.diabetesjournals.org/misc/ econcosts.pdf

Cerrito, P. (2007) Introduction to Data Mining Using SAS Enterprise Miner. Cary, NC: SAS publishing.

Kishore, P. (2008, June). *Diabetes Mellitus.* Retrievedfrom http://www.merck.com/mmhe/sec13/ ch165/ch165a.html

Mountford, W. K., Soule, J. B., Lackland, D. T., Lipsitz, S. R., Colwell, J. A., & Mountford, W. K. (2007). Diabetes-related lower extremity amputation rates fall significantly in South Carolina. *Southern Medical Journal, 100*(8), 787–790.

Nathan, D. M. (1993, June). Long-term complications of diabetes mellitus. *The New England Journal of Medicine, 328*(23). doi:10.1056/ NEJM199306103282306

Scanlon, D. P., Hollenbeak, C. S., Beich, J., Dyer, A. M., Gabbay, R. A., & Milstein, A. (2008). Financial and clinical impact of team-based treatment for medicaid enrollees with diabetes in a federally qualified health center. [Research Support, Non-U.S. Gov't]. *Diabetes Care, 31*(11), 2160–2165. doi:10.2337/dc08-0587

Slaughter, S. J., & Delwiche, L. D. (2006) The Little SAS Book for Enterprise Guide 4.1. Cary, NC: SAS publishing.

Chapter 9
An Example of Defining Patient Compliance

Christiana Petrou
University of Louisville, USA

ABSTRACT

This case examines the issue of compliance by patients at the University of Louisville School of Dentistry (ULSD). The focus is defining compliance and constructing a measurement scale. Confidence interval estimation and bootstrapping were explored to assist with the allocation of patients to compliance levels. Patients who were within the 95% confidence interval of the median for visit intervals at least 80% of the time were defined as fully compliant, with decreasing levels of compliance as the percentage decreases. Research on compliance has developed over the past few years, but a lot of work still needs to be done. A new measure of compliance could assist in understanding the patients' needs and concerns other than the obvious financial, fear and psychological reasons as well as shedding some light on the way dentists operate and how that affects compliance. A new way of defining and measuring compliance is proposed in this research study.

BACKGROUND

Formally, compliance is defined to be "either a state of being in accordance with established guidelines, specifications, or legislation, or the process of becoming so" (Data Management, 2005). In 1980, 30 practicing orthodontists were asked to list specific behaviors of patients (mostly adolescents) that they viewed as indicative of compliance or noncompliance. The result was a list of 10 patient behaviors that were frequently considered in evaluating patient cooperation:

1. arrives late and/or breaks appointments
2. has parents who are observed to be indifferent to treatment
3. acts withdrawn; shows no interest in treatment
4. has poor oral hygiene

DOI: 10.4018/978-1-61520-723-7.ch009

Copyright © 2010, IGI Global. Copying or distributing in print or electronic forms without written permission of IGI Global is prohibited.

5. if patient has braces and the wires are distorted or has loose bands
6. complaints about treatment procedure
7. fails to cooperate in the use of headgear and/or elastics
8. demonstrates behavior that is hostile or rude
9. speaks of family problems or poor relationship with family; and
10. complains about mouth pieces for restorative purposes (Robertson and Maddux, 1986)

Although the above list pertains primarily to orthodontic treatment, it captures the essentials for a patient to be compliant. In a general aspect, the major variables that associate with compliance are age, sex, family, personality, attitude and education.

To define compliance is challenging; to measure it is even more challenging. Placing an evaluation number on how compliant a patient is requires a deep analysis of behavioral factors and unbiased attitudes. The more traditional approach to measuring compliance has been, as described by Demetriou, Tsami-Pandi and Parashis (Demetriou et al., 1995), to classify patients into groups (mainly four). The first group consists of patients who fail to return for a treatment or annual/semiannual checkup, the second group consists of patients who were in complete compliance based upon attendance for more than 80% of the recommended appointments, the third group includes erratic attendees; that is, they presented themselves less than 80% of the time for appointments. The fourth group consists of patients who showed up at least once, but then discontinued attendance.

Several groups can be added, if necessary, to increase the thoroughness of a study; for example, groups can be refined to examine patients' compliance if they attended 60%, 40% and 20% of the scheduled appointments. Degree of compliance is estimated by adding the total number of appointments during the total time frame of a study and dividing by the number of scheduled

visits the patient should have attended over the time period (Demetriou et al., 1995). There are also some general definitions that can be utilized. For example, patients who missed less than 30% of all prescribed maintenance visits were classified as complete compliers. Another definition is patients who went less than 2 years without a maintenance visit who are classified as complete compliers (Miyahoto et al., 2006).

A measure of compliance has been developed through the use of several questionnaires that are answered by patients. For example, Albrecht and Hoogstraten, (Albrecht and Hoogstraten, 1998) measured compliance at the general level and the dental level. General complianc, that is, the general tendency to adhere to medical recommendations, was determined with the General Adherence Scale, which is a five item questionnaire. Compliance on the dental level was measured by a questionnaire on oral health behavior (Albrecht and Hoogstraten, 1998). Research studies have also used a measure of compliance by which the dentists rate the patients on a scale with typically 1 being a poor complier and 9 being a very good complier (Robertson and Maddux, 1986). This definition; however, this does not offer an objective definition since the compliance measure relies solely on the opinion of a dentist and not on behavioral data. This chapter will attempt to define a new definition of compliance that eliminates the factor of personal biasness.

SETTING THE STAGE

In most statistics studies, the central theme is to learn new information from the data. Data are generated daily in many fields such as healthcare and manufacturing, and they are in the form of numbers or text that can be useful in statistical analysis projects. What the statistician is interested in are the patterns, associations and relationships that exist within the data in order to make new statements regarding unknown facts and to provide further information to validate original assumptions. Vast amounts of data are available for exploration. The rate at which data are produced and stored is proportional to the technological advancement of today's society. "Since so many paper transactions are now in paperless digital form, lots of "big" data are available for further analysis" (Weis et.al., 2005).

The naked eye of a statistician might take a while to detect patterns in a data set, and in a world where time is money, it is not effective to spend days looking at data merely for pattern recognition. The answer to pattern detection is data mining. Generally, data mining (also referred to as knowledge-discovery in databases) is the process of analyzing data from different perspectives and summarizing it into useful information.

For this project, the use of SAS 9.1.3 and more specifically Base SAS was the vital tool that allowed for the compliance variable construction once the definition was established.

Confidence interval theory will be the central component in the definitions for patient compliance. One of the main themes in statistics is to make general statements about a population based on information that is extracted from a sample. We want to make inferences about parameters. Parameters are characteristics of the population. They are constants that appear in the probability function of a distribution. For example, the parameters of a normal distribution are μ, the population mean and σ, the population variance (Cugnet, 1997).

In most cases, the numerical value of a parameter cannot be determined because we cannot measure all units in the population. We have to estimate the parameter using sample information. A statistic is a characteristic of a sample that estimates a parameter. In order to estimate a parameter, a random sample from the population is taken and used to calculate a sample statistic that estimates the parameter. There are two procedures for parameter estimation: point estimation and interval estimation. Both procedures use an

estimator for the parameter estimate, where "an estimator is a rule that tells how to calculate the value of an estimate based on the measurements contained in a sample" (Upton and Cook, 2004). Point estimation uses the information in the sample to find a number that should be close to the true parameter value, while interval estimation uses the sample information to get two numbers that determine the range that contains the parameter of interest.

The measure of compliance will be defined on the data set provided by ULSD. The data set contains information such as demographics, treatment codes (ICD-9 codes), date of visit, as well as physician and clinic. The database contains well over 30,000 patient visits. With the use of SAS 9.1.3 software, data mining techniques will be used to analyze and define compliance.

The data are entered by treatment and identification codes; hence, the data from one visit and treatment must be linked to all other visits and treatments by patient. The definition for measure of compliance will be directly from the data. The patient habits and performance will indicate their level of compliance. There will be no need for any questionnaires to be answered by patients or dentists. The time interval between visits will be computed from visit dates. Median treatment intervals will be estimated from the data (median is used to avoid the influence of outliers). Then, patients who are within the 95% confidence interval of the median at least 80% of the time will be defined as fully compliant, with decreasing levels of compliance as the percentage decreases to 60%, 40%, 20% and 0%. The 80% cutoff for compliance has been used in the past, so it is a reasonable cutoff point.

The dental data contain the visit intervals as well as the median interval visit for each patient. The median was employed to avoid the undue influence of any outliers. An assumption had to be made in regards to visit intervals. Typically, patients on a maintenance regimen go to the dentist every 6 to 12 months. A patient, however, in active treatment can have a visit interval of 1 to 3 weeks. So, a patient exceeding a 12 month visit interval can be considered as an outlier. By employing the use of the median statistic, we eliminate the influence of outliers primarily because the median is a robust statistic. After ordering the median interval visits of individual patients, we note that the 50th percentile for the data set of visit intervals is 14; what we are interested in is the interval for the median in which the parameter exists. When the interval is obtained, then the visit intervals for the patients will be classified in levels of compliance based on how many visit intervals fall within the parameter interval.

The interval estimator is a rule that determines a method for using the sample data to calculate two numbers that result in the endpoints of the interval (Upton and Cook, 2004). The formal name for the interval estimator is confidence interval. The endpoints of the confidence interval will vary depending on the sample taken from the population since they are functions of the selected samples. When computing a confidence interval, certain criteria need to be satisfied. First and foremost, the interval should contain the parameter of interest and secondly, the interval should be as narrow as possible. The aim is to find an interval that is narrow enough but has a high probability of enclosing the parameter.

More formally, a $100(1-\alpha)\%$ confidence interval for an unknown population parameter, θ, is an interval between two numbers with an associated probability $(1-\alpha)$ that is generated from a random sample of an underlying population such that if the sampling were repeated numerous times, and the confidence interval recalculated from each sample according to the same method, a proportion $(1-\alpha)$ of the confidence intervals would contain the population parameter in question (Wickedly et al., 2002).

Definition 1: Let X_1, X_2, ..., X_n be a random sample of size n from a population X with density $f(x, \theta)$, where θ is an unknown parameter. The interval estimator of θ is called the $100(1-\alpha)\%$ confidence interval for θ if $P(L \leq \theta \leq U) = 1 - \alpha$ (Sahoo, 2002).

The random variable L is the lower confidence endpoint (or limit), and U is the upper confidence endpoint (or limit). The $(1-\alpha)$ value is called the confidence coefficient or degree of confidence. There are several methods for constructing a confidence interval. Some examples are Pivotal Quantity, Maximum Likelihood Estimator and Bootstrapping.

A pivotal quantity is a function of the data whose distribution does not depend on unknown parameters and, in effect, the confidence interval can be constructed from the distribution by solving for the parameter. The maximum likelihood estimator approach can be used for a population parameter by using its maximum likelihood estimator. By the asymptotic property of the maximum likelihood estimator, if the expected value of the estimator is subtracted from it and divided by the variance of the estimator, then the distribution of the estimator approaches a standard normal distribution. Using that fact, the confidence interval can be derived easily (Sahoo, 2002). Finally, the bootstrap procedure takes a nonparametric approach towards estimating a confidence interval.

Two of the above methods will be explored in more detail: the Pivotal Quantity and Bootstrapping. Originally, bootstrapping was employed in the attempt to compute the 95% median confidence interval. However, the bootstrapping procedure, outlined in the next section, is too intense for a computer to handle given the return on time required since vast amounts of data are generated by small computations. The final attempt was to use a more traditional approach with the pivotal quantity.

The Bootstrap Method

In statistics, we usually make a priori assumptions as to whether to choose a parametric or nonparametric statistical test. What is the difference between the two? Parametric inferential statistical methods are mathematical procedures for statistical hypothesis testing that follow the assumption that the variables included in the analysis come from a known family of probability distributions. For example, in order for the Student's t-test to be performed; that is, to check whether the means of two populations are equal, the assumption that the data are normally distributed is necessary.

Nonparametric statistics, also known as distribution-free statistics, make no underlying assumptions about the data. Non-parametric statistics, unlike parametric statistics, do not assign a distribution to the variables used in a hypothesis testing model. Making assumptions about the data can be cumbersome. What happens when the distribution of data tends to be skewed, and the assumption of normality is not appropriate? Sometimes, depending on the statistic that is estimated, there is a nonparametric test available with a corresponding counterpart to a parametric test. For example, the Wilcoxon Signed Rank test can be used for the paired t-test. This availability could lead to a conclusion that we can just use nonparametric tests and avoid the decisions about the assumptions on the distributions of the variables in a study. It is not that simple since one of the biggest disadvantages of nonparametric statistics over parametric statistics is that they do not have as much information to use in order to determine the significance of a statistic; so in that sense, they are less powerful.

Even though nonparametric estimation has some disadvantages over parametric estimation, very recently, statisticians have worked with the technique of "re-sampling". Re-sampling is the construction of a sampling distribution by repeatedly sampling, with replacement, from the actual sample of data. Therefore, re-sampling allows one to approximate the distribution of a statistic by using only the active data set in use. This revolutionary method is simple to understand, but "very computationally intensive, so it is only with the

age of modern computers that it has been a viable technique" (Barker, 2005). Some commonly used methods of re-sampling are the bootstrap and the jackknife.

"Bootstrapping is a statistical method for estimating the sampling distribution of an estimator by sampling with replacement from the original sample" One of the first statisticians to consider bootstrapping was Bradley Efron. "The bootstrap was introduced in 1979 as a computer based method for estimating the standard error of θ" (Efron and Tibshirani, 1998), where θ is an estimate of a parameter of interest. The main theme of the bootstrap method is to use "the data collected for a single experiment to stimulate what the results might be if the experiment was repeated over and over with a new sample" (Miller, 2004). The new experiments are called bootstrap samples and they are obtained from the original dataset through the procedure of resampling. The sampling distribution is the probability distribution generated by the resampling of a population for a given statistic. If θ is a parameter of a probability distribution from some population, then θ was estimated by means of an estimator $\hat{\theta}$ using a sample drawn from the population. The sampling distribution of an estimate $\hat{\theta}$ for θ "can be thought of as the relative frequency of all possible values of $\hat{\theta}$ calculated from an infinite number of random samples of size n drawn from the population" (Cugnet, 1997).

When Efron initiated the bootstrap procedure, the underlying goal was to randomly draw a large number of observations, or "re-samples" from the population. Each re-sample will have the same number of elements, and due to the replacement that takes place, some elements may be included one time, more than once, or not at all. Hence, each one of these samples will vary in the observations included in it. For each re-sample, the statistic $\hat{\theta}_i$ will be calculated, where i refers to the number of the sample. Due to the slight differences from sample to sample, each $\hat{\theta}_i$ will have a slightly different value.

The central assertion of the bootstrap method is that the relative frequency distribution of the $\hat{\theta}$'s is an estimate of the sampling distribution of $\hat{\theta}$ (Cugnet, 1997). The origin of the bootstrap procedure is merely the conceptual notion that the empirical distribution estimates the population distribution. Having a random sample of size n from a probability distribution f, the empirical distribution is defined to be the discrete distribution that

puts probability $\dfrac{1}{n}$ on each value of the sample. So, if a random sample of size n approaches the population size, then the empirical distribution approaches the population distribution. If the sample increases in size, then it contains more and more information about the population until it reaches the population size. Also, if the sample is large enough, then as the number of re-samples increases to infinity, the sampling distribution approaches the distribution of θ.

The outline of the bootstrap estimate can be illustrated through the description of the bootstrap estimate of the standard error, since after all, that was what initiated the study on bootstrapping. According to Efron & Tibshirani (Efron and Tibshirani, 1998), we let $\hat{f}$ be the empirical distribution. A bootstrap sample is defined to be a random sample of size n from $\hat{f}$ such that $\mathbf{x}^{*} = (x^{*}_{1}, x^{*}_{2}, ..., x^{*}_{n})$, where $\mathbf{x}^{*}$ indicates that we are not referring to the actual data set $\mathbf{x}$ but to a re-sample from the population $\mathbf{x} = (x_{1}, x_{2}, ..., x_{n})$. For each bootstrap data set $\mathbf{x}^{*}$, there is a bootstrap replication of $\hat{\theta}$; that is, $\hat{\theta}^{*} = s(\mathbf{x}^{*})$.

To estimate the standard error, the standard deviation of a statistic, we use the plug-in estimate of the empirical distribution since the true population distribution is unknown,

$$\hat{se}_{B} = \left\{ \sum_{i=1}^{B} [\hat{\theta}^{*}(i) - \hat{\theta}^{*}(\cdot)]^{2} / (B-1) \right\}^{\frac{1}{2}}$$

where $\hat{\theta}^{*}(\cdot) = \sum_{b=1}^{B} \hat{\theta}^{*}(b) / B$ and B is the number of total bootstrap samples. The number of

samples, B, needed for the procedure should be large. In a data set with n observations, there are a total of n^{n} possible subsets of size n where the order matters, and this number grows exponentially. For re-sampling, one can assume that the order of the observations is irrelevant. Ideally, B should approach infinity, but realistically, can only be as large as n^{n}; hence, depending on the CPU capabilities, we settle for B being at least as large as 100.

"The bootstrap algorithm above works by drawing many independent bootstrap samples, evaluating the corresponding bootstrap replications, and estimating the standard error of $\hat{\theta}$ by the empirical standard deviation of the replications" (Efron and Tibshirani, 1998). To generate bootstrap samples in SAS, the following code is used:

```
data bootsamp;
do sampnum =1 to 10000;
do i = 1 to nobs;
x = round(ranuni(0)*nobs);
set dataset nobs=nobs point = x;
output;
end;
end;
stop;
run;
```

The number of bootstrap samples was set to 10,000. For this project, the goal was to compute the median for each sample, and the code for SAS was

```
proc means data=bootsamp noprint nway;
class sampnum;
var median;
output out=bootmedian median=median;
run;
```

Standard errors are needed for the computation of a confidence interval. For example, given an estimate $\hat{\theta}$ and an estimated standard error $\hat{se}$, the usual 95% confidence interval is

$\hat{\theta} \pm 1.96\ s\hat{e}$. This comes from the assumption that $Z = (\hat{\theta} - \theta)/s\hat{e} \sim N(0,1)$. The advantage of bootstrapping is that these assumptions can be avoided. There are several methods that employ bootstrapping and avoid any parametric assumption that results in confidence interval estimation. We will briefly mention three such methods: the percentile method, the bootstrapped t-method and the BCa method.

The percentile method is the simplest of all the methods for calculating bootstrap confidence intervals. The procedure will be outlined in reference to the estimation of a confidence interval for medians since this is the ultimate goal for this section. We generate B bootstrap samples, and for each, we compute the sample median, M_i for $i = 1, ..., B$. The values of the B median estimates represent the sampling distribution of the median. We then sort the sample medians from low to high. In SAS, the command is

```
proc sort data=bootsamp;
by median;
run;
```

Once the data are sorted, the relevant percentiles are estimated. For the 95% confidence interval, we simply select the bootstrap estimates that lie on the 2.5th percentile and the 97.5th percentile (Barker, 2005). In general, to estimate the (1-α) % confidence interval for the sorted data, the upper and lower cutoffs are the $\frac{\alpha}{2}$ and $1 - \frac{\alpha}{2}$ percentiles of the data set. The code to use in SAS is given as follows,

```
data sasuser.bootsamp;
do sampnum =1 to 100000;
do i = 1 to nobs;
x = round(ranuni(0)*nobs);
set sasuser.charges6 nobs=nobs point = x;
output;
```

```
end;
end;
stop;
run;
proc means data=sasuser.bootsamp noprint
nway;
class sampnum;
var median;
output out=sasuser.bootmedian
median=median;
run;
proc sort data=sasuser.bootmedian;
by median;
run;
data sasuser.ci_perc;
set sasuser.bootmedian end=eof;
retain conf_lo conf_hi;
if _n_=12500 then conf_lo=median;
if _n_=87500 then conf_hi=median;
if eof then output;
keep conf_lo conf_hi;
run;
```

For the dental data, the percentile method yielded a confidence interval of (14, 16).

The next method is the bootstrapped t-method that attempts to estimate the distribution of the statistic $Z = \left(\dfrac{\hat{\theta} - \theta}{s\hat{e}}\right)$ directly from the data. Once again, the generated bootstrap samples will be used to estimate the value of Z in the following way: compute $\hat{\theta}_i^*$, the estimate of $\hat{\theta}$ for the ith bootstrap sample and $s\hat{e}_i^*$, the standard error of $\hat{\theta}_i^*$ for the ith bootstrap sample. Then $Z_i^* = \left(\dfrac{\hat{\theta}_i^* - \theta}{s\hat{e}_i^*}\right)$ for $i = 1, ..., B$ where B is the number of bootstrap samples. All of the Z*'s will constitute the sampling distribution of Z.

Under ideal conditions, the sampling distribution of Z must be the Student's t-distribution [Howell, 2002]. The αth percentile of Z_i^* is estimated as the $\hat{t}^{(a)}$, the αth percentile of the t-distribution on n-1 degrees of freedom, such that $\#\dfrac{\left\{Z_i^* \le \hat{t}^{(a)}\right\}}{B} = a$. Then the confidence interval is

$(\hat{\theta} - \hat{t}(1-\alpha)s\hat{e}, \hat{\theta} - \hat{t}(\alpha)s\hat{e}\,)$ (Barker, 2005).

The problem with the bootstrap t-method is that it requires a great deal of intensive computation to calculate the standard error, since for each bootstrap sample, we need to perform resampling in order to estimate the standard error for each $\hat{\theta}_i^*$.

The BCa method is the best method for constructing confidence intervals using bootstrap samples compared to the previous two methods encountered. BCa stands for Bias-corrected and accelerated. Some knowledge regarding bias and jackknife is essential in understanding the method. Bias is said to measure the average accuracy of an estimator. Formally, Bias $(\hat{\theta}) = E(\hat{\theta})-\theta$. Ideally, the bias should be as small as possible because the smaller the magnitude of the bias, the better the estimator tends to be.

The BCa confidence interval endpoints, just like the percentile interval method, are calculated from percentiles of the bootstrap distribution. The percentiles used depend upon two values, the acceleration and the bias-correction, denoted by $\hat{\alpha}$ and $\hat{z}_0$ respectively. The confidence interval is of the form $(\hat{\theta}^{*(\alpha 1)}, \hat{\theta}^{*(\alpha 2)})$, where

$\alpha_1 = \Phi\left(\hat{z}_0 + \dfrac{\hat{z}_0 + z^{(\alpha)}}{1 - \hat{\alpha}(\hat{z}_0 + z^{(\alpha)})}\right)$

and

$\alpha_2 = \Phi\left(\hat{z}_0 + \dfrac{\hat{z}_0 + z^{(1-\alpha)}}{1 - \hat{\alpha}(\hat{z}_0 + z^{(1-\alpha)})}\right).$

Note that Φ is the standard normal distribution function and $z^{(\alpha)}$ is the 100 x α^{th} percentile point of the standard normal distribution (Efron and Tibshirani, 1998). To calculate the bias- correction, we first append the bootstrap samples to the original data set and find the proportion of samples that have a sample statistic less than the statistic calculated from the original data set.

For example, in the case of the dental data, the median was 14; we are looking for the samples that have a median less than 14. Hence, $\hat{\theta}$ is the original data statistic, $\hat{\theta}_i^*$ is the statistic calculated from the ith bootstrap sample, and B is the number of bootstrap samples with $\hat{z}_0 = \Phi^{-1}(\#\{\hat{\theta}_i^* \le \hat{\theta}\}/B)$, where $\Phi^{-1}(x)$ indicates the inverse function of a standard normal distribution. This procedure can be done very quickly using SAS in utilizing the following code:

```
data bootsamp;
do sampnum =1 to 10000;
do i = 1 to nobs;
x = round(ranuni(0)*nobs);
set dataset nobs=nobs point = x;
output;
end;
end;
stop;
run;
proc means data=bootsamp noprint nway;
class sampnum;
var median;
output out=bootmedian median=median;
run;
data bootdata;
set dataset (in=a) bootsamp;
if a then sampnum=0;
run;
data proportionless;
set bootmedian;
retain origmedian;
if sampnum=0 then origmedian=median;
```

```
if median lt origmedian then lessthan=1;
else lessthan=0;
retain nless 0;
if sampnum gt 0 then
nless=nless+lessthan;
if sampnum ne 0 then output proportion-
less;
run;
data bias;
set proportionless;
by sampnum;
if last.sampnum then do;
propless=nless/sampnum;
bias=probit(propless);
output bias;
end;
run;
```

The acceleration statistic $\hat{\alpha}$ represents the rate of change of the standard error of the estimate of the sample statistic with respect to the true value of the statistic (Efron and Tibshirani, 1998).

Efron and Tibshirani suggest calculating the acceleration using the jackknife procedure. The jackknife method bears a great deal of similarity with the bootstrap procedure in the notion of re-sampling and is actually what initiated the study on bootstrapping. The goal of the procedure is to estimate the bias and standard error of an estimate by focusing on the samples that leave out one observation at a time. So, ultimately, we are gathering information on how much each individual record influences the estimate. The statistic of a jackknife sample is denoted by $\hat{\theta}_{(i)}$, and the mean of n jackknife samples is denoted by $\hat{\theta}_{(\cdot)} = \sum_{i=1}^{n} \frac{\hat{\theta}_{(i)}}{n}$. The acceleration is calculated by the following equation:

$$\hat{\alpha} = \frac{\sum_{i=1}^{n} (\hat{\theta}_{(\cdot)} - \hat{\theta}_{(i)})^3}{6\{(\sum_{i=1}^{n} (\hat{\theta}_{(\cdot)} - \hat{\theta}_{(i)})^2\}^{\frac{3}{2}}}$$

The proof for the above formula is located in Efron (Efron and Tibshirani, 1998). Once again, the code for SAS programming is as follows:

```
data origjack;
set dataset end=eof;
obsnum=_n_;
if eof then call
symput('nobs',put(obsnum,2.));
run;
%macro jackdata;
data jackdata;
set %do i=1%to 307;
sasuser.origjack (in=in&i where=(obsnum
ne &i)) %end;;
%do i=1%to 307;
if in&i then repeat=&i;
%end;
run;
%mend;
%jackdata;
proc means data=work.jackdata noprint
nway;
class repeat obsnum;
var median;
output out=sasuser.jacksum median=median;
run;
proc sql noprint;
select median(median)
into:medianjack from sasuser.jacksum;
quit;
data jacksum1;
set sasuser.jacksum;
cubed=(&medianjack - median)**3;
squared=(&medianjack - median)**2;
run;
proc means data=jacksum1 noprint;
output out=jacksum2 sum(cubed)=sumcube
```

```
sum(squared)=sumsquar;
run;
data accel;
set jacksum2;
accel=sumcube/(6*(sumsquar**1.5));
keep accel;
run;
```

Having both the acceleration and the bias correction estimates, we can find the values for α_1 and α_2. The final step is to order the random variable of interest and compute the value $N_1 = \alpha_1*B$ as well as $N_2 = \alpha_2*B$. The N_1^{st} order value of the random variable will be the lower endpoint of the confidence interval while the N_2^{nd} order value will be the upper endpoint of the confidence interval. The SAS code to use is

```
data ciends;
part1=(2.17 +probit(0.125))/
(1-(-0.000071647*(2.17+probit(0.125)))));
part2=(2.17 +probit(0.875))/
(1-(-0.000071647*(2.17+probit(0.875)))));
alpha1=probnorm(2.17+part1);
alpha2=probnorm(2.17+part2);
n1=alpha1*1000;
n2=alpha2*1000;
call symput ('n1',put(floor(n1),5.));
call symput ('n2',put(floor(n2),5.));
run;
proc sort data=sasuser.bootmed;
by median;
run;
data ci_bca;
set sasuser.bootmed end=eof;
retain conf_lo conf_hi;
if _n_=&n1 then conf_lo=median;
if _n_=&n2 then conf_hi=median;
if eof then output;
keep conf_lo conf_hi;
run;
```

When this procedure was performed for the Dental data, the confidence interval derived was (14, 14). The reason for this outcome is primarily due to the statistic of interest within the dental data. The median is not a "smooth" statistic. A smooth function is one that is continuous and has its first derivative continuous. The median function is continuous in definition, but the rate of change is not continuous, being zero over an interval of the real number line, then some constant over a subsequent interval followed by zero again. "The lack of smoothness causes the jackknife estimate of standard error to be inconsistent for the median" (Efron and Tibshirani, 1998).

There is a way to fix this inconsistency. Instead of leaving one observation at a time, we can leave out two or three, or even more observations. The procedure is known as the deleted-d jackknife (Efron and Tibshirani, 1998). The rule of thumb, according to Efron and Tibshirani, is to leave out d observations at a time, where $d = \sqrt{n}$ and n is the total number of observations in a data set. This rule is applied merely to achieve consistency for the jackknife estimate of standard error. With all the computer capabilities that we have, this can still be quite a challenging task, since the more data values deleted, the more the resulting table of appended jackknife samples grows exponentially.

For example, the dental data set consisted of 307 observations. Deleting one observation at a time resulted in a jackknife sample of 306, repeated 307 times, and the resulting merged tables for the jackknife data set had 93,942 records. In the case of deleting two observations, each sample had 305 records, and there were 46,971 possible combinations for deleting 2 values at a time. The result was a data set with 4,398,129,585 records! Once that was done, the confidence interval was still (14, 14). It gets worse with deleting three observations, which was too much for the computer to handle.

The bootstrap confidence interval methodology, in theory, relieves a statistician from making any parametric assumption and is conceptually straightforward to understand. However, in view of the fact that vast amounts of data are generated from the procedure, which inevitably is challenging for the CPU to manage with no significant change occurring in the confidence interval, a more traditional approach was utilized involving pivotal quantities for this work.

Pivotal Quantity

The pivotal quantity method is a very well known approach towards constructing confidence intervals. The main goal is to define a function of the sample and the unknown parameter, where the unknown parameter is the only one in the function, and the probability distribution function does not depend on the unknown parameter (Upton and Cook, 2004). The logic behind this method is that for a random variable X, the probability $P(a \leq X \leq b)$ is unaffected by a change of scale or translation on X. Therefore, if we know the probability distribution of a pivotal quantity, we may be able to use operations such as scaling and translation to create an interval estimator.

Definition 2: A random variable $Q(\mathbf{X}, \theta) = Q(X_1, X_2, ..., X_n, \theta)$ is a pivotal quantity (or pivot) if the distribution of $Q(\mathbf{X}, \theta)$ is independent of all parameters. That is, if $\mathbf{X} \sim F(x|\theta)$, then $Q(\mathbf{X}, \theta)$ has the same distribution for all values of θ (Sahoo, 2002)

There is no general rule for finding a pivotal quantity for a parameter. The work of finding one is ad hoc and relies mainly on guesswork. There is, however, a systematic way to find pivots if the probability density function belongs to the location scale family.

Definition 3: Let $g: \mathfrak{R} \rightarrow \mathfrak{R}$ be a probability density function. Then, for any μ and any $\sigma > 0$, the family of functions, $F = \left\{ f(x; \mu, \sigma) = \dfrac{1}{\sigma} g\left(\dfrac{x - \mu}{\sigma}\right) \mid \mu \in (-\infty, \infty), \sigma \in (0, \infty) \right\}$ is called the location scale family with standard probability density $f(x, \theta)$. The parameter μ is called the location parameter

and the parameter σ is called the scale parameter. If $\sigma = 1$, then F is called the location family. If $\mu = 0$, then F is called the scale family (Sahoo, 2002).

The widest known probability density function that belongs to the location scale family is the normal distribution. If we can identify a distribution that belongs to a location scale family, then the guesswork is minimized. In general, differences are pivotal for location problems while ratios or products are pivotal for scale problems (Sahoo, 2002). To construct the confidence interval, we proceed as follows:

1. Let $X_1, X_2, ..., X_n$ be a random sample from the population X with probability density function (pdf), $f(x; \theta)$, where θ is an unknown parameter.
2. Consider the pdf to see if a pivot exists and determine the pivotal quantity $Q(X, \theta)$.
3. For a specific value of α, we can find numbers a and b that do not depend on θ, to satisfy $P(a \leq Q(X, \theta) \leq b) \geq 1 - \alpha$.
4. Algebraically manipulate the inequalities to isolate θ in the middle,

$P(L \leq \theta \leq U) = 1 - \alpha$ where $L = L(X_1, X_2, ..., X_n)$ and $U = U(X_1, X_2, ..., X_n)$.

Then the limits of the form (L, U) are a subinterval of the real line, $\mathfrak{R}$. Therefore, we conclude that if we take a "large number of samples from the underlying population and construct all the corresponding $(1 - \alpha)$% confidence intervals, then approximately $(1 - \alpha)$% of these intervals would include the unknown value of the parameter θ (Sahoo, 2002). To illustrate the above theory, let $\hat{\theta}$ be a statistic that is normally distributed with mean θ and standard error $\sigma_{\hat{\theta}}$. Then we want to find a confidence interval for $\hat{\theta}$ that possesses a confidence coefficient equal to $1 - \alpha$.

The quantity $Z = (\hat{\theta} - \theta)/\sigma_{\hat{\theta}} \sim N(0, 1)$. We select two values from the tails of the normal distribu-

Figure 1. Two tails of the normal distribution with probability α

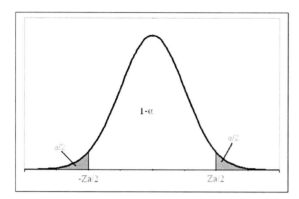

tion, namely -$z\dfrac{\alpha}{2}$ and $z\dfrac{\alpha}{2}$ such that

$$P(-z_{\frac{\alpha}{2}} \leq Z \leq z_{\frac{\alpha}{2}}) = 1-\alpha.$$

Figure 1 displays the graph of a normal curve, and indicates the proportion of the graph for which

-$z\dfrac{\alpha}{2}$ and $z\dfrac{\alpha}{2}$ can be possible estimates.

Substitute for Z in the probability statement to get

$$P(-z\frac{\alpha}{2} \leq (\hat{\theta}-\theta)/\sigma_{\hat{\theta}} \leq z\frac{\alpha}{2}) = 1-\alpha.$$

Multiplying by $\sigma_{\hat{\theta}}$ to get

$$P(-z\sigma_{\hat{\theta}\frac{\alpha}{2}} \leq \hat{\theta}-\theta \leq z_{\frac{\alpha}{2}}\sigma_{\hat{\theta}}) = 1-\alpha.$$

Subtracting $\hat{\theta}$ from both terms of the inequality to obtain

$$P(-\hat{\theta} - z_{\frac{\alpha}{2}}\sigma_{\hat{\theta}} \leq -\theta \leq -\hat{\theta} + z_{\frac{\alpha}{2}}\sigma_{\hat{\theta}}) = 1-\alpha.$$

Finally, multiplying each term by -1 and changing the directions of the inequalities, we have

$$P(\hat{\theta} - z_{\frac{\alpha}{2}}\sigma_{\hat{\theta}} \leq \theta \leq \hat{\theta} + z_{\frac{\alpha}{2}}\sigma_{\hat{\theta}}) = 1-\alpha.$$

Hence, the confidence endpoints for a (1-α)% confidence interval for θ are

$$L = \hat{\theta} - z_{\frac{\alpha}{2}}\sigma_{\hat{\theta}} \text{ and } U = \hat{\theta} + z_{\frac{\alpha}{2}}\sigma_{\hat{\theta}} \text{ (Upton and}$$

Cook, 2004).

Now, this theory can be applied to construct the confidence interval for the median. First, we state the following theorem.

Theorem 1. For a random sample of size n from an infinite population having values x and density function f(x), the probability density of the rth order statistic Y_r is given by

$$g_r(y_r) = \frac{n!}{(r-1)!(n-r)!}\left(\int_{-\infty}^{y_r} f(x)dx\right)^{r-1} f(y_r)$$

$$\left(\int_{y_r}^{\infty} f(x)dx\right)^{n-r} \text{ (Gasella and Berger, 2002).}$$

A detailed proof for this theorem can be found in the paper by Merberg and Miller "*The Sampling Distribution of the Median*". From the above theorem, we can proceed to the Median Theorem to determine the sampling distribution of the median. The proof of the Median Theorem will be outlined below, but an interested reader can refer to Merberg and Miller (Merberg and Miller, 2006) for detailed work.

Median Theorem. Let a sample of size n=2m+1, with n large, be taken from a density function f ($\tilde{x}$) that is nonzero at the population median $\tilde{\mu}$ and continuously differentiable in a neighborhood of $\tilde{\mu}$. The sampling distribution of the median is approximately normal with mean $\tilde{\mu}$ and variance

$$\frac{1}{8f\left(\tilde{\mu}\right)m}$$ (Merberg and Miller, 2006).

Proof. For a random sample of size *n* from an infinite population having values *x* and density

$f(x)$, the probability density of the rth order statistic Y_r as stated in the previous theorem is given by

$$g_r(y_r) = \frac{n!}{(r-1)!(n-r)!} \left[\int_{-\infty}^{y_r} f(x)dx \right]^{r-1} f(y_r) \left[\int_{y_r}^{\infty} f(x)dx \right]^{n-r}$$

We will let the median random variable $\tilde{X}$ have a value of $\tilde{x}$ and density $g(\tilde{x})$ and denote the population median by $\tilde{\mu}$. If F is the cumulative distribution function of f then $F'=f$ and by definition the population median satisfies $\int_{-\infty}^{\tilde{\mu}} f(x)dx = \frac{1}{2}$, which becomes $F(\tilde{\mu}) = \frac{1}{2}$. Since the sample is of size $2m+1$, the median is the $(m+1)^{th}$ order statistic. Therefore, its distribution is

$$g(\tilde{x}) = \frac{(2m+1)!}{m!\,m!} \left[\int_{-\infty}^{\tilde{x}} f(\tilde{x})dx \right]^{m} f(\tilde{x}) \left[\int_{\tilde{x}}^{\infty} f(\tilde{x})dx \right]^{m}$$

The first step is to find an approximation of the constant term in the equation above. This is accomplished by employing Stirling's approximation where we conclude that $n! = n^n e^{-n} \sqrt{2\pi n}(1 + O(n^{-1}))$. The big-O notation is used primarily to characterize the residual term of a truncated infinite series. That is when $A(x)=O(B(x))$. It is interpreted that there is a $C>0$ and an x_0 such that for all $x \geq x_0$, $|A(x)| \leq CB(x)$. Sufficiently large values will be considered so that the terms of order $\frac{1}{n}$ can be ignored. Hence

$$\frac{(2m+1)!}{m!\,m!} = \frac{(2m+1)(2m)!}{(m!)^2} \approx$$

$$\frac{(2m+1)(2m)^{2m}e^{-2m}\sqrt{2\pi(2m)}}{(m^m e^{-m}\sqrt{2\pi m})^2} = \frac{(2m+1)4^m}{\sqrt{\pi m}}.$$

Since F is the cumulative distribution function, then $F(\tilde{x}) = \int_{-\infty}^{\tilde{x}} f(x)dx$; this implies that

$$g(\tilde{x}) \approx \frac{(2m+1)4^m}{\sqrt{\pi m}} \left[F(\tilde{x}) \right]^{m} f(\tilde{x}) \left[1 - F(\tilde{x}) \right]^{m.}$$

The Taylor series expansion will be incorporated for $F(\tilde{x})$ about $\tilde{\mu}$ in the following manner

$$F(\tilde{x}) = F(\tilde{\mu}) + F'(\tilde{\mu})(\tilde{x}-\tilde{\mu}) + O((\tilde{x}-\tilde{\mu})^2).$$

Since $\tilde{\mu}$ is the population median as stated earlier, $F(\tilde{\mu}) = \frac{1}{2}$ and the above equation becomes $F(\tilde{x}) = \frac{1}{2} + f(\tilde{\mu})(\tilde{x}-\tilde{\mu}) + O((\tilde{x}-\tilde{\mu})^2)$. We need $\lim_{n\to\infty} |\tilde{x}-\tilde{\mu}| = 0$ to make $F(\tilde{x})$ a useful approximation. This result will be stated in this work, but its proof can be found in the paper by Merberg and Miller. We let $t = \tilde{x}-\tilde{\mu}$, which is small and tending to 0 as $m\to\infty$. Substituting into the Taylor series expansion of $g(\tilde{x})$, we get

$$g(\tilde{x}) \approx \frac{(2m+1)4^m}{\sqrt{\pi m}} \left[\frac{1}{2} + f(\tilde{\mu})t + O(t^2) \right]^m$$

$$f(x) \left[1 - \left(\frac{1}{2} + f(\tilde{\mu})t + O(t^2) \right) \right]^m.$$

Rearranging and combining factors, we get

$$g(\tilde{x}) \approx \frac{(2m+1)4^m}{\sqrt{\pi m}} f(\tilde{x}) \left[\frac{1}{4} - (f(\tilde{\mu})t)^2 + O(t^3) \right]^m$$

$$= \frac{(2m+1)f(\tilde{x})}{\sqrt{\pi m}} \left[1 - \frac{4m(f(\tilde{\mu})t)^2}{m} + O(t^3) \right]^m.$$

Recall that $e^x = \exp(x) = \lim_{n\to\infty} \left(1 - \frac{x}{n} \right)^n$. Using this fact and ignoring higher powers of t, we get that for large m,

$$g(\tilde{x}) \approx \frac{(2m+1)f(\tilde{x})}{\sqrt{\pi m}} \exp\left(-4m f(\tilde{\mu})^2 t^2 \right)$$

$$\approx \frac{(2m+1)f(\tilde{x})}{\sqrt{\pi m}} \exp\left(-\frac{\tilde{x}-\tilde{\mu}}{\frac{1}{4m f(\tilde{\mu})^2}} \right).$$

Since $\tilde{x}$ can be assumed to be arbitrarily close to $\tilde{\mu}$, then we can also assume that $f(\tilde{x}) \approx f(\tilde{\mu})$ such that

$$g(\tilde{x}) \approx \frac{(2m+1)f(\tilde{\mu})}{\sqrt{\pi m}} \exp\left(- \frac{\tilde{x} - \tilde{\mu}}{\frac{1}{4mf(\tilde{\mu})^2}}\right),$$

observing the exponential part of the expression that appears to be a normal density with mean $\tilde{\mu}$ and $\sigma^2 = \dfrac{1}{8mf(\tilde{\mu})^2}$.

CASE DESCRIPTION

At this point, we can use pivotal quantities to construct the confidence interval for the population median. We will assume that the population variance is unknown. Let $X_1, X_2 \ldots X_n$ be a random sample from a population whose probability density function is continuous and unimodal. First of all, we need a pivotal quantity $Q(X_1, X_2 \ldots X_n, \tilde{\mu})$ where $\tilde{\mu}$ is the population median. By the Median Theorem, we get that the distribution of the sample median is given by $X\tilde{m} \sim N\left(\tilde{\mu}, \dfrac{1}{8f(\tilde{\mu})m}\right)$. Because the population distribution equation is unknown, we will employ the Maritz-Jarrett method to find the variance.

Maritz and Jarrett (1978) derived an estimate of the standard error (standard deviation) of the sample median, which in theory can be extended to the more general case involving x_q (Wilcox, 2005). For any q, $0 < q < 1$, x_q refers to the qth quantile. For a continuous random variable X, x_q is defined by $P(X \le x_q) = q$ and $x_q = X_{(m)}$; the mth observation after the data are placed in ascending order. The median $x_{0.5}$ is also known as the 50th percentile. The Maritz-Jarrett method for estimating the standard error of an order statistic is based on the fact that $E(x_q)$ and $E(x_q^2)$ can be related to a beta distribution.

The pdf of a beta distribution is $f(x) = \dfrac{(a+b+1)!}{a!b!} x^a(1-x)^b$ where a and b are positive

integers and $0 \le x \le 1$. (Sahoo, 2002). The outline of the method is as follows:

1. Sort the X in ascending order.
2. Let $m = [q*n + 0.5]$ (i.e., round down to the nearest integer).
3. $A = m - 1$
4. $B = n - m$
5. $W_i = $ BETCDF($i/n,A,B$) - BETCDF($(i-1)/n,A,B$) where BETCDF is the beta cumulative distribution function with shape parameters A and B.
6. $C_k = \sum_{i=1}^{n} W_i X_i^k$
7. $MJ = \sqrt{C_2 - C_1^2}$ [DataplotNationalInstitute of Standards and Technology](Statistical Engineering Divisian; Dataplot National Institute of Standards and Technology)

The University of Louisville Dental Clinic advertises the following services in addition to offering emergency care: cosmetic bleaching, on site lab, crowns and bridges, periodontal services, dentures and partials, relines, implant dentistry and repairs. Therefore, ULSD has a rich database containing information on a wide variety of treatments and care options. The data are entered by treatment and identification codes; hence, the data from one visit and treatment must be linked to all other visits and treatments by patient identifier code. The data set contains information such as demographics, treatment code (ICD-9 code), date of visit, as well as physician and clinic for over 30,000 patient visits. As a result, there are a total of 320 distinct patients with their corresponding visit intervals and median visit intervals derived. A total of 307 out of 320 patients have a nonzero entry as their median visit. Those patients were selected as a sample to determine the Maritz-Jarrett estimate of standard error. This procedure was performed using SAS 9.1 and the code used is

```
data sasuser.mj1;
set sasuser.charges7;
%let i=obsnum;
y=cdf('BETA',(&i/307),153,154)-
cdf('BETA',((&i-1)/307),153,154);
run;
quit;
data sasuser.mj2;
set sasuser.mj1;
c1=y*median;
c2=y*(median**2);
run;
```

Once the code runs successfully, we get that the standard error (or standard deviation) of the sample median is equal to 1.023878934. Hence, the sampling distribution of the median for this study is approximately normal with mean $\tilde{\mu}=14$ and variance 1.048328071.

If we standardized $X_{0.5}$, then we get $\dfrac{X_{\tilde{m}} - \tilde{\mu}}{\sigma_{MJ}} \sim$ N (0, 1). The distribution of the standardized $X_{0.5}$ is independent of $\tilde{\mu}$. The standardized $X_{0.5}$ is the pivotal quantity since it is a function of the population median $\tilde{\mu}$ and its probability distribution is independent of $\tilde{\mu}$. Using the pivotal quantity, we construct the confidence interval the same way we did earlier:

$$1 - \alpha = P(z_{\frac{\alpha}{2}} \leq \frac{X_{\tilde{m}} - \tilde{\mu}}{\sigma_{MJ}} \leq z_{\frac{\alpha}{2}})$$

$$1 - \alpha = P(X_{\tilde{m}} - \sigma_{MJ} z_{\frac{\alpha}{2}} \leq \tilde{\mu} \leq X_{\tilde{m}} + \sigma_{MJ} z_{\frac{\alpha}{2}})$$

Hence, the (1-α)% confidence interval for $\tilde{\mu}$ is

$$(X_{\tilde{m}} - \sigma_{MJ} z_{\frac{\alpha}{2}}, X_{\tilde{m}} + \sigma_{MJ} z_{\frac{\alpha}{2}})$$

Therefore, the confidence interval for the sample that consists of all nonzero visit intervals for the dental school turned out to be (11.99, 16.007).

The patients were then classified into the different compliance level groups. Some work was done in Excel in regards to finding out how many visits each patient had that were within the confidence interval endpoints, and from that, the percentage was estimated. Then in SAS 9.1, the following SAS code was used to classify the patients in compliance levels:

```
data sasuser.dependentvar;
set sasuser.compliance;
by compliance;
if compliance lt 20 then level=5;
if compliance ge 20 lt 40 then level=4;
if compliance ge 40 lt 60 then level=3;
if compliance ge 60 lt 80 then level=2;
if compliance ge 80 lt 100 then level=1;
run;
```

Hence, a patient that had less than 20% of their visit intervals within the confidence interval was classified in the lowest compliance group. A patient that had more than 80% of their visit intervals in the confidence interval was classified in the compliance level group 1, which means that they are more likely to continue attending the Dental School and are fully compliant. Table 1 describes the allocation of patients in the different Compliance levels based on approximately 30,000 visits in the data set.

It is evident that the majority of the patients that attend the Dental School are not compliant.

Table 1. Frequency counts for compliance levels

Compliance Level	Frequency	Percentage
1	0	0
2	1	0.31
3	14	4.38
4	43	13.44
5	262	81.88

A severity variable was also derived by performing text mining on the dental codes, ICD-9. The most obvious relation that emerged from the interaction of severity and compliance is that all the patients who are listed in the least severe cluster belong in the least compliant level group. In general, there is a pattern of patients being moderately compliant (20%) across all severity groups. Patients who are classified in the second to last group in terms of severity indicate a higher percentage of compliance than any other severity group. The pattern seems to be that the most severe patients tend to be the least compliant ones.

The relationship of compliance to severity will be explored to gain a better understanding of what type of patients attend the Dental school more often. The relationship between the levels of compliance and severity is illustrated in Table 2 through a table analysis.

The most obvious relation that emerges from the above table is that all the patients who are listed in the least severe cluster belong in the least compliant level group. In general, there is a pattern of patients who are compliant at most 20% of the time in all severity groups. Patients who are classified in the second to last group in terms of severity indicate a higher percentage of compliance than any other severity group; to be specific, they are complaint on an interval at least 20% of the time and at most 40%. Similarly, patients in the 3rd severity group tend to belong in the compliance level group of attending their

regular visits at least 40% and at most 60% of the time. For the highest levels of compliance, there is at most 1 patient belonging to both groups, which does not convey enough information. A visual interpretation of Table 2 is given in Figure 2 with the bivariate kernel density estimation of the severity level by compliance level.

Computing the kernel density plot of the compliance levels by the severity levels, Figure 3 is obtained.

The different compliance levels are compared based upon the severity ranking of the ICD-9 codes that were recorded at the Dental School. Patients belonging in compliance level 3 have the lowest probability of belonging in the two most severe clusters, unlike compliance levels 4 and 5. In fact, patients have the highest probability of being least compliant when they suffer from conditions that are the most severe. However, patients in the 3rd level of compliance have the highest probability of belonging in the 3rd cluster in terms of severity. Patients in the 4th compliance level group have the higher probability when being in the second to last severity cluster while patients in compliance level 5 have a higher probability of being in the least severe cluster.

Variables that could affect compliance level are also age and socioeconomic status. The age of each patient was computed up until the year 2005 (which was when the data became available), and the median household income was also imported into the data set by means of the Tapestry files.

Table 2. Table analysis of compliance by severity indicating frequency and column percentage

Severity(→) Compliance(↓)	1	2	3	4	5	Total
2	0 0.00	1 1.10	0 0.00	0 0.00	0 0.00	1
3	4 3.96	2 2.20	6 13.64	2 4.00	0 0.00	14
4	17 16.83	13 14.29	3 6.82	10 20.00	0 0.00	43
5	80 79.21	75 82.42	35 79.55	38 76.00	34 100.00	262
Total	101	91	44	50	34	320

The tapestry segmentation is provided by ESRI (Environmental Systems Research Institute) and classifies U.S. neighborhoods into 65 segments based on their socioeconomic and demographic composition. The dental school patients were classified into median household income groups. The kernel density distribution of compliance was estimated depending on age and median household income. The results are provided in figures 4-7.

It seems that patients who are between 55 and 65 years old have a higher probability of being in the higher compliance group out of the three. Furthermore, patients between the ages of 20 to 30 and 75 to 85 have a higher probability of belonging in compliance level 5, the least compliant. While for compliance level 4, the most probable patients are those of age 35 to 45 and 85 and over.

For the median household income kernel density plot, patients who make under $20,000 seems to have a higher probability of being in the most compliant group; however, the probability density indicates an overlap of compliance levels 3 and

Figure 2. Bivariate kernel density

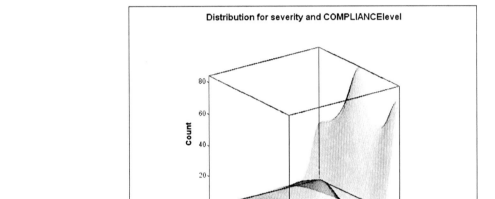

Figure 3. Kernel density estimation of compliance by severity

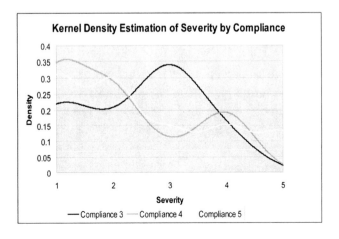

Figure 4. Kernel density estimation of compliance by age

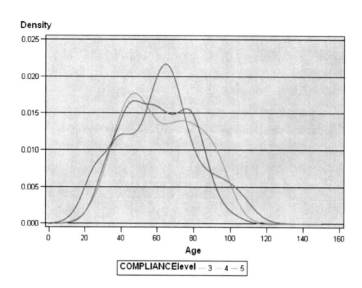

Figure 5. Kernel density estimation of compliance by income

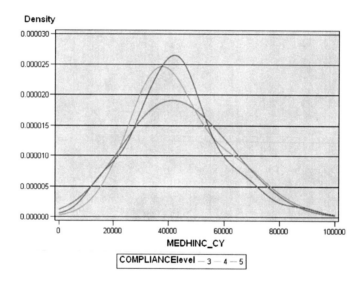

5, meaning that there is also a high probability of not being compliant as well. Therefore patients who make under $20,000 can go either way on compliance level. Patients who have a median household income between $20,000 and $38,000 have greater chances of belonging to compliance group 4. If the median household income of a patient is between $38,000 and $58,000, then there is a high probability of them being in the least compliant group. The most compliant patients of the three levels indicated a higher probability when they are in the income range of $58,000 to $63,000 while patients with any income above that amount exhibit a higher probability of belonging to the two least compliant groups.

The striking conclusions from the kernel density plot in Figure 7 is that patients who are between 18 to 30 are probably experiencing the

Figure 6. Kernel density estimation of severity by age

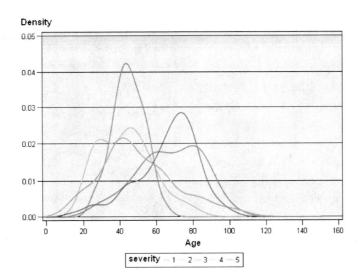

Figure 7. Kernel density estimation of severity by income

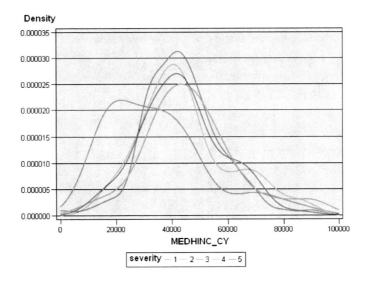

most severe cases, while patients between 30 to 60 years old have greater chances of being in the second most severe cluster of dental procedures needed. On the other hand, patients 60 and above have a higher probability of experiencing the least severe conditions.

Patients having median household income less than $30,000 have a higher probability of experiencing the most severe dental needs. Pa-tients with median household income between $30,000 and $55,000 are probably experiencing conditions that are borderline serious since they tend to belong into severity cluster 3. Higher income patients tend to have a higher probability of interchangeably being in the second and fourth most severe cluster.

CURRENT AND FUTURE CHALLENGES FACING THE ORGANIZATION

Bootstrapping is a method that simulates multiple data sets equivalent to the original. Even though in theory it is a nonparametric approach to the confidence interval estimation for the median; in practicality, however, it is unattainable unless a good CPU is available. If a CPU is not attainable, then we are handicapped in using a more traditional approach of interval estimation. The benchmark of this work was the ability to quantify compliance.

Compliance is a behavioral variable that depends on social and economic factors that vary greatly from person to person. This research attempted to consider earlier versions of compliance definitions and to improve them by developing an objective classification of patients in compliance levels based on the mathematical theory of confidence intervals. To define compliance is challenging; to measure it is even more challenging. Placing an evaluation number on how compliant a patient is requires deep analysis of behavioral factors and unbiased attitudes. In general, research on compliance has developed over the past few years, but a lot of work still needs to be done. A new measure of compliance could assist in understanding the patients' needs and concerns other than the obvious financial, fear and psychological reasons as well as shedding some light on the way dentists operate and how that affects compliance. The majority of the attempts in research done thus far, in defining compliance, introduce a form of bias that ranges from doctors' perceptions of their patients' compliance to the patients themselves ranking their compliance level through questionnaires. A new way of defining and measuring compliance was proposed in this chapter that offers a more objective quantifier.

REFERENCES

Barker, N. (2005). *A Practical Introduction to the Bootstrap Using the SAS System.* In Proceedings of SAS Conference, Oxford Pharmaceutical Science.

Cugnet, P. (1997). *Confidence Interval Estimation for Distribution Systems Power Consumption By using the Bootstrap Method.* Virginia Tech University.

Demetriou, N., Tsami-Pandi, A., & Parashis, A. (1995). Compliance with suportive periodontal treatment in private Periodonatal Practice. A 14 year retrospective study. *Journal of Periodontology*, *66*(2), 145–149.

Howell. (2002). *Bootstrapping Medians.* Burlington, VT: University of Vermont.

Merberg, A., & Miller, S. (2006). *The Sampling Distribution of the Median. Efron, B., & Tibshirani, R. J. (1998). An Introduction to the Bootstrap.* Boca Raton, FL: CRC Press LLC.

Miller, D. P. (n.d.). Bootstrap 101: Obtain Robust Confidence Intervals for Any Statistic. In *Proceedings of SUGI 29, Ovation Research Group* (pp.193-229).

Miyamoto, T., Kumagai, T., Jones, J. A., Van Dyke, T. E., & Nunn, M. E. (2006). Compliance as a Prognostic Indicator: Retrospective Study of 505 Patients Treated and Maintained for 15 Years. *Journal of Periodontology*, *77*(2), 223–232. doi:10.1902/jop.2006.040349

Robertson, S., & Maddux, J. (1986). Compliance in Pediatric Orthodontic Treatment: Current Research and Issues. *Children's Health Care*, *15*(1), 40–48. doi:10.1207/s15326888chc1501_7

Sahoo, P. (2002). *Probability and Mathematical Statistics.* Louisville, KY: Department of Mathematics, University of Louisville.

Upton, G., & Cook, I. (2004). *Dictionary of Statistics*. Oxford, UK: Oxford University Press.

Weis, S. M., Indurkhya, N., Zhang, T., & Damerau, F. J. (2005). *Text Mining: Predictive Methods for Analyzing Unstructured Information*. New York: Springer.

Wickedly, D. D., Mendenhall, W. III, & Scheaffer, R. L. (2002). *Mathematical Statistics with Applications.* Sixth Edition. Casella, G., & Berger, R. (2002). *Statistical Inference.* Second Edition. Albrecht, G., & Hoogstraten, J. (n.d.). *Satisfacion as a determinant of Compliance.* (1998). *Community Dentistry and Oral Epidemiology, 26*(2), 139–146.

Wilcox, R. R. (2005). Introduction to Robust Estimation and Hypothesis Testing. Second Edition.

ADDITIONAL READING

Robertson, S., & Maddux, J. (1986). Compliance in Pediatric Orthodontic Treatment: Current Research and Issues. *Children's Health Care, 15*(1) Brodeur, P. (2001). *Improving Dental Care.* In To Improve Health and Health Care, IV. Michalowicz, B. S., Gunsolley, J. C., Sparks, B. S., Brooks, C. N., Koertge, T. E., Califano, J. V., Burmeister, J. A., & Schenkein, H. A. (2000). Evidence of a Substantial Genetic Basis for Risk of Adult Periodontitis. *Journal of Periodontology, 71*(11).

Sahoo, P. (2002). *Probability and Mathematical Statistics. Louisville, KY: Department of Mathematics, University of Louisville. Efron, B., & Tibshirani, R. J. (1998). An Introduction to the Bootstrap. Boca Raton, FL: CRC Press LLC. Cugnet, P. (1997). Confidence Interval Estimation for Distribution Systems Power Consumption By using the Bootstrap Method.* Virgina, USA: Virginia Tech University.

Satcher, D. (n.d.). *Oral Health in America: A Report of the Surgeon General. In* 2000 *. National Institute of Dental and Craniofacial Research.*

Chapter 10
Outcomes Research in Gastrointestinal Treatment

Pedro Ramos
University of Louisville, USA

ABSTRACT

This case study describes the use of SAS technology in streamlining cross-sectional and retrospective case-control studies in the exploration of the co-morbidity of depression and gastrointestinal disorders. Various studies in Europe and America have documented associations between irritable bowel syndrome and psychological conditions such as depression and anxiety disorders; however, these were observational studies. Because it is impossible to randomize symptoms, it is difficult to isolate patients with these co-morbidities for randomized trials. Therefore, studies will continue to use observational data. In this study, all steps are conducted electronically in a rapid development environment provided by SAS technology. In addition, it examines the potential rate of health-care utilization particularly for GI disorders among individuals with depressive symptoms and anxiety disorders. We find that the proportion of patients with gastrointestinal problems and psychological disorders is typically higher than the proportion of patients with only gastrointestinal problems.

BACKGROUND

It has been previously reported that depressive symptoms are highly prevalent in the inpatient population with current gastrointestinal symptoms and vice versa. Inadomi et al (2003) reports that in the United States and Europe, one of the major reasons to visit a gastroenterologist is irritable bowel

syndrome. Moreover, Drossman D. et al (2002) report that between fifty and sixty percent of IBS patients in gastroenterology clinics suffer from psychiatric disorders that exacerbate the patients' poor quality of life, causing them to seek more medical help. This has led to theories that patients with depressive symptoms have an increased use of health care services and work absenteeism because of abdominal complaints. According to Hillilä et al (2008), symptoms of depression are common in

DOI: 10.4018/978-1-61520-723-7.ch010

Copyright © 2010, IGI Global. Copying or distributing in print or electronic forms without written permission of IGI Global is prohibited.

the general population and are associated with symptoms in the gastrointestinal system; in turn, these cause an increase in the use of the health care system.

Other theories indicate that patients with severe irritable bowel syndrome may increase their health-related quality of life by following psychological treatments. Jackson R. et al (2000)'s review of data concludes that patients with irritable bowel syndrome found that symptoms improved with the use of antidepressants as much as four times more compared to the use of a placebo. Similarly, Creed F. et al (2005) supports the idea that IBS patients, even those without psychological disorders who do not respond positively to the usual treatment may find improvement from psychological treatment. Another hypothesis in the matter is that irritable bowel syndrome is induced by stress (Whitehead W, 1994). A study conducted by Blanchard et al (2008) measured a significant correlation between some gastrointestinal symptoms, such as IBS and dyspepsia. They found that some life stressors exist over an extended period of time. They concluded that the data support a reciprocal relation between stress and gastrointestinal symptoms rather than a relation of cause and effect. These results concur with those of an earlier study by Levy R. (1997). A great deal of literature supports the important associations between psychiatric illness and chronic medical conditions in a clinical setting.

However, the perspective of risk may be based upon erroneous information, or because what is known is incomplete, and that may bias both diagnosis and treatment. A very good example of this is in the treatment of ulcers. For many years, it was assumed that ulcers were caused by stress. The immediate ulcer was treated using antacids, but prescribed long-term treatment was generally psychological to help the patient reduce stress. Because there was a general perspective that bacteria could not survive in the acid environment of the stomach, infection was not even considered as a possibility. Yet we know now that infection by the *H.pylori* bacterium is the primary cause of most

ulcers, with the use of NSAIDs responsible for almost all others.(Huang, Sridhar, & Hunt, 2002; Soll & Gastroenterology, 1996)

SETTING THE STAGE

The data set for the year 2005 was obtained from the National Inpatient Sample (NIS), the largest all-payer inpatient care database in the United States. A ten percent sample was obtained with a sampling module from SAS Enterprise Miner. It contains data on 7,995,048 hospital stays from approximately one-thousand hospitals. From it, a random ten per cent sample from the data set for the year 2005 was obtained.

First, this set was filtered to contain the records of patients having a digestive condition as the primary reason for being in a hospital. The dataset was created by filtering on the field, DRG, diagnosis related group, on the basis of DRG values related to non-infectious conditions on the digestive systems such as irritable bowel disease, chronic diarrhea, peptic ulcers, chronic constipation, and so on. For a more complete list of the relevant codes, see Table 1. A second subset was defined for those individuals experiencing psychological disorders as the main reason for visiting a hospital. Similarly, the original set was filtered based on DRG values related to psychological conditions such as anxiety disorders, several types of depression, and so on. For a more complete list of the relevant codes, see Table 2. From these two subsets, we obtained a frequency count for hospital visits related to non-infectious digestive diseases and for hospital visits related to the psychological conditions described above.

From these frequencies, we obtained the proportion of hospital visits due to such digestive disorders and due to such psychological ailments respectively.

The second phase of the preprocessing involved determining conditional proportions with the previously built subsets. To do this, the first subset

Table 1.DRG codes related to digestive conditions

Table of DRG's	
DRG Value	**Description**
152	MINOR SMALL and LARGE BOWEL PROCEDURES W CC'
154	MINOR SMALL and LARGE BOWEL PROCEDURES W/O CC'
155	STOMACH, ESOPHAGEAL and DUODENAL PROCEDURES AGE >17 W
156	STOMACH, ESOPHAGEAL and DUODENAL PROCEDURES AGE >17 W/O
157	STOMACH, ESOPHAGEAL and DUODENAL PROCEDURES AGE 0-17'
158	ANAL & STOMAL PROCEDURES W CC'
159	ANAL & STOMAL PROCEDURES W/O CC'
170	OTHER DIGESTIVE SYSTEM O.R. PROCEDURES W CC'
171	OTHER DIGESTIVE SYSTEM O.R. PROCEDURES W/O CC'
174	G.I. HEMORRHAGE W CC'
175	G.I. HEMORRHAGE W/O CC'
172	DIGESTIVE MALIGNANCY W CC'
173	DIGESTIVE MALIGNANCY W/O CC'
176	COMPLICATED PEPTIC ULCER'
177	UNCOMPLICATED PEPTIC ULCER W CC'
178	UNCOMPLICATED PEPTIC ULCER W/O CC'
179	INFLAMMATORY BOWEL DISEASE'
182	ESOPHAGITIS, GASTROENT & MISC DIGEST DISORDERS
184	ESOPHAGITIS, GASTROENT & MISC DIGEST DISORDERS AGE 0-17
183	ESOPHAGITIS, GASTROENT & MISC DIGEST DISORDERS
188	OTHER DIGESTIVE SYSTEM DIAGNOSES AGE >17 W CC'
189	OTHER DIGESTIVE SYSTEM DIAGNOSES AGE >17 W/O CC'
190	OTHER DIGESTIVE SYSTEM DIAGNOSES AGE 0-17'
202	CIRRHOSIS & ALCOHOLIC HEPATITIS'

Table 2. DRG codes related to psychological disorders

Table of DRG's	
DRG Value	**Description**
425	ACUTE ADJUST REACT & DISTURBANCES OF PSYCHOSOCIAL DYSFUNCTION
426	DEPRESSIVE NEUROSES
427	NEUROSES EXCEPT DEPRESSIVE
428	DISORDERS OF PERSONALITY & IMPULSE CONTROL
430	PSYCHOSES
432	OTHER MENTAL DISORDER DIAGNOSES
433	ALCOHOL/DRUG ABUSE OR DEPENDENCE, LEFT AMA

was filtered for the presence of psychological conditions. The D*X* variables were used; these contain ICD9 codes for diagnosis 1 through 15. Using SQL statements from SAS, the observations were filtered for those containing an ICD9 code related to psychological afflictions, such as various kinds of depressions and anxiety disorders within any of the D*X* fields. A binary variable, DIGESTIVE, was computed to mark these records (Figure 1).

Likewise using a SAS SQL code module, the second subset was filtered for the presence of ailments of the digestive system on the D*X* fields on ICD9 values that correspond to digestive systems conditions such as irritable bowel disease, chronic diarrhea, peptic ulcers, and chronic constipation (Figure 2). Within this query and filter process, a binary variable, PSYCHOLGICAL, was created to identify these records. Subsequently, the *SAS merge* procedure was used to merge these subsets to their *parent* sets respectively. At this point, those records from the *parent* sets that did not make it into the queries had blank values in the computed fields, DIGESTIVE and PSYCHOLGICAL. These blank values were replaced with values of 0. At this point, the *one-way frequency* method from *SAS* was used on each of the *parent sets* to determine the wanted conditional probabilities.

Moreover, these subsets were merged using SAS code to obtain summary statistics and analytic graphs. SAS Enterprise Guide was also used to build a relative frequency bar chart based on the subset of those patients visiting a hospital for a digestive condition.

Figure 1.

```
PROC SQL;

CREATE TABLE Q_DRG_PSYCHOLOGICAL AS SELECT KEY FORMAT=Z14,
AGE,DRG,DX1,DX2,DX3,DX4,DX5,DX6,DX7,DX8,DX9,DX10,DX11,DX12,DX13,DX14,DX1
5,FEMALE,LOS,TOTCHG FROM NISGASTRIC AS  NISGASTRIC

WHERE DRG IN (425, 426, 427, 428, 432, 430, 431, 433) ORDER BY KEY
```

Figure 2.

```
PROC SQL;

CREATE TABLE PEDRO.Q_DRG_PSY_DX_DIGEST AS SELECT Q_DRG_PSYCHOLOGICAL.KEY
Q_DRG_PSYCHOLOGICAL.AGE,Q_DRG_PSYCHOLOGICAL.DRG,

Q_DRG_PSYCHOLOGICAL.DX1,Q_DRG_PSYCHOLOGICAL.DX2,Q_DRG_PSYCHOLOGICAL.DX3,

Q_DRG_PSYCHOLOGICAL.DX4,Q_DRG_PSYCHOLOGICAL.DX5,Q_DRG_PSYCHOLOGICAL.DX6,

Q_DRG_PSYCHOLOGICAL.DX7,Q_DRG_PSYCHOLOGICAL.DX8,Q_DRG_PSYCHOLOGICAL.DX9,

Q_DRG_PSYCHOLOGICAL.DX10,Q_DRG_PSYCHOLOGICAL.DX11,Q_DRG_PSYCHOLOGICAL.DX12,

Q_DRG_PSYCHOLOGICAL.DX13,Q_DRG_PSYCHOLOGICAL.DX14,

Q_DRG_PSYCHOLOGICAL.DX15,Q_DRG_PSYCHOLOGICAL.FEMALE,Q_DRG_PSYCHOLOGICAL.LOS
,

Q_DRG_PSYCHOLOGICAL.TOTCHG,Q_DRG_PSYCHOLOGICAL.MDC,

FROM PEDRO.Q_DRG_PSYCHOLOGICAL AS Q_DRG_PSYCHOLOGICAL

WHERE Q_DRG_PSYCHOLOGICAL.DX1 IN ("53300", "53301", "53310", "53311",
"53320", "53321", "53330", "53331", "53340", "53341", "53350", "53351",
"53360", "53361", "53370", "53371", "53390", "53391", "00867", "00869",
"5550", "5551", "5552", "5559", "5560", "5561", "5562", "5563", "5568",
"5581", "5582", "5583", "9570", "9571", "5589", "56400", "56401", "56402",
"56409", "6540 ", "5641 ", "5643 ", "5644 ", "5645 ", "5646 ", "5648 ",
"56481", "56489", "5649 ", "5692 ", "5691 ", "56942", "56949", "56982",
"56984", "56985", "56989", "5699 ")53320", "53321", "53330", "53331",
"53340", "53341", "53350", "53351", "53360") OR

Q_DRG_PSYCHOLOGICAL.DX2 IN ("53300", "53301", "53310", "53311", "53320",
```

It identifies the patients having a psychological condition, namely condition 2. Finally, the SAS Kernel Density function was used to compute the distribution of *Length of Stay* and *Total Charges* by the presence of psychological conditions given that a digestive condition was the reason to visit a hospital.

CASE DESCRIPTION

First, the proportion of patients attending a hospital for digestive conditions is rather high at about eighty per cent while the proportion of people looking for assistance in a hospital for psychological disorders is about twenty-five per cent (Figure 3). The proportion of patients with a psychological condition given that the diges-

tive condition was first diagnosed is twenty per cent (Figure 4). The proportion of patients with a digestive condition given that the psychological disorder was first diagnosed is ten per cent. Similarly, the proportion of patients having both conditions is ten percent.

We also found that that distribution of Length of Stay and Total Charges is different if a psychological condition was present (Figure 5 & 6). These differences may indicate that a relationship between some gastrointestinal disorders and some psychological conditions may exist.

We also use kernel density estimation to investigate the data.

Patients with these conditions generally spend a short period of time in the hospital; the costs are generally low compared to other patient conditions.

Figure 3.

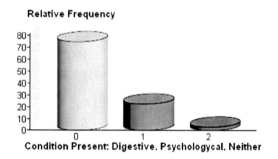

Figure 4.

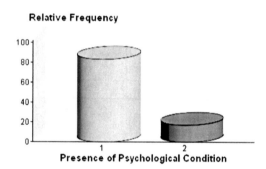

Figure 5.

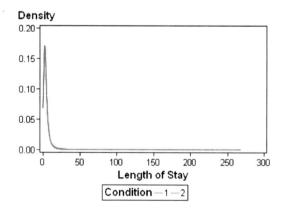

Figure 6.

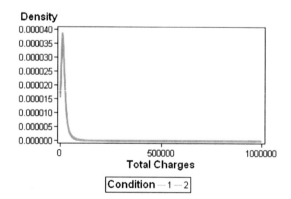

CURRENT AND FUTURE CHALLENGES FACING THE ORGANIZATION

With this information, it is possible to identify a cohort of patients who require aggressive treatment for both gastrointestinal complaints and mental disorders simultaneously. Currently, this treatment is disjoint rather than unified. In the end, treating the patient as a cohestive unit rather than a collection of disjoint parts will enhance healing in this area.

REFERENCES

Blanchard, E. (2001). *Irritable bowel syndrome: psychosocial assessment and treatment.* Washington, DC: American Psychological Association. doi:10.1037/10393-000

Blanchard, E., Lackner, J., Carosella, A., Jaccard, J., Krassner, S., & Kuhn, E. (2008). The role of stress in symptom exacerbation among IBS patients. *Journal of Psychosomatic Research, 64,* 119–128. doi:10.1016/j.jpsychores.2007.10.010

Creed, F. (1999). The relationship between psychosocial parameters and outcome in irritable bowel syndrome. *The American Journal of Medicine, 107,* 74S–80S. doi:10.1016/S0002-9343(99)00083-2

Creed, F., Guthrie, E., Ratcliffe, J., Fernandes, L., Rigby, C., & Tomenson, B. (2005). Does psychological treatment help only those patients with severe irritable bowel syndrome who also have a concurrent psychiatric disorder? *The Australian and New Zealand Journal of Psychiatry, 39,* 807–815.

Drossman, D., Camilleri, M., Mayer, E., & Whitehead, W. (2002). AGA technical review on irritable bowel syndrome. *Gastroenterology, 123,* 2108–2131. doi:10.1053/gast.2002.37095

Hillilä, M., Hämäläinen, J., Heikkinen, M., & Färäkkilä, M. (2008). Gastrointestinal complaints among subjects with depressive symptoms in the general population. *Alimentary Pharmacology & Therapeutics, 28,* 648–654. doi:10.1111/j.1365-2036.2008.03771.x

Huang, J.-Q., Sridhar, S., & Hunt, R. H. (2002). Role of helicobacter pylori infection and non-steroidal anti-inflammatory drugs in peptic-ulcer disease: a meta-analysis. *Lancet, 359*(9300), 14,19.

Inadomi, J., Fennerty, M., & Bjorkman, D. (2003). Systematic review: the economic impact of irritable bowel syndrome. *Alimentary Pharmacology & Therapeutics, 18,* 671–682. doi:10.1046/j.1365-2036.2003.t01-1-01736.x

Jackson, J., O'Malley, P., Tomkins, G., Balden, E., Santoro, J., & Kroenke, K. (2000). Treatment of functional gastrointestinal disorders with anti-depressants: a meta-analysis. *The American Journal of Medicine, 108,* 65–72. doi:10.1016/S0002-9343(99)00299-5

Levy, R., Cain, K., Jarrett, M., & Heitkemper, M. (1997). The relationship between daily life stress and gastrointestinal symptoms in women with irritable bowel syndrome. *Journal of Behavioral Medicine, 20,* 177–193. doi:10.1023/A:1025582728271

Roy-Byrne, P., Davidson, K., Kessler, R., Asmundson, G., Goodwin, R., & Kubzansky, L. (2008). Anxiety disorders and co morbid medical illness. *General Hospital Psychiatry, 30,* 208–225. doi:10.1016/j.genhosppsych.2007.12.006

Soll, A. H., & Gastroenterology, C. A. C. o. (1996). Medical treatment of peptic ulcer disease: practice guidelines. *Journal of the American Medical Association, 275*(8), 622–629. doi:10.1001/jama.275.8.622

Whitehead, W. (1994). Assessing the effects of stress on physical symptoms. *Health Psychology, 13*, 99–102. doi:10.1037/0278-6133.13.2.99

ADDITIONAL READING

Blanchard, E. (2001). *Irritable bowel syndrome: psychosocial assessment and treatment.* Washington, DC: American Psychological Association. doi:10.1037/10393-000

Blanchard, E., Lackner, J., Carosella, A., Jaccard, J., Krassner, S., & Kuhn, E. (2008). The role of stress in symptom exacerbation among IBS patients. *Journal of Psychosomatic Research, 64*, 119–128. doi:10.1016/j.jpsychores.2007.10.010

Cerrito, P. B. (2009a). *Data Mining Healthcare and Clinical Databases.* Cary, NC: SAS Press, Inc.

Cerrito, P. B. (2009b). *Text Mining Techniques for Healthcare Provider Quality Determination: Methods for Rank Comparisons.* Hershey, PA: IGI Global Publishing.

Cerrito, P. B. (n.d.). *A Casebook on Pediatric Diseases.* Oak Park, IL . *Bentham Science Publishing.*

Rodriguez, F., Nguyen, T. C., Galanko, J. A., Morton, J., Rodriguez, F., & Nguyen, T. C. (2007). Gastrointestinal complications after coronary artery bypass grafting: a national study of morbidity and mortality predictors. *Journal of the American College of Surgeons, 205*(6), 741–747. doi:10.1016/j.jamcollsurg.2007.07.003

Soll, A. H., & Gastroenterology, C. o. t. A. C. o. (1996). Medical treatment of peptic ulcer disease: practice guidelines. *Journal of the American Medical Association, 275*(8), 622–629. doi:10.1001/jama.275.8.622

Chapter 11
Outcomes Research in Hydrocephalus Treatment

Damien Wilburn
University of Louisville, USA

ABSTRACT

Hydrocephalus is a disorder where cerebrospinal fluid (CSF) is unable to drain efficiently from the brain. This paper presents a set of exploratory analyses comparing attributes of inpatients under one-year old diagnosed with hydrocephalus provided by the Agency for Healthcare Research and Quality (AHRQ) as part of the National Inpatient Sample (NIS). The general methods include calculation of summary statistics, kernel density estimation, logistic regression, linear regression, and the production of figures and charts using the statistical data modeling software, SAS. It was determined that younger infants show higher mortality rates; additionally, males are more likely to present hydrocephalus and cost slightly more on average than females despite the distribution curves for length of stay appearing virtually identical between genders. Diagnoses and procedures expected for non-hydrocephalic infants showed a negative correlation in the logistic model. The study overall validates much of the literature and expands it with a cost analysis approach.

BACKGROUND

The rising cost of healthcare in America is a frequent issue raised by various media outlets as well as politicians. In 2007, the total spending on healthcare reached $2.3 billion, and that number is estimated to reach $3 billion by 2011. In 2006, the total cost accounted for 16% of the United States'

gross domestic product (GDP) (Poisal, Truffer, & Smith, 2007). These figures represent the national totals, but costs of individual patients must also be considered. Particularly for infants, the costs can be especially high due to the requirement of more sophisticated techniques and equipment.

Hydrocephalus, literally meaning "water head", is a disorder that can occur at any age, but experts predict that it affects approximately 1 in 500 infants. It is characterized by an excess of cerebrospinal fluid

DOI: 10.4018/978-1-61520-723-7.ch011

Copyright © 2010, IGI Global. Copying or distributing in print or electronic forms without written permission of IGI Global is prohibited.

(CSF) filling the ventricles of the brain and not draining efficiently. Most early models presume that resistance to CSF is pressure-independent, and thus, will be constant regardless of secretion rates (Meier, Zeilinger, & Kintzel, 1999). Most newer models are built around Hakim *et al.*'s hypothesis that the brain acts as an open submicroscopic sponge of viscoelastic matter (Hakim, Venegas, & Burton, 1976). In particular, Nagashima *et al.* constructed a model using the finite element method to predict the dynamic flow of CSF in cases of hydrocephalus (Nagashima, Tamaki, Matsumoto, & Seguchi, 1986); combined with pressure dependent models of draining and arterial resistance/compliance (Meier et al., 1999), a positive feedback loop could influence the progression of the disease. The exact causes of the disorder are not well understood and are believed to vary from case to case. Several hypothesized causes include inherited genetic abnormalities, developmental disorders, meningitis, tumors, traumatic head injury, or subarachnoid hemorrhage. Multiple forms of hydrocephalus exist, including congenital, acquired, communicating, or obstructive. Two other forms that primarily affect adults are hydrocephalus ex-vacuo and normal pressure hydrocephalus ((NINDS), 2008).

The symptoms also vary between patients, but in infants, it is normally accompanied by an enlarged head via their soft skulls, expanding to compensate for the increased CSF pressure. Other symptoms can include vomiting, sleepiness, irritability, downward deviation of the eyes, and seizures. Hydrocephalus is regularly diagnosed by some form of advanced cranial imaging, including ultrasonography, computed tomography (CT), magnetic resonance imaging (MRI), or pressure-monitoring techniques. The normal treatment for hydrocephalus is surgically inserting a shunt system to redirect the flow of CSF to other parts of the body, where it can eventually be recycled or excreted ((NINDS), 2008). The two common shunt systems for infants include ventriculoatrial (VA) and ventriculoperitoneal (VP), but follow-up

studies demonstrate that, on average, VA systems require more adjustments, present with more complications, and complications are more serious (Keucher & Mealey, 1979).

Data mining is the analytical practice designed to explore large and complex data sets in search of patterns, systematic relationships between variables, and eventually validating relationships with new subsets of data. Thus, the three major steps of data mining involve data exploration, model construction, and validation. For a study such as this, the objectives will rely principally on exploration and model construction. Exploration involves primarily summary statistics: mean, median, mode, and frequency calculations on different subsets of the data, presented in simple graphical or tabular formats. Kernel density estimation is an extension of these techniques by interpolating frequencies for continuous variables to produce an approximate probability density curve. Based on both initial and final results obtained during exploration, the data must also be "cleaned" or formatted in a matter conducive to further statistical analysis and modeling. A simple example is the division of age into groups to allow a reasonable number of values per group for significant calculations. A particular consideration that needs to be made in rare-occurrence events for diseases such as hydrocephalus is proper controls. If one were to use a full dataset and the event only occurs 1% of the time, simply assuming all cases to be non-occurrence yields 99% accuracy by default. Thus, an effective technique in cleaning the data to circumvent this is to only include a random subset of non-occurrence cases equal in size to the subset that is occurrence cases (StatSoft, 2007).

Linear regression is a popular and powerful technique used in multivariate modeling. Utilizing multiple independent variables and calculating coefficients to weight their individual and independent impact, the likelihood of a single continuous dependent variable can be predicted.

$$y=b_0+b_1x_1+b_2x_2+\ldots+b_nx_n$$

Despite a linear function being produced naturally in multivariate cases, we cannot visualize the result in two-dimensions. Two large assumptions must be made when employing this technique: the relationship between variables is linear and the residuals, the difference between observed and predicted values, are distributed normally. These assumptions can be tested by examining the R^2-values and performing the F-test, respectively. The standard practice is to reject values failing to meet the 95% confidence limit for either of these values. A large limitation to multiple regressions, not exclusively linear regression, is the establishment of relationship only, but not causation; thus, one must interpret the results with hesitance and reservation (StatSoft, 2007). Additionally, too few observations relative to the number of variables can exploit the law of large numbers in randomly identifying a variable with a relationship without any real causation: Freedman and Pee, in a simulation study, demonstrated that over-fitting would occur in linear regression if the Events per Variable (EVP) ratio is less than 0.25 (L. S. Freedman & Pee, 1989).

Logistic regression is a second form of modeling commonly used primarily for multivariate analysis.

$$y = \frac{e^{b_0 + b_1 x_1 + \dots + b_n x_n}}{1 + e^{b_0 + b_1 x_1 + \dots + b_n x_n}}$$

Analogous to linear modeling, by assuming a fit to a logistic curve, numerous independent variables can be used in calculating the likelihood of a dependent variable value, but it must be transformed such that it will never be less than zero nor greater than one. However, a large and extremely seductive characteristic relative to linear modeling is removal of the limitation that the dependent variable must be continuous; any numeric type is acceptable as a dependent variable. A practical application utilizes the indicator function as the dependent variable and

thus, the regression equation effectively serves as a multivariate probability density function. By performing a logit transformation, a logistic regression can be expressed as a linear function, thus making it an extension of the general linear model (StatSoft, 2007). Again, utilizing simulated studies, the minimum threshold determined for EVP values in logistic regressions is 10; anything less than 10 can readily result in bias in both positive and negative directions. The 90% confidence intervals about the estimated values may not have adequate coverage; the Wald statistic could be highly conservative under the null hypothesis, and the frequency of paradoxical associations might increase (Peduzzi, Concato, Kemper, Theodore R. Holford, & Feinstein, 1996).

The purpose of this chapter is to provide an exploratory analysis of a sample of infants suffering from hydrocephalus matched to an equally large control sample, and similarly analyze the relative costs of their treatment. It will be demonstrated that within particular subgroups of the infants with hydrocephalus, utilizing numerous statistical methods and techniques; there are distinctions and anomalies compared to counterparts both in frequency and relative cost.

SETTING THE STAGE

This study analyzed a relatively large group of infants less than one year old who were diagnosed with hydrocephalus (N=2130) versus an equally large, randomly selected control group of infants also less than one year old. The data set is from the National Inpatient Sample (NIS), part of the Healthcare Cost and Utilization Project (HCUP) sponsored by the Agency for Healthcare Research and Quality (AHRQ) for the year 2005 (Quality, 2000). The data from the NIS is publicly available and all inpatients included have been de-identified. Analysis of the data was performed using the statistical software package, SAS, including cleaning the data, performing descriptive statistics, kernel density estimation, and production of tables and figures. Any patients lacking values for a specific variable were removed from calculations involving that variable.

Descriptive statistics were performed to compare race, gender, age at admission, mortality, length of stay, and total charges between infants with hydrocephalus versus the control group. Kernel density estimates were likewise performed using length of stay and total charges, with categorical variables including race, gender, age at admission, and diagnosis of hydrocephalus. These data are presented as pie charts, bar graphs, or line

plots as deemed appropriate to best represent the comparisons.

Included in the data from the NIS is up to 15 ICD-9 diagnosis codes and procedure codes per inpatient. Diagnosis codes are normally 3 characters long, but can include decimal values that further describe the diagnoses. Similarly, procedure codes are 2 characters long with further descriptors as decimals. Because of the inconsistency of reporting between hospitals, the top twenty five diagnosis and procedure codes were examined for infants with hydrocephalus. Based on the 3 or 2 digit base codes for diagnoses and

Table 1. Top 25 ICD-9 diagnoses codes for infants with hydrocephalus

Diagnoses Code	Description	Frequency	Percent
331.4*	Obstructive hydrocephalus (acquired)	1190	5.91
331	Other cerebral degenerations	1059	5.26
741*	Spina bifida	751	3.73
769*	Respiratory distress syndrome	379	1.88
765*	Disorders relating to short gestation and low birthweight	346	1.72
996*	Complications peculiar to certain specified procedures	319	1.58
770*	Other respiratory conditions of fetus and newborn	285	1.42
741.03	Spina bifida, with hydrocephalus, lumbar region	281	1.40
V30*	Single liveborn	280	1.39
V45.2*	Presence of cerebrospinal fluid drainage device	279	1.39
770.7	Chronic respiratory disease arising in the perinatal period	253	1.26
772*	Fetal and neonatal hemorrhage	247	1.23
996.2	Mechanical complication of nervous system device, implant, and graft	233	1.16
530.81*	Esophageal reflux	220	1.09
780	General symptoms	219	1.09
780.39	Other convulsions	213	1.06
741.00	Spina bifida, with hydrocephalus, no specific region	190	0.94
V30.01	Single liveborn, in hospital by cesarian delivery	185	0.92
779	Other and ill-defined conditions originating in the perinatal period	184	0.91
741.93	Spina bifida, without mention of hydrocephalus, lumbar region	181	0.90
774.2	Neonatal jaundice associated with preterm delivery	176	0.87
779.3	Feeding problems in newborn	156	0.77
771.81	Septicemia [sepsis] of newborn	152	0.75
772.14	Grade IV	141	0.70
742	Other congenital anomalies of nervous system	140	0.70

procedures, respectively, 10 indicator functions were created for the top codes (an asterisk is used in the following tables to represent the codes for which indicator functions were defined). They are listed in Tables 1 and 2. Combined with total charge, length of stay, age, gender, and survival; these variables were compiled into a model using step-wise logistic regression. All variables failing to meet 95% confidence were removed from the model.

As an extension to the kernel density estimation for length of stay and total charges relative to the common descriptors, linear models were constructed for both variables. Independent vari-

ables initially included age, race, gender, survival, presence of hydrocephalus, income quartile of patients, reported disease indicator functions, and all procedure and disease indicator functions created above. Crosses between these variables and the presence of hydrocephalus were also tested. Because of the relatively small size of the data set and the inclusion of several more classification variables to quantitative variables, many variables would result in the Post Hoc tests becoming non-estimable. These variables, along with any that did not meet at least 95% confidence in a Type III SS test, were removed from the model.

Table 2. Top 25 ICD-9 procedure codes for infants with hydrocephalus

Procedure Code	Description	Frequency	Percent
02.34*	Ventricular shunt to abdominal cavity and organs	524	29.64
38.93*	Venous catheterization, not elsewhere classified	332	18.78
96.04*	Insertion of endotracheal tube	118	6.67
96.72	Continuous mechanical ventilation for 96 consecutive hours or more	111	6.28
02.42	Replacement of ventricular shunt	52	2.94
02.2	Ventriculostomy	51	2.88
03.52*	Repair of spinal myelomeningocele	47	2.66
03.31	Spinal tap	34	1.92
96.71	Continuous mechanical ventilation for less than 96 consecutive hours	34	1.92
01.02*	Ventriculopuncture through previously implanted catheter	34	1.92
99.15*	Parenteral infusion of concentrated nutritional substances	33	1.87
99.04	Transfusion of packed cells	31	1.75
38.91	Arterial catheterization	29	1.64
88.91*	Magnetic resonance imaging of brain and brain stem	27	1.53
02.43	Removal of ventricular shunt	22	1.24
87.03*	Computerized axial tomography of head	22	1.24
38.92	Umbilical vein catheterization	18	1.02
01.09	Other cranial puncture	14	0.79
99.83	Other phototherapy	10	0.57
64.0*	Circumcision	9	0.51
02.39	Other operations to establish drainage of ventricle	8	0.45
93.90*	Continuous positive airway pressure [CPAP]	7	0.40
54.95	Incision of peritoneum	7	0.40
96.6	Enteral infusion of concentrated nutritional substances	6	0.34
38.85	Other surgical occlusion of other thoracic vessels	6	0.34

CASE DESCRIPTION

The initial descriptive statistics include the distribution of race and gender of the treatment and control groups. The comparison can be readily visualized using pie charts and numerically interpreted via tables summarizing the data. It should be noted that a large number of values are missing for race from the patient's profiles for both the control and treatment groups.

Figure 1 diagrams the frequency of inpatients of a particular race for both the control and treatment groups. There is minor variation between the two groups, but the percentages are relatively consistent between the control and the treatment, and what variation exists is likely due to random chance. Of the total sample of 2130 inpatients per group, 550 from the control and 770 from the treatment did not have their race reported and thus were removed from the calculation of these percentages.

Figure 2 shows the ratio of inpatients of each gender for both the control and treatment groups. For both groups, all members are less than one year old. Considering that the human sex ratio is 51.3% (105 males to 100 females), these per-

centages appear consistent for the control group (Jacobsen, Møller, & Mouritsen, 1999). For the treatment group with a ratio of ~4:3 male to female, this significantly deviates from both the control group and human sex ratio, signifying a higher occurrence of hydrocephalus in infant males. Of the 2130 inpatients in each group, 3 in the control group and 2 in the treatment group did not have their gender reported, and thus were removed from the calculation of these percentages.

Table 3 demonstrates a distribution difference between infants in the control group and those afflicted with hydrocephalus. In the control group, virtually all the infant inpatients are less than 73 days old, likely implying complications at birth. However, although the majority of infants with hydrocephalus are still admitted at that same age, there is a broader distribution across the first year.

Figure 3 displays the frequency of mortality for infants less than one year old who are part of either the control or treatment groups. In the control group, with only 10 out of 2130 inpatients dying, this low morality rate is almost negligible. In the treatment group, with a mortality rate approximately eight-fold that of the control group, there

Figure 1. Race (frequency, control and treatment groups)

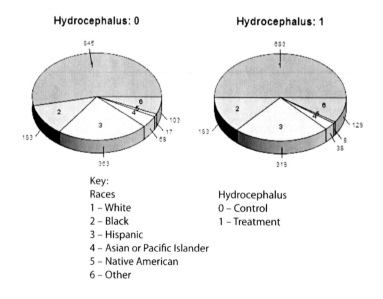

is clearly a significant difference, implying that hydrocephalus is life-threatening. One inpatient's mortality was not reported in the treatment group and was therefore removed from calculations. No inpatients from the control group were removed from these percentage calculations.

Figure 2. Gender (frequency, control and treatment groups)

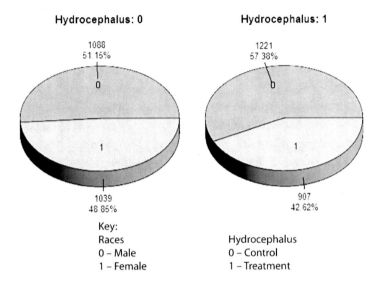

Key:
Races
0 – Male
1 – Female

Hydrocephalus
0 – Control
1 – Treatment

Table 3. Infants with hydrocephalus by age in days at admittance

Hydrocephalus	Age (Days)					
	0-73	**74-146**	**146-219**	**220-292**	**293-365**	**Total**
control	2046 96.06%	24 1.13%	23 1.08%	15 0.70%	22 1.03%	2130
treatment	1351 63.43%	273 12.82%	208 9.77%	170 7.98%	128 6.01%	2130
Total	3397	297	231	185	150	4260

Figure 3. Mortality (frequency, control group)

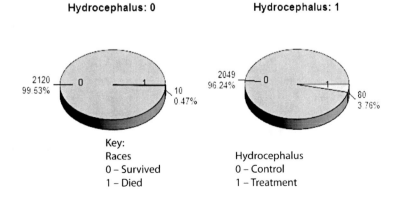

Key:
Races
0 – Survived
1 – Died

Hydrocephalus
0 – Control
1 – Treatment

Figure 4 shows the number of infants with hydrocephalus in the treatment group who die subdivided into different age of admittance brackets (the same that were used to compare age of admittance versus treatment or control group). Clearly, the largest percentage of the infants who die are in the youngest age bracket, but this is also the largest bracket to be diagnosed with hydrocephalus. One inpatient from the treatment group was missing the mortality information, and was therefore removed from calculation.

Table 4 elucidates the ratios of the number of infants who die versus survive per age bracket. Figure 4 revealed that the youngest bracket was where the highest mortality occurred, but it did not reveal whether it was greater over the other brackets or if simply more infants were diagnosed

in the youngest bracket, which would account for more deaths as well. With only one death in the 220-292 days bracket and a morality rate ~1/9 that of the 0-73 bracket, it is clear that the highest mortality rate is in the youngest bracket. One inpatient in the treatment group did not have its mortality reported, and it was therefore removed from these calculations.

Figure 5 displays a kernel density estimation plot comparing the length of stay for inpatients in the control group versus those diagnosed with hydrocephalus. The mode for both plots is at ~2.5 days; however, the magnitude of the control is roughly four times that of the treatment group. The treatment group shows a much more severe left-skew, with multiple inpatients staying greater than one month.

Figure 4. Mortality by age at admittance (frequency, treatment group)

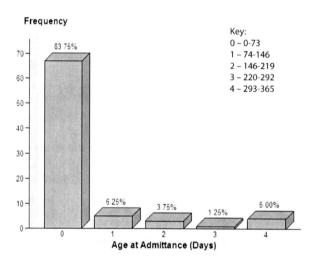

Table 4. Mortality for infants with hydrocephalus by age of admittance

Hydrocephalus	Age at Admittance (Days)					Total
	0-73	74-146	146-219	220-292	293-365	
control	1283 95.04%	268 98.17%	205 98.56%	169 99.41%	124 96.88%	2049
treatment	67 4.96%	5 1.83%	3 1.44%	1 0.59%	4 3.13%	80
Total	1350	273	208	170	128	2129
Frequency Missing = 1						

Figure 6 presents a kernel density estimation comparing the total charges for an inpatient between the control group and the treatment group. Unlike the KDE plot in Fig.5, the modes for the control and treatment groups are not equivalent, with a shift to the right for those with hydrocephalus. The left-skew is even more prevalent in this descriptor for the treatment group relative to the control when compared to the kernel density for the length of stay.

Figure 7 shows a plot of the kernel density estimate for the length of stay for inpatients afflicted with hydrocephalus subdivided into brackets based on the infant's age in days at admittance. All five brackets share a common mode of approximately a length of stay of 2 days, but the highest percentage staying the least amount of time are those admitted when between 220 and 292 days old. The first bracket, from 0 to 73 days old, has the broadest distribution

Figure 5. Length of stay (density by group)

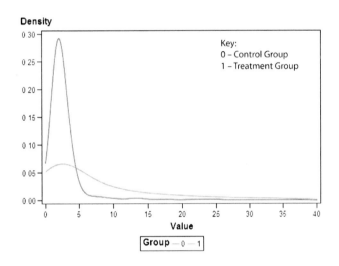

Figure 6. Total charges (density by group)

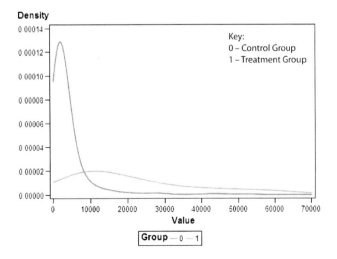

Figure 7. Length of stay (density by age bracket)

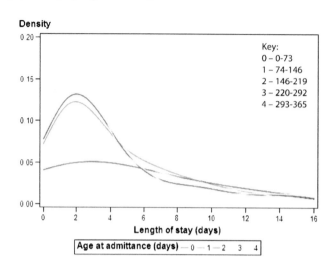

Figure 8. Total charges (density by age bracket)

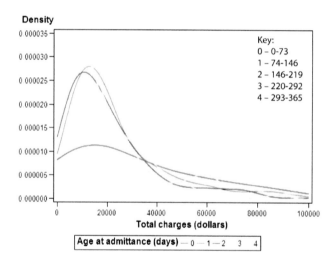

curve and consequently averages the longest length of stay.

Figure 8 displays a plot for a kernel density estimation of total charges for inpatients with hydrocephalus, divided into the same age brackets as previously described. Similar to the length of stay densities, all the age brackets have approximately the same mode with the 220-292 days bracket having the steepest peak and the 0-73 days the least. However, an anomaly at ~$60,000 shows the probability is higher in the 220-292 days bracket

despite the 0-73 having the greatest probability of any bracket beyond ~$40,000. Otherwise, the data remain consistent with the length of stay density plot in Figure 7.

Figure 9 presents a plot of the density of the length of stay for infants afflicted with hydrocephalus subdivided by race (excluding inpatients whose race was not reported). Although the mode for almost all races is ~2.5 days, the variation in each race's distribution curve should be noted. White infants have both the highest mode and

Figure 9. Length of stay (density by race)

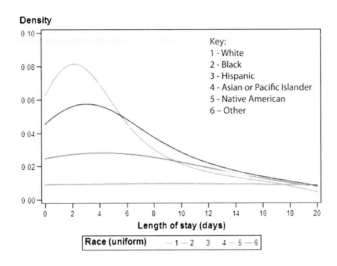

Figure 10. Total charges (density by race)

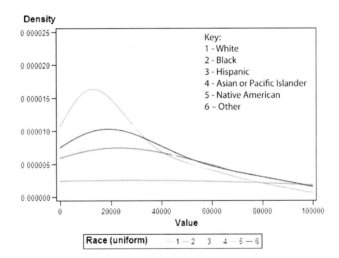

the sharpest decline on the right down-slope; because of limited numbers in the dataset, the Native American group has an almost uniform distribution.

Figure 10 shows the density plot of the total charges for the inpatients separated by race. When compared with the same groupings analyzing length of stay, the order of the plots remains consistent with an inversion between Asian or Pacific islander and "other," implying that on average, Asian or Pacific islander inpatients cost

less but spend more days in the hospital. This could possibly be due to a bias in the locations sampled and the actual cost in that particular region. Again, as with the length of stay, the distribution for Native American inpatients is practically uniform.

Figure 11 displays a kernel density estimation plot comparing the length of stay between inpatients with hydrocephalus separated by gender. Despite males having a slightly higher mode, the plots are virtually identical, signifying no real dif-

Figure 11. Length of stay (density by gender)

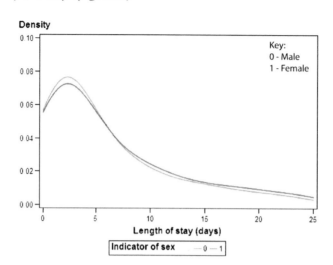

Figure 12. Total charges (density by gender)

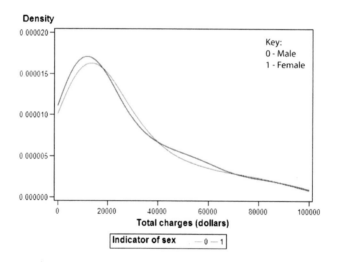

ference in their distributions. Inpatients missing the gender value were not included.

Figure 12 presents the kernel density estimate plots of total costs for inpatients afflicted with hydrocephalus separated by gender. Unlike in the density plots for length of stay, the modes are not exactly equal, and the male density's curve is virtually the same as the female's just shifted down and to the right by ~$2000. This implies a slightly higher average cost for males, and when coupled to the density plot for length of stay, there is no

clear explanation for this. Based on Figure 12, there are more males in the sample, so this could possibly have influenced the density calculations producing the down-shift. Any inpatients whose gender was not reported are not displayed.

A stepwise logistic regression was performed to construct a model correlating the presence of hydrocephalus with multiple demographics (age, gender, race, and mortality), total charges, length of stay, and diagnoses/procedures. Because a stepwise regression was used, only the variables

Table 5a. Analysis of maximum likelihood estimates

Parameter	DF	Estimate	Standard Error	Wald Chi-Square	Pr > ChiSq
Intercept	1	-5.5380	0.7781	50.6517	<.0001
Total charges	1	-5.4E-6	1.523E-6	12.5612	0.0004
Age (in days at admittance)	1	-0.00706	0.00120	34.8628	<.0001
Mortality	1	0.9853	0.3081	10.2258	0.0014
Nonoperative intubation and irrigation (PR 96)	1	0.5184	0.1519	11.6411	0.0006
Operations on spinal cord and spinal canal structures (PR 03)	1	1.2541	0.1339	87.7556	<.0001
Other nonoperative procedures (PR 99)	1	-0.2968	0.1091	7.4043	0.0065
Other diagnostic radiology and related techniques (PR 88)	1	1.0891	0.2522	18.6531	<.0001
Operations on penis (PR 64)	1	-0.4632	0.1326	12.1948	0.0005
Complications peculiar to certain specified procedures (DX 996)	1	1.8958	0.5083	13.9111	0.0002
Other respiratory conditions of fetus and newborn (DX 770)	1	0.2719	0.1144	5.6521	0.0174
Single liveborn (DX V30)	1	-0.7996	0.0974	67.3870	<.0001
Other postprocedural states (DX V45)	1	1.2036	0.3062	15.4513	<.0001
Fetal and neonatal hemorrhage (DX 772)	1	1.0433	0.1860	31.4562	<.0001
Respiratory distress syndrome (DX 769)	1	-0.5325	0.2212	5.7930	0.0161

Table 5b. Odds ratio estimates

Effect	Point Estimate	95% Wald Confidence Limits	
Total charges	1.000	1.000	1.000
Age (in days at admittance)	0.993	0.991	0.995
Mortality 0 vs 1	7.176	2.144	24.012
Nonoperative intubation and irrigation (PR 96) 0 vs 1	2.820	1.555	5.117
Operations on spinal cord and spinal canal structures (PR 03) 0 vs 1	12.282	7.267	20.757
Other nonoperative procedures (PR 99) 0 vs 1	0.552	0.360	0.847
Other diagnostic radiology and related techniques (PR 88) 0 vs 1	8.831	3.286	23.731
Operations on penis (PR 64) 0 vs 1	0.396	0.235	0.666
Complications peculiar to certain specified procedures (DX 996) 0 vs 1	44.325	6.044	325.046
Other respiratory conditions of fetus and newborn (DX 770) 0 vs 1	1.723	1.100	2.697
Single liveborn (DX V30) 0 vs 1	0.202	0.138	0.296
Other postprocedural states (DX V45) 0 vs 1	11.103	3.343	36.875
Fetal and neonatal hemorrhage (DX 772) 0 vs 1	8.057	3.886	16.705
Respiratory distress syndrome (DX 769) 0 vs 1	0.345	0.145	0.821

listed in Table 5a were calculated to be significant to the model.

Table 5b shows the odds ratio estimates for all variables that were deemed significant. Because of the total charges point estimate of 1.000, it is effectively a constant in the model. For age at admittance in days, infusions (PRcode99), circumcision (PRcode64), live birth (DXcodeV30),

Table 5c. Association of predicted probabilities and observed responses

Percent Concordant	93.1	**Somers' D**	0.872
Percent Discordant	5.9	**Gamma**	0.881
Percent Tied	1.1	**Tau-a**	0.427
Pairs	773937	**c**	0.936

and respiratory distress syndrome (DXcode769), both the point estimate and the 95% confidence interval of the odds ratio estimate are less than 1, signifying a decrease in the probability of hydrocephalus as the odds of these variables increase. For age, this is consistent with Table 3, since the largest percentage of infants with hydrocephalus was in the first age bracket. Since the diagnoses and procedures are fairly common among regular infants, it is logical that those admitted because of, or related to hydrocephalus would not necessarily be diagnosed with or receive treatment for them. The remaining variables show a positive correlation with the presence of hydrocephalus.

Table 5c shows that when testing all possible disparate pairs (773937), the model was accurate 93.1% of the time, inaccurate 5.9%, and tied 1.1%. This is highly consistent with the Somers' D and c scores being close to 1, and thus showing high agreement between the pairs and the model.

Linear models were constructed for both length of stay (Tables 6a and 6b) and total charges (Tables 7a and 7b) based upon all the descriptive variables used until now, the diagnosis and procedure indicator functions, and the indicator function for the reported diseases by HCUP. Any variables

resulting in non-estimable Post Hoc tests or failing to meet the 95% confidence in a Type III SS test were removed from the model.

A variable that warrants further analysis is Hydrocephalus*Disorders relating to short gestation and low birthweight (DX 765). The average length of stay for patients with hydrocephalus and DX 765 was ~80 days, roughly 9 times the model's mean. Comparison of the means for the four possibilities in this cross showed $P < 0.001$ for all combinations except for no hydrocephalus with and without DX 765. This further implies significance of complications that can arise due to hydrocephalus.

In comparing the two linear models, certain variables are shared; yet, there are some missing in one that would be expected to be critical in both. Examples of the former include Single liveborn (DX V30) and Fetal and neonatal hemorrhage (DX 772), both having appeared in the logistic regression. However, age at admittance, which was demonstrated significant to the disease by the logistic regression, would expect to be negatively correlated to both total charges and length of stay based on the density plots in Figures 7 and 8. While significant in the length of stay linear regression, it

Table 6a. Influence of general descriptors, diagnoses, and procedures on length of stay analysis of variance

Source	DF	Sum of Squares	Mean Square	F Value	Pr > F
Model	25	516561.1818	20662.4473	93.23	<.0001
Error	1777	393839.9175	221.6319		
Corrected Total	1802	910401.0993			

Note that the mean of this model is 9.614 days and the R-square is 0.5674.

Table 6b. Statistical significance of variables in linear model for length of stay

Source	DF	Type III SS	Mean Square	F Value	Pr > F
Age (in days at admittance)	1	3522.11521	3522.11521	15.89	<.0001
Race	3	4702.09136	1567.36379	7.07	0.0001
Mortality	1	1425.61384	1425.61384	6.43	0.0113
Congestive Heart Failure	1	882.01855	882.01855	3.98	0.0462
Severe Liver Disease	1	2328.19296	2328.19296	10.50	0.0012
Hydrocepahlus*Race	3	3443.56801	1147.85600	5.18	0.0015
Incision, excision, and occlusion of vessels (PR 38)	1	7146.63516	7146.63516	32.25	<.0001
Hydrocephalus*Nonoperative intubation and irrigation (PR 96)	2	5129.04859	2564.52430	11.57	<.0001
Incision and excision of skull, brain, and cerebral meninges (PR 01)	1	7765.17658	7765.17658	35.04	<.0001
Operations on penis (PR 64)	1	2192.27043	2192.27043	9.89	0.0017
Hydrocephalus*Operations on penis (PR 64)	1	1813.04056	1813.04056	8.18	0.0043
Respiratory distress syndrome (DX 769)	1	36740.38080	36740.38080	165.77	<.0001
Hydrocephalus*Respiratory distress syndrome (DX 769)	1	3904.04059	3904.04059	17.61	<.0001
Disorders relating to short gestation and low birthweight (DX 765)	1	6385.00961	6385.00961	28.81	<.0001
Hydrocephalus*Disorders relating to short gestation and low birthweight (DX 765)	1	1402.85728	1402.85728	6.33	0.0120
Other respiratory conditions of fetus and newborn (DX 770)	1	4359.01841	4359.01841	19.67	<.0001
Single liveborn (DX V30)	1	11095.29033	11095.29033	50.06	<.0001
Hydrocephalus*Single liveborn (DX V30)	1	3721.62651	3721.62651	16.79	<.0001
Fetal and neonatal hemorrhage (DX 772)	1	4619.97872	4619.97872	20.85	<.0001

did not meet the set criterion to be included in the linear model for total charges. While this may be a result of complications in the modeling, such as producing non-estimable means, it does raise the question of significance in recovery time versus expensive treatments.

CURRENT AND FUTURE CHALLENGES FACING THE ORGANIZATION

The presented data in this exploratory study show clear distinctions in infants suffering from hydrocephalus compared to the control study of equal sample size (N=2130). The various plots directly comparing the two, between mortality, length of

Table 7a. Influence of general descriptors, diagnoses, and procedures on total charges analysis of variance

Source	DF	Sum of Squares	Mean Square	F Value	Pr > F
Model	22	2.1032871E13	956039595322	160.86	<.0001
Error	2757	1.6385835E13	5943356866.9		
Corrected Total	2779	3.7418706E13			

Note that the mean of this model is $47,379 and the R-square is 0.5621.

Table 7b. Statistical significance of variables in linear model for total charges

Source	DF	Type III SS	Mean Square	F Value	Pr > F
Mortality	1	226843672225	226843672225	38.17	<.0001
Congestive Heart Failure	1	198866842358	198866842358	33.46	<.0001
Renal Disease	1	176533955233	176533955233	29.70	<.0001
Cancer	1	26483754063	26483754063	4.46	0.0349
Severe Liver Disease	1	215368977217	215368977217	36.24	<.0001
Hydrocephalus*Congestive Heart Failure	1	40156839374	40156839374	6.76	0.0094
Other operations on skull, brain, and cerebral meninges (PR 02)	1	194330663898	194330663898	32.70	<.0001
Incision, excision, and occlusion of vessels (PR 38)	1	430958727746	430958727746	72.51	<.0001
Nonoperative intubation and irrigation (PR 96)	1	106695156057	106695156057	17.95	<.0001
Hydrocephalus*Nonoperative intubation and irrigation (PR 96)	1	113351655132	113351655132	19.07	<.0001
Operations on spinal cord and spinal canal structures (PR 03)	1	74668399532	74668399532	12.56	0.0004
Incision and excision of skull, brain, and cerebral meninges (PR 01)	1	115750108744	115750108744	19.48	<.0001
Other nonoperative procedures (PR 99)	1	207363647142	207363647142	34.89	<.0001
Hydrocephalus*Other nonoperative procedures (PR 99)	1	107325070808	107325070808	18.06	<.0001
Hydrocephalus*Physical therapy, respiratory therapy, rehabilitation, and related procedures (PR 93)	2	44541610344	22270805172	3.75	0.0237
Respiratory distress syndrome (DX 769)	1	722868227369	722868227369	121.63	<.0001
Hydrocephalus*Respiratory distress syndrome (DX 769)	1	137019557476	137019557476	23.05	<.0001
Hydrocephalus*Disorders relating to short gestation and low birth-weight (DX 765)	1	111642120675	111642120675	18.78	<.0001
Single liveborn (DX V30)	1	155468081069	155468081069	26.16	<.0001
Fetal and neonatal hemorrhage (DX 772)	1	569220637747	569220637747	95.77	<.0001

stay, and total costs all make clear that it is a life threatening disease. With the most common treatment being surgery to insert a ventricular shunt to drain the buildup of CSF ((NINDS), 2008), the elevated costs of surgery, risk of complications, and extended recovery times likely explain all of these variables. However, because older treatments presented many more frequent complications (McLaughlin, Loeser, & Roberts, 1997), many questions should be raised to the exact forms of treatment used.

Although there is no clear distinction between the distributions of race between the two samples, there is some discrepancy between the length of stay and the total costs for the inpatients. The clearest is the shift between Native Americans and all other races listed as "other" between the two density plots. However, with only 38 inpatients listed as Native Americans, this cannot be considered a large enough sample to develop a true density plot spread across $100,000, and these data are likely a product of a small sample size. Likewise, the uniform density for Asian and Pacific islanders is unusual when compared to all other races' density functions resembling a Chi-squared distribution. However, with only 8 inpatients in that particular sample, it is far too small to attempt to calculate a probability density function.

The comparison of the gender of infants with hydrocephalus also displayed peculiarities. Not suffering from the same limited samples as some of the races, based upon the nearly identical density curves for length of stay, total costs would have been expected to follow the same pattern. However, the male curve appears shifted both down and right, raising the average male cost. With more males suffering from the disease, it is possible that there is a greater risk of complications arising. However, this is not the first report of predominately males suffering from hydrocephalus being reported, and the trend applies at least to those under 18 (Shah et al., 2008).

The logistic modeling used presents another method to compare several of the aforementioned variables used in the summary statistics with the presence of hydrocephalus, along with a means of analyzing the relevance of several prevalent diagnoses and procedures. Multiple procedures and treatments should come as no surprise as positively correlating with the presence of hydrocephalus, such as "complication of nervous system device, implant, and graft," (DX 996) since the primary treatment of hydrocephalus is shunt insertion ((NINDS), 2008). For the variables that were found to be statistically significant, but show negative correlation, it was concluded that because of their relative prevalence in non-hydrocephalus patients, they are not issues that will likely be treated or bothered with while an infant is admitted for hydrocephalus. Other variables that remain consistent with summary statistics include mortality and age.

The inclusion of the linear models continues to emphasize the relevance of some of the aforementioned variables, particularly age. However, the failure of age at admittance to meet significance in the model for total charges raises the question of recovery time versus cost to recover. For patients with hydrocephalus, the required surgery should greatly increase the cost, but since this should be relatively uniform for all infants, young age may present the need for longer recovery times versus those slightly older who have more developed and acclimated bodies. The models also allowed the opportunity to explore interactions between certain variables and their influence on length of stay or total costs. Disorders related to gestation or low birth weight (DX 765) was one of particular value, since the differences in mean estimates for length of stay were not significant between afflicted infants without hydrocephalus, but those with hydrocephalus were highly significant. A similar phenomenon was observed in total charges for the same interaction.

These initial exploratory analyses present multiple anomalies between various reference groups and helped to demonstrate the changes in relative medical costs between them. Although relative to the total costs in America, those suffering from hydrocephalus represent a very small portion; but, as clearly seen in Figure 6, the total costs for infants with hydrocephalus can fairly easily reach or exceed $100,000 compared to most infants in the control costing one fifth of that. All of these data should serve as the foundation for more expansive studies that will couple the current data with analyses of specific diagnoses and treatments, further density estimation based on such data, and construction of regression models around determined correlations.

Americans claim one of the top political issues is the concern of rising healthcare costs, and what Washington will do in the coming years to answer these cries has yet to be seen. Healthcare is a sector of the economy that suffers from inflation at a faster rate than the national average, and so the already present disparity in healthcare equality of Americans could continue to increase. Diseases such as hydrocephalus, which incur exorbitant costs that those without insurance could more than likely not afford, are going to be the earliest to see reductions in the number of patients treated or appearance of shortcuts to reduce costs, likely at the expense of quality. These costs are further compounded in infants, who are on average more expensive than adults. Studies such as this can serve as powerful models of not only methods to processing large databases of inpatient data but also provide insight into potential problems the healthcare industry is likely to face in coming years. There are three critical, clear lessons that can be taken from this study: regression modeling is a set of powerful techniques for finding less obvious trends that cannot be readily detected with summary statistics, infants can present with greater recovery times at little to minimal additional costs, and hydrocephalus is a disease with a relatively low mortality rate but has many complications that are likely to be compounded by gender and common newborn illnesses.

REFERENCES

Freedman, L. S., & Pee, D. (1989). Return to a note on screening regression equations. The American Statistician, 43, 279–282. doi:10.2307/2685389doi:10.2307/2685389

Hakim, S., Venegas, J. G., & Burton, J. D. (1976). The physics of the cranial cavity, hydrocephalus and normal pressure hydrocephalus: mechanical interpretation and mathematical model. Surgical Neurology, 5(3), 187–210. PubMed

Jacobsen, R., Møller, H., & Mouritsen, A. (1999). Natural variation in the human sex ratio. Human Reproduction (Oxford, England), 14, 3120–3125. PubMeddoi:10.1093/humrep/14.12.3120doi:10.1093/humrep/14.12.3120

Keucher, T. R., & Mealey, J. (1979). Long-term results after ventriculoatrial and ventriculoperitoneal shunting for infantile hydrocephalus. Journal of Neurosurgery, 50(2), 179–186. PubMeddoi:10.3171/jns.1979.50.2.0179doi:10.3171/jns.1979.50.2.0179

McLaughlin, J. F., Loeser, J. D., & Roberts, T. S. (1997). Acquired hydrocephalus associated with superior vena cava syndrome in infants. Child's Nervous System, 13, 59–63. PubMeddoi:10.1007/s003810050042doi:10.1007/s003810050042

Meier, U., Zeilinger, F. S., & Kintzel, D. (1999). Diagnostic in Normal Pressure Hydrocephalus: A Mathematical Model for Determination of the ICP-Dependent Resistance and Compliance. Acta Neurochirurgica, 141, 941–948. PubMeddoi:10.1007/s007010050400doi:10.1007/s007010050400

Nagashima, T., Tamaki, N., Matsumoto, S., & Seguchi, Y. (1986). Biomechanics and a theoretical model of hydrocephalus: application of the finite element method. In J. D. Miller (Ed.), Intracranial Pressure VI (pp. 441–446). New York: Springer.

(NINDS), N. I. o. N. D. a. S. (2008, August 1). Hydrocephalus Fact Sheet. Retrieved September 14, 2008, from http://www.ninds.nih.gov/disorders/hydrocephalus/detail_hydrocephalus.htm

Peduzzi, P., Concato, J., Kemper, E., Holford, T. R., & Feinstein, A. R. (1996). A Simulation Study of the Number of Events per Variable in Logistic Regression Analysis. Journal of Clinical Epidemiology, 49(12), 1373–1379. PubMeddoi:10.1016/S0895-4356(96)00236-3doi:10.1016/S0895-4356(96)00236-3

Poisal, J. A., Truffer, C., & Smith, S. (2007). Health Spending Projections Through 2016: Modest Changes Obscure Part D's Impact. Health Affairs, 26(2), 242–253. doi:10.1377/hlthaff.26.2.w242doi:10.1377/hlthaff.26.2.w242

Quality, A. H. R. a. (2000). Healthcare Cost and Utilization Project (HCUP) Retrieved September 14, 2008, from www.hcup-us.ahrq.gov/nisoverview.jsp

Shah, S. S., Hall, M., Slonim, A. D., Hornig, G. W., Berry, J. G., & Sharma, V. (2008). A multicenter study of factors influencing cerebrospinal fluid shunt survival in infants and children. Neurosurgery, 2008, 1095–1103. doi:10.1227/01.neu.0000325871.60129.23doi:10.1227/01.neu.0000325871.60129.23

StatSoft. (2007). Electronic Statistics Textbook. Tulsa, OK: StatSoft.

ADDITIONAL READING

Cerrito, P. B. (2009). A Casebook on Pediatric Diseases. Park, IL: Bentham Science:Oak.

Keucher, T. R., & Mealey, J. (1979). Long-term results after ventriculoatrial and ventriculoperitoneal shunting for infantile hydrocephalus. Journal of Neurosurgery, 50(2), 179–186. PubMeddoi:10.3171/jns.1979.50.2.0179doi:10.3171/jns.1979.50.2.0179

Peduzzi, P., Concato, J., Kemper, E., Holford, T. R., & Feinstein, A. R. (1996). A Simulation Study of the Number of Events per Variable in Logistic Regression Analysis. Journal of Clinical Epidemiology, 49(12), 1373–1379. PubMeddoi:10.1016/S0895-4356(96)00236-3doi:10.1016/S0895-4356(96)00236-3

Poisal, J. A., Truffer, C., & Smith, S. (2007). Health Spending Projections Through 2016: Modest Changes Obscure Part D's Impact. Health Affairs, 26(2), 242–253. doi:10.1377/hlthaff.26.2.w242doi:10.1377/hlthaff.26.2.w242

Quality, A. H. R. a. (2000). *Healthcare Cost and Utilization Project (HCUP)* Retrieved September 14, 2008, from www.hcup-us.ahrq.gov/nisoverview.jsp

Shah, S. S., Hall, M., Slonim, A. D., Hornig, G. W., Berry, J. G., & Sharma, V. (2008). A multicenter study of factors influencing cerebrospinal fluid shunt survival in infants and children. Neurosurgery, 1095–1103. PubMeddoi:10.1227/01.neu.0000325871.60129.23doi:10.1227/01.neu.0000325871.60129.23

Section 2
Case Studies in Healthcare Delivery

Chapter 12
Analyzing Problems of Childhood and Adolescence

Patricia B. Cerrito
University of Louisville, USA

Aparna Sreepada
University of Louisville, USA

ABSTRACT

The study presents the analysis of the results of a health survey that focuses on the health risk behaviors and attitudes in adolescents that result in teenage obesity. Predictive models are built and charts are plotted to map variations in childhood physical health with respect to their weight behavior and to compare the impact of each weight control plan. The analysis provides many useful observations and suggestions that can be helpful in developing child health policies. We also investigate another aspect of child health by examining the severity of immediate risk from disease versus the immediate risk from childhood vaccination by comparing mortality rates from the disease to the mortality rates from the vaccination. Results show that for some individuals, the risk from the vaccine can be higher than the risk from the disease. Therefore, individual risk should be taken into consideration rather than uniform risk across the population.

BACKGROUND

Obesity is a serious problem among teenage children. In fact one in every five children is obese. Children who are obese are at risk of developing high blood pressure, high cholesterol, diabetes, asthma, and other psychological problems. Overweight children are at high risk of becoming overweight adolescents and adults. Some of the main reasons for teenage obesity include overeating, reduced physical activity, sedentary lifestyles and increased TV viewing. (Anonymous-Teenage Obesity-ygoy, 2007) It can cause psychological distress, isolation, low self-esteem, and negative self-image. The current study details a Data Mining approach to analyze and uncover the likely causes and effective measures necessary to prevent teenage obesity.

Body Mass Index is the diagnostic tool to identify obesity problems. BMI is useful to estimate the overall health in comparison with the person's

DOI: 10.4018/978-1-61520-723-7.ch012

Copyright © 2010, IGI Global. Copying or distributing in print or electronic forms without written permission of IGI Global is prohibited.

weight and height. BMI can be influenced by the different weight control behaviors such as exercise, drinking more water, eating low fat food, etc. The purpose of this project is to analyze various weight control measures tried by the students and their impact on their Body Mass Index.

Predictive analytics include a variety of techniques from data mining that analyze the statistical data to make predictions about future events. This paper has also utilized the key features of SAS® Enterprise Miner™ to choose the best predictive model for the study using the student health survey data that records children's attitudes and experiences concerning a wide range of health related behaviors and lifestyle issues. This paper can be a working example to understand the various steps involved in the process of predictive modeling and model assessment.

Every medical treatment has risk that must be compared to the risk of the disease. It is important to calculate the actual risk rather than to make treatment recommendations based upon perceived risk. In addition, risk needs to be re-evaluated as it can change over time. Medical risk also is generally assumed to be uniform across the population; however, risk is individual and treatment must be considered in relationship to individual risk. In addition, only short term risks of treatment are known; long-term risks are not investigated and remain unknown.

There is some disagreement in the general community as to the safety of vaccines, resulting in lower rates of vaccination, particularly for MMR (measles, mumps, and rubella) vaccination under the belief that the vaccine is related to the development of autism. Prior to the start of vaccination, death and occurrence were much higher compared to 2000-2008. (O'Reilly, 2008) Pre-vaccine levels of death from pertussis, for example, were approximately 4000 per year. However, the vaccine has been available since the early 1940's prior antibiotic use and the risk of death cannot be considered the same were the vaccine to be eliminated. Pre-vaccine deaths

were few for measles (440), mumps (39), and rubella (17).

Various states are making personal exemptions from vaccinations easier, and in those states, individual opt-out is increasing. Twenty eight states have a religious exemption only, but another 20 have a personal belief exemption. Fifteen states require just one parental signature to opt out. Only West Virginia and Mississippi do not allow either a religious or personal exemption. Some states such as New York regulate the religious exemption, making it very difficult to acquire. There are calls to make the exemptions more difficult, or to eliminate them altogether for some diseases. (O'Reilly, 2008) However, such decisions should be made with respect to current rather than to historical risk.

SETTING THE STAGE

Childhood Obesity

The data set under study is taken from a survey that was conducted by the Health Behavior in School-Aged Children (HBSC). HSBC data are the result of the United States survey conducted on 11 to 15 year old school children, who are in early adolescence, during the 2001-2002 school years. This is a large collection of data on a wide range of health behaviors and health indicators, and factors that may influence them. A fraction of the data is used for the present study, which primarily concentrates on the students' weight control attitudes.

As the first step to investigate obesity, the data have been cleaned and all the missing values are removed from the observations. The variables that are considered for the study are kept and listed below. A sample with 2000 observations is selected for the analysis.

The following series of variables related to the weight control behaviors are used to study their impact on BMI_COMP:

Gender

BMI_COMP

Q36A - Weight Control Behavior – Exercise

Q36B - Weight Control Behavior - Skip Meals

Q36C - Weight Control Behavior – Fasting

Q36D - Weight Control Behavior - Eat Fewer Sweets

Q36E - Weight Control Behavior - Eat Less Fat

Q36F - Weight Control Behavior - Drink Fewer Soft Drinks

Q36G - Weight Control Behavior - Eat Less

Q36H - Weight Control Behavior - Eat More Fruits/Veggies

Q36I - Weight Control Behavior - Drink More Water

Q36J - Weight Control Behavior - Restrict to 1 Food Group

Q36K - Weight Control Behavior – Vomiting

Q36L - Weight Control Behavior - Use Pills

Q36M - Weight Control Behavior - Smoke More

Q36N - Weight Control Behavior - Under Professional

The variable 'BMI_COMP' takes values 2 and 4, which denote healthy weight and overweight respectively. The variable 'Gender' takes values 1 and 2, which denote 'boy' and 'girl' respectively. The variables in the 'Q36' series take values 1 and 2, which denote the students who adopt it as the primary weight control measure and who do not consider it as a weight control measure, respectively.

BMI_COMP is calculated using not only the child's height and weight but also their age and the other children's statistics that are of the same age and sex. The Bar graphs are plotted for each weight control behavior against gender and BMI_COMP to understand the association between the different weight control measures that are employed by the students and their recorded BMI. Multiple charts are plotted to show the variations in the BMI with respect to students' gender and their primary weight control behavior

to enable comparisons between boys and girls. A grouped Kernel Density Estimation is generated to find and compare the relative impact of each weight control plan on students' weight.

A Kernel Density Estimator is generated using the SAS code node for better visualization and to enable the comparison between the different weight control variables. Kernel Density Estimation is particularly useful to understand which of the weight control measures are more effective on BMI and which measures are most popular in the student community.

As the second step of investigation into teenage obesity, the predictive models, Decision Tree, Neural network and Regression are built to study the effects of other variables on BMI_COMP (Body Mass Index), which is considered to be the pointer towards being physically healthy.

These are the steps followed for the analysis.

1. Pre-Processing the Data
2. Sample
3. Data partition
4. Data analysis
5. Model Assessment

Before launching the dataset for predictive modeling, the irrelevant data elements are eliminated. These include name, school, month, class-id, dist-id, school-id, (student-id is retained to avoid confusion) and many such variables that have no effect on the target variable. The variables that directly contribute to target variable such as weight, height and age are also not included in the analysis.

Since the study is particularly about the health behaviors and attitudes resulting in childhood obesity, the target variable has been changed from nominal to binary by eliminating irrelevant values such as missing and unanswered. Only the variables related to a child's eating habits, physical activity and social behavior are observed for the study. The dataset originally contained 563 variables, but has been reduced to 95 variables. The dataset has nearly 16% of students classified as overweight in a sample size of 10,000.

Childhood Vaccination

Data mining techniques allow us to investigate details to identify risk rather than to depend upon perceptions of risk. In addition, there are now many large healthcare databases that are available to examine using data mining techniques. For this case study, we examined the National Inpatient Sample, available from the Healthcare Cost and Utilization Project. (Anonymous-NIS, 2007) This is a stratified sample from 1000 hospitals across 37 different states. The dataset contains observation weights so that the results can be generalized to the entire US population. While the dataset is incomplete and does not record all cases of the disease, it records those that require hospitalization, or those cases that are the most severe.

To examine the impact of the vaccine, there is only a voluntary reporting system, called VAERS, or the Vaccine Adverse Event Reporting System(Anonymous-VAERS, 2008), sponsored by the Centers for Disease Control (CDC). It is strictly voluntary, so it is not known how representative the information is of the general public. Each report contains a text field describing the

adverse event. In addition, there are multiple columns to list symptoms. There are multiple columns to list the vaccine administered, since there are combinations of vaccines that are often given simultaneously. Therefore, we can examine general patterns, and then examine patterns with respect to a specific vaccine. In addition, there is a field to identify whether the patient recovered from the adverse event, or did not. We can use this information as a target variable in relationship to the patterns of adverse reporting. To be inclusive, we need to add patient demographic information available in the dataset. Attorneys looking for cases use the VAERS (and AERS) reports to find the potential for clients. Therefore, pharmaceutical companies need to be diligent in their investigations as well.

The datasets in VAERS are small enough to be saved in Excel spreadsheets in comma delimited format. It is possible to append multiple years for investigation; however, the reporting forms can change from year to year so that care must be taken to ensure that the files will append properly. In our first examination, we will look at the years 1999 and 2000 restricted to the rotavirus vaccine. Because of the changes in the variables reported, we filter down to report identifier, demographic fields, description of adverse events, columns of symptoms, and vaccine fields. We then look

Figure 1. The effect of 'exercise' on BMI_COMP for boys and girls

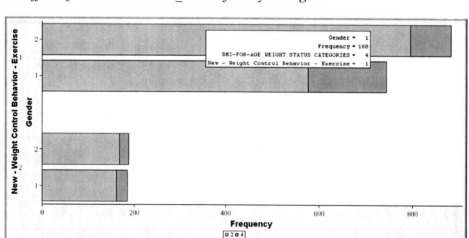

at more general reporting across multiple vaccines.

There were approximately 100,000 reports for the most common childhood vaccinations. Moreover, this reporting system is concerned with immediate adverse effects of the vaccines; therefore, it will not examine the issue of autism and MMR. However, it will have information on death and hospitalization within a short period of time following vaccination.

CASE DESCRIPTION

Childhood Obesity

All the comparisons are shown using bar charts and kernel density estimators.

Weight Control Behaviors

In Figure 1, the X_axis shows frequency, which denotes the number of students. The Y_axis of the graph is classified based on 'Gender' and Weight Control Behavior – Exercise. The bars are subgrouped according to the values taken by BMI_COMP. The blue part denotes the students having healthy weight (2) and the pink part denotes the students having overweight.

The upper part of the graph shows the statistics of boys and the lower part of the graph shows the statistics of girls. The values 1 and 2 denote the students who did exercise to control weight and the students who did not.

According to Figure 1, it can be understood that Exercise, as a weight control measure, is very effective on improving BMI and it is also one of the popular weight control measures taken by boys rather than girls. Out of 750 boys, approximately 580 boys, who did exercise for keeping off extra weight, succeeded in improving their BMI. For girls, even though Exercise is not popular, there is a very small group of them who do not benefit by the Exercise.

The bar chart of the weight control behavior, 'Skip Meals,' (Figure 2) shows that girls tend to Skip Meals more than boys, even though it does not seem to be as effective as Exercise. Approximately 75% of students who adapted this measure have healthy weight.

From the bar chart of Fasting (Figure 3), it is clear that this is one of the least favored weight control behaviors tried by the students. Surprisingly, girls who adapt this measure are more numerous than boys.

It can be noticed from Figure 4 that Eating fewer sweets resulted in healthy BMI for the students. It seems this measure is favored more

Figure 2. The effect of 'skip meals' on BMI_COMP for boys and girls

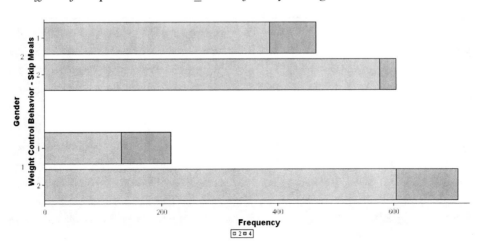

Figure 3. The effect of 'fasting' on BMI_COMP for boys and girls

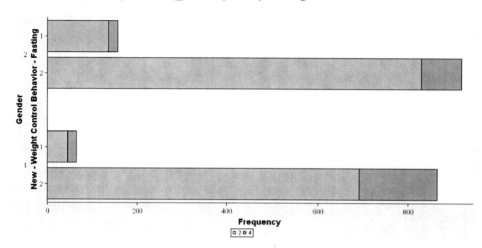

Figure 4. The effect of 'eat fewer sweets' on BMI_COMP for boys and girls

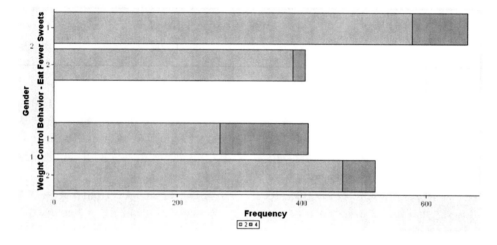

by the girls than the boys and also as high as 80% (approximately) of the girls are found with healthy weight.

Eat Fewer Sweets can be considered to be one of the best weight control measures.

Figure 5 shows the bar chart of the effect of eating less fat on the students' health. Girls who take up this measure are more in number than boys and their results are also impressive. Almost 85% of girls have healthy weight whereas 65% of boys have good results. When considered for girls, this weight control behavior seems to be effective in improving BMI.

Figure 6 shows more than 85% of girls who drank fewer soft drinks kept healthy weight. The pink part of the graph shows 25% of the boys who drank fewer soft drinks in order to control weight gain are overweight. This shows that drinking fewer soft drinks to control weight is not very effective for the boys.

Figure 7 shows another measure that is effective for girls to keep off extra weight.

The graph also shows that there are more students who did not consider it as a weight control option. 'Eat Less' can be considered as moderately effective since, even though it yielded good

Figure 5. The effect of 'eat less fat' on BMI_COMP for boys and girls

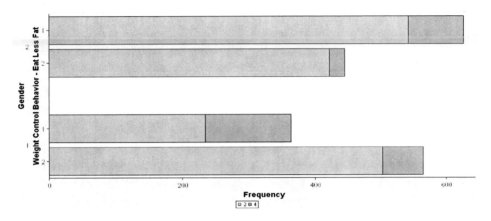

Figure 6. The effect of 'drink fewer soft drinks' on BMI_COMP for boys and girls

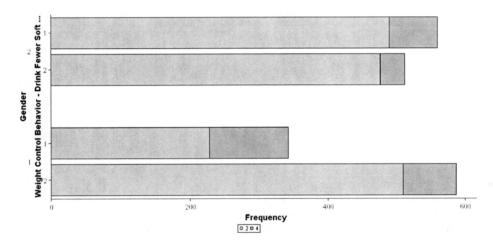

Figure 7. The effect of 'eat less' on BMI_COMP for boys and girls

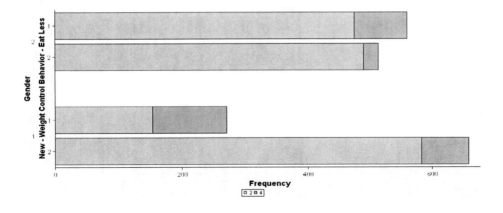

results for girls, approximately 45% of boys were overweight in spite of eating less.

'Restrict to 1 Food Group' (Figure 8) has been the least favored weight control measure taken by the students so far. The results are not considerable even though there are slightly more girls than boys who maintained healthy weight.

According to Figure 9, Eating more fruits and vegetables is one of the best weight control behaviors that gave good results for boys and girls to maintain good health. Almost 90% of the girls and more than 85% of the boys had healthy weight. Also, the results show an improvement over the results yielded by other weight control behaviors such as Eat Fewer Sweets, Eat less Fat and Drink Fewer Soft Drinks with respect to the students with overweight.

Figure 10 shows the bar chart for the variable, 'Drinking More Water'. Almost 90% of the girls who drank more water in order to control their weight had healthy weight. Approximately 80% of boys had healthy weight by drinking more water. The graph also shows that the girls are more inclined to drink more water for weight control than boys.

Figure 11 clearly says that Vomiting is the least opted weight control behavior of the students. There are more students who did not want to try it than the students who tried.

Figure 12 shows that 'Use of pills' is also one of the least opted weight control measures. Although the graph shows that a small number of girls who used pills have healthy weight, the number in the case of boys is even smaller.

Figure 8. The effect of 'restrict to 1 food group' on BMI_COMP for boys and girls

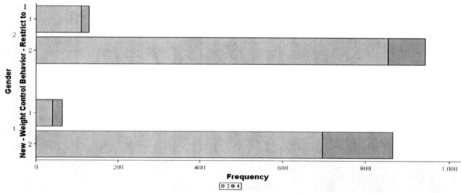

Figure 9. The effect of 'eat more fruits/veggies' on BMI_COMP for boys and girls

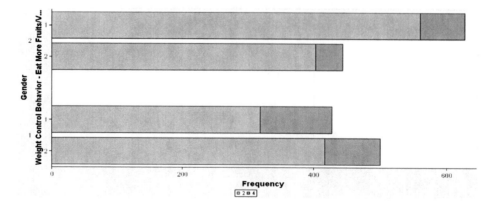

The number of boys and girls who smoke more to be in a healthy weight category are almost the same (Figure 13). Also, there is an equal number of boys and girls who maintained healthy weight using Smoking More as a weight control measure.

Smoke More also is considered to be one of the least favored options to weight control.

Professional Training for weight control is not considered by many students (Figure 14). The girls who were trained under professionals

Figure 10. The effect of 'drinking more water' on BMI_COMP for boys and girls

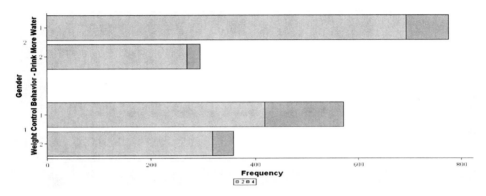

Figure 11. The effect of 'vomiting' as a weight control measure for boys and girls

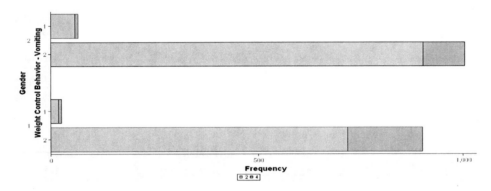

Figure 12. The effect of ' use of pills' to control weight for boys and girls

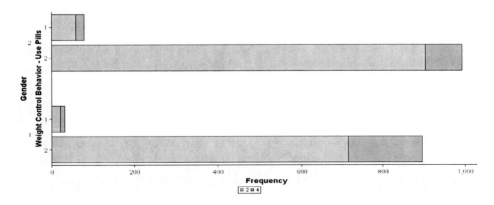

Figure 13. The effect of 'smoking' on bmi_comp for boys and girls

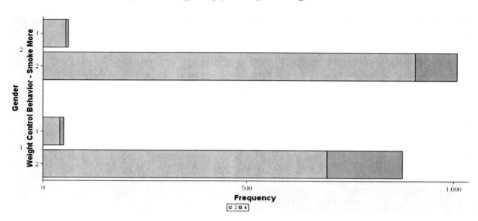

Figure 14. The effect of professional training on bmi_comp for boys and girls

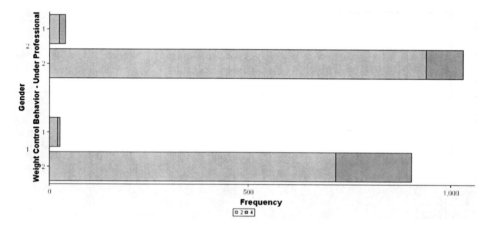

had almost equal numbers of healthy and obese girls. This shows that the weight control measure, Professional Training, did not yield good results. Although the graph shows that a number of girls who used pills have healthy weight when the total population is taken into consideration, it does not provide a significant number.

Figure 15 shows the grouped kernel density estimations of the Q36 series of questions that deal with the different weight control behaviors shown by the students. Figure 15 shows smooth curves for all the variables with two significant peaks, which are around 1 and 2 values simultaneously. The peak at the value 1 shows the density of the population who tried a weight control option and

the peak at value 2 shows the density of population who did not.

As a part of the data analysis, the predictive models have been developed using the Decision Tree, Artificial Neural Networks, Dmine and Logistic Regression nodes. The Model Comparison node is used to compare the results from the modeling nodes and to understand cross-model comparisons and assessments. Figure 16 gives the process flow diagram of the entire project.

Regression predicts the probability that a binary target variable will acquire the event of interest as a function of one or more independent inputs. Logistic regression is the default model since the target variable of the project, Body Mass Index

Figure 15. Overlay of kernel density estimators

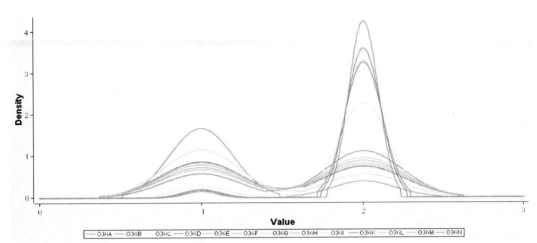

Figure 16. Process flow diagram

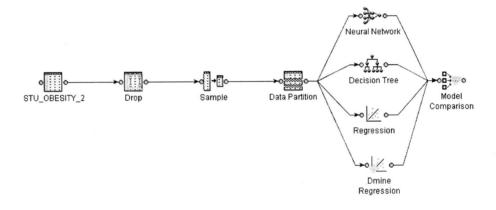

(BMP_COMP), is binary. It has two levels that are represented by healthy weight and overweight, or 2 and 4.

For this analysis, the stepwise selection model is chosen for selecting the variables. The Entry Significance Level is set to 0.01 and Stay Significance Level is set to 0.05. The Validation Misclassification Rate is considered as the Model Selection Criterion.

The results of the Decision node are shown in Figure 17. Here, the leaf with the least intensity of color denotes the highest rate of healthy students who are not considered obese.

The Tree in Figure 17 is a collection of hierarchical rules that divide the data into segments. The root node is the entire dataset and the terminal nodes denote a decision made and applied to the observations. The Decision rules give many insights on the effects of the variables on the target variable, BMI_COMP. Here, the Tree is classified based on the two variables 'Think about Body', 'Watch TV Weekdays', 'New-Weight Control Behavior - Eat less', 'Time Homework Weekdays' and 'Gender'.

The variable, 'Think about Body,' takes values 1, 2, 3, 4 and 5.

Figure 17. Complete view of the decision tree

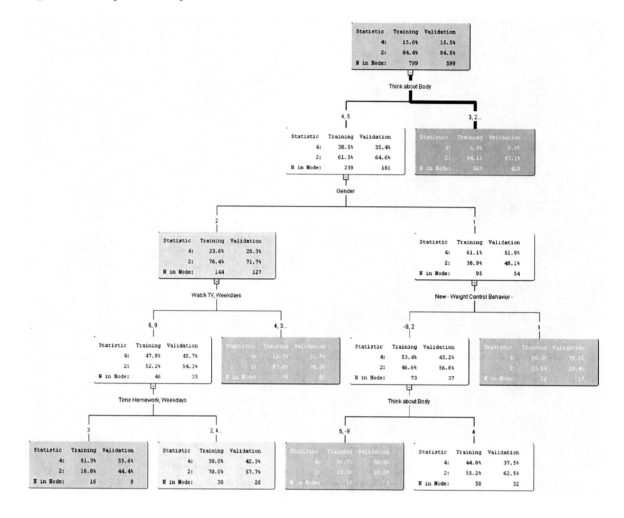

1 Much too thin
2 A bit too thin
3 About the right size
4 A bit too fat
5 Much too fat

'Gender' takes values 1 and 2, which indicates boy and girl respectively.

Here each segment contains both healthy weight and overweight students. The following rule illustrates that the girls who think they are overweight but control watching T.V. for less than 1 hr during weekdays have a healthy weight. On the contrary, girls who spend more than 3 hours watching T.V. have a close proximity to become obese.

```
IF Watch TV, Weekdays IS ONE OF: 4 3
AND Gender EQUALS 2
AND Think about Body IS ONE OF: 4 5
THEN
4: 21.7%
2: 78.3%
```

Another rule classifies boys, who think that they are overweight and do not eat less as follows.

Figure 18. ROC for the models

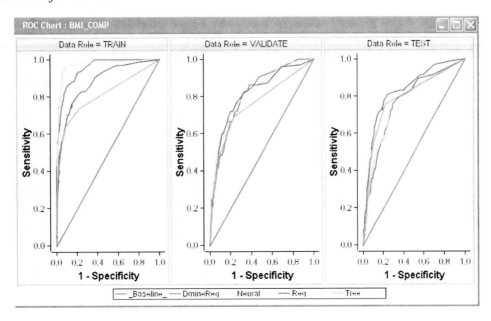

```
IF 'Think about Body' is 4
AND New - Weight Control Behavior - Eat
Less IS ONE OF: -9 2
AND Gender EQUALS 1
THEN
4: 44.8%
2: 55.2%
```

The models developed are compared for their performance using the Model Comparison node. The validation Misclassification Rate is taken as the selection criterion property. If the students, overweight or healthy weight are correctly classified as overweight or healthy weight, then there would not be any misclassification; otherwise, there will be a misclassification. The model with the smallest misclassification rate should beconsidered as the best fit.

The Figure 18 shows Regression, Dmine Regression, Neural Network and Decision Tree models together for the training, validation and test datasets.

The above ROC charts map the sensitivity of the test and indicates the accuracy of the model. Here, the ROC charts for the test dataset are considered to compare the models. For the test data, Logistic Regression and Decision Tree show more accurate results. By the outcome of ROC charts, LR seems to be the right fit for the data.

According to the results in Figure 19, Regression clearly has the best cumulative lift, which is slightly higher than Decision Tree. Both the ROC Chart and the lift curves show Regression as the better model than Decision Tree.

From Table 1, the Dmine Regression node and Neural Network nodes have the highest misclassification rate at 18%. Also, they have the highest Average Error Function. Thus, Dmine Regression and ANN do not provide good models for the data.

Decision Tree has the lower misclassification than Regression. The lower misclassification rate indicates a higher accuracy in the model classification. The ROC curves in Figure 18 reflect that Regression and Decision Tree are the first and second good models for considering the best. Also, the Regression and Decision Tree results are very close with 0.83 and 0.80 of ROC Index respectively from Table 1. Regression also has the average error function at 0.41.

Figure 19. Lift curves for the models

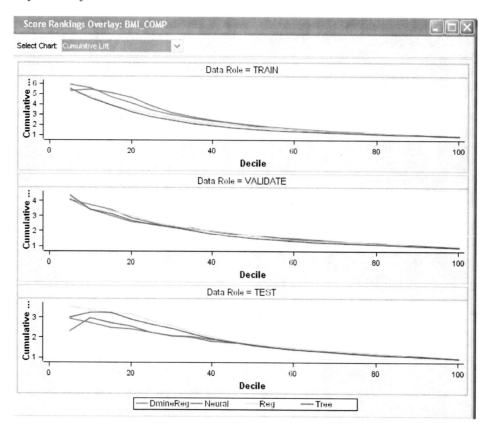

Hence, considering the misclassification rate and ROC index from the Fit Statistics of the Model Assessment node and ROC curves in Figure 18, the Decision Tree model has been understood as the best predictive model for the student health survey data.

Childhood Vaccinations

Rotavirus

We start with the adverse events reported for the rotavirus in 1999 and 2000 (the dataset for 2000 reports on 1999 administration of the vaccine). There were 143 adverse reports in 1999 and 26 reported in 2000 when the rotavirus, RotaShield was removed from the market because of a risk of Intussusceptions, or a blockage of the intestine that required surgery to repair. It is also a life-threatening condition. There were 23 reports of the symptom in the VAERS database (16% of total reports). The vaccine was only available on the market for 9 months prior to removal. The rate of the event was estimated as 1 in 10,000 to 1 in 32,000, with the highest risk occurring between 3 to 14 days after the first dose. (Bines, 2005) There were just 15 cases that motivated market removal. (Anonymous-MMWR, 2004) A second study found an occurrence rate of 35 per 100,000. (O'Ryan, Lucero, Pena, & Valenzuela, 2003) As it turned out, there was an association of intussusceptions to infants more than 90 days old, suggesting that the problem could have been avoided by earlier administration of the first dose. (Simonsen, Viboud, Elixhauser, Taylor, & Kapikian, 2005)

Two new vaccines without the risk of intussusceptions, Rotarix and RotaTeq, were approved

Table 1. Fit statistics for test data set

Statistic	Dmine Reg	Neu	Reg	Tree
Kolmogorov-Smirnov Statistic	0.47	0.44	0.57	0.54
Average Squared Error	0.14	0.14	0.12	0.11
Roc Index	0.77	0.78	0.83	0.80
Average Error Function.	0.51	0.57	0.41	.
Frequency of Classified Cases	602	.	.	.
Divisor for TASE	1204	1204	1204	1204
Error Function.	618.3	692.19	497.25	.
Gini Coefficient	0.53	0.55	0.66	0.58
Bin-Based Two-Way Kolmogorov-Smirnov Statistic	0.45	0.43	0.57	0.53
Maximum Absolute Error	1	1	1	0.94
Misclassification Rate	0.18	0.18	0.15	0.14
Lower 95% Conf. Limit for TMISC.	.	.	0.12	.
Upper 95% Conf. Limit for TMISC.	.	.	0.18	.
Mean Squared Error.	.	0.14	0.12	.
Sum of Frequencies	602	602	602	602
Root Average Squared Error	0.37	0.38	0.34	0.34
Root Mean Squared Error.	.	0.38	0.34	
Sum of Squared Errors	167.25	173.9	138.87	136.18
Sum of Weights Times Freqs	.	1204	1204	1204
Number of Wrong Classifications.	108	107	.	.

in 2006. (Rotavirus, 2008) Using data from 2007 and 2008, there are 975 total adverse event reports for the rotavirus vaccines, of which 79 were for intussusceptions (8% of total reports), half of the previous rate. If 16% is too many, why is 8% acceptable? It must, however, be recalled that these percentages are with respect to the adverse event reporting and not to the general population of infants who received the vaccines. Should the new vaccines be examined more carefully for the rate of occurrence, which is clearly not zero? It is also known that an avoidance of day care and/or full time nursing results in a virtually zero likelihood of acquiring the rotavirus. Given the nonzero probability of a rare, life-threatening occurrence, should physicians make universal recommendations in favor of the vaccine, or recommend based upon the child's risk?

Table 2 shows the text clusters identified for the rotavirus vaccine in 1999-2000. Table 3 shows the text clusters for the years 2007-2008 with the modified rotavirus vaccine. Because of the manner in which text symptoms are entered, there are some clusters that provide no real information. These are clusters 4, 5, 8, 9, 11, and 12; Intussusceptions are identified in cluster 7.

Because there are six clusters that do not convey any information concerning adverse events, we filter out all of the observations from these clusters, and then re-cluster, yielding a total of four clusters from the remaining 6 original clusters (Table 4).

Intussusception is now in cluster 4, which contains 146 observations with diarrhea and vomiting in the remaining three clusters. Intussusception is related to a symptom of bleeding. These clusters

Table 2. Text clusters for early rotavirus vaccine

Cluster #	Descriptive Terms	Frequency	Percentage
1	Viral, +,do, constipation, +experience, + test, positive, bowel, + not, rotavirus, recv	10	0.059
2	+ child, mom, mild diarrhea, mild, evening, same, same evening, diarrhea, recv, + resolve	9	0.053
3	High, fever, pt recv vax, devel, vax, territory representative, territory, rash, recv, p/vax pt devel	42	0.248
4	+ enema, barium, + reduce, surgery, intussusceptions, + barium enema, bloody, hosp, + bloody stool, + stool	26	0.213
5	Physician, old, + report, + infant, + receive, + mother, shield, rota, information, + develop	32	0.189
6	Exp, + rotavirus antigen, + antigen, + last, diarrhea, severe, p/vax, w/in, positive, + stool	40	0.237

Table 3. Text clusters for modified rotavirus vaccine

Cluster #	Descriptive Terms	Frequency	Percentage
1	+ vaccine, + develop, + not, + day, + have, + month, rotateq, + report, + old, + patient	112	0.1149
2	+ stool, + day, + diarrhea, + experience, + have, first, rotate, + patient, + request, additional	127	0.1302
3	+ stool, other, + experience, medical, + month, + old, + patient, + product, + attention, quality	114	0.1169
4	+ register, + week, nurse, first,+ dose, rotate, + vaccinate, + receive, + seek, additional	122	0.1252
5	+ obtain, + individual, identifying, distinguish, + mention, + attempt, + make, + provide, + report, + week	13	0.0133
6	Hospital, rotavirus, + diarrhea, + recover, + old, + month, quality, + complaint, + product, + patient	57	0.0585
7	Intussusceptions, important, + consider, + event, other, + recover, + experience, medical, + patient, + complaint	63	0.0646
8	+ twin, source, several, + symptom, same, + report, + month, + old, + request, + have	13	0.0133
9	+ involve, + month, quality, + complaint, + product, + old, first, + request, additionalm + experience	146	0.1497
10	+ outcome, unknown, po, + report, + attention, + seek, + vomit, medical, + develop, unspecified	111	0.0038
11	+ register, + problem, nurse, + week, + involve, + seek, + attention, + product, quality, + not	39	0.04
12	Live, rotavirus, human-bovine, + vaccine, + month, + report, + patient, + receive, + request, + attention	58	0.0595

suggest that, while the severe adverse effect does not occur as often, it is not yet a completely safe vaccine.

Common Vaccinations

We next examine the data more generally, independent of vaccine, to see if the patterns of adverse events can predict the vaccine. This type of analysis can be used prospectively to find potential problems with medications. Because of the size of the dataset, we limit our analysis to the following vaccines:

- DTAP (Diptheria, etc.) 32,833 reports
- Flu 20,079 reports
- Varicella (Chicken Pox) 14,924 reports
- HPV4 (Gardasil) 10,798 reports

Table 4. Filtered clusters for modified rotavirus vaccine

Cluster #	Descriptive Terms	Frequency	Percentage
1	History, diagnostic, + perform, + lab, + allergy, rotavirus, concomitant, + recover, + old, + week, quality, + complaint, + product, + diarrhea, male, female, + month, + vomit, + day, first	139	0.2945
2	Assistant, source, same, several, + vaccine, + note, po, + report, + vomit, concomitant, + vaccinate, rotate, unknown, + time, female, + outcome, + dose, first, + receive, + request	65	0.1801
3	Unknown, + attention, + diarrhea, + outcome, + seek, nurse, + register, severe, unspecified, + time, + report, po, + develop, + vomit, + dose, subsequently, + request, rotate, + receive, + vaccinate	102	0.2161
4	+ stool, bloody, + event, + review, internal, blood, other, + consider, important, + determine, intussusceptions, + involve, + week, medical, + month, + not, + old, + have, male, + day	146	0.3093

- HEP (Hepatitis) 11,110 reports
- MMR 8,178 reports

The first clustering in SAS Text Miner (Table 5) has some unnecessary clusters that focus on the reporting rather than on the adverse event. We filter these out, and re-cluster.

It is clear that most of the reports are fairly mild, except for cluster 1 that discusses death and autopsy. Clusters 2, 3, and 4 suggest an allergic reaction to the vaccine. Other concerns suggested occur in cluster 7 with developmental delays and autism, although the connection to the vaccine is not clear. Cluster 11 suggests seizures that are also of concern. Table 6 gives the relationship of vaccine to cluster.

DTAP appears in clusters 2, 4, and 12 in considerably higher proportions compared to the total number of adverse events. Clusters 2 and 4 indicate swelling and rash at the injection site; cluster 12 is more serious indicating that the patient was admitted. The MMR vaccine appears in much higher proportion in cluster #7, listing the possibility of developmental disorders and autism. There have been numerous studies conducted that indicate MMR is not related to autism; however, anecdotal stories continue to persist. The new HPV4 vaccine (Gardasil) appears higher in cluster 11, indicating an adverse event of seizures. This side effect has not yet been discussed in the medical literature, although an article in MMWR discusses a problem of syncope, or general weak-ness.(Anonymous-MMWR, 2008) However, the attorneys have already started soliciting clients based upon the reports of seizures. (Anonymous-attorney, 2008)

The flu vaccine, too, appears to have a high proportion of reports in cluster 11 with seizures. However, reports in the medical literature suggest that these adverse reports are not real. (Tosh, Boyce, & Poland, 2008) Another report for flu that is much larger than expected is cluster 8. This is for a rash or lesion at the injection site, and similar to cluster 3, which also has a high proportion of Flu vaccine reports. A high proportion of reports for the HEP vaccine occur in clusters 8, 9, and 16. Clusters 8 and 9 focus mostly on irritation, swelling, and rash at the injection site. Cluster 16 is more serious with nausea and vomiting. In this group, there is a danger of dehydration, particularly since the vaccine is administered to infants.

Pertussis

We look at a number of diseases for which childhood vaccinations are available, and look to the risk of the disease. The first we want to examine is pertussis. In 1985, the recommendations were immunizations at 2,4, and 6 months, 12-15 months, and 6 years, but none beyond 10 years of age. (Anonymous-1985, recommendations, 1985) Those guidelines were still in place in 2002. (Gardner, Pickering, Orenstein, Gershon, & Nichol, 2002) However, by 2007, the recom-

Table 5. Clustering of VAERS, 1999-2008

Cluster Number	Descriptive Terms	Percentage
1	Unresponsive, information, + death, + report, + reveal, autopsy, report, + sid, + infant, + die, + old, sudden, + find, certificate, + autopsy	1
2	Er, + erport, + call, + do, Tylenol, + not, + have, + state, + give, + red, + child, + leg, +swell, + mom, + see	7
3	+ face, neck, + start, + red, + trunk, + body, + back, popular, + low, + itch, + fever, + chest, + leg, + extremity, + develop	7
4	+ body, + give, + develop, + minute, Benadryl, + symptom, + vaccine, + itch, + fever, + chest, + leg, + extremity, + develop	7
5	+ shoot, + receive, + vaccine, + last, er, + throat, + state, + not, + flu, + back, + call, + minute, + symptom, feel, have	10
6	+ swell, + deltoid, + elbow, + pain, + right arm, upper + leave, + leave arm, + shoot, erythema, + red, + arm, + shoulder, + right, + upper arm	9
7	+ follow, + eye, + do, language, + month, + not, developmental, + disorder, + age, speech, autism, + diagnose, + contact, + behavior, + delay	1
8	Exp, + rash, chickenpox, pt exp, pt recv vac, devel, same, + lesion, inj, rxn, approx, pi, + late, + day, rpt	5
9	+ deltoid, + raise, + tender, + site, + red, Benadryl, + area, redness, + arm, + leave, + inch, + compress, + induration, upper, + warm	6
10	+ call, + receive, + complain, + report, + give, + vaccine, + symptom, + develop, + state, + have, + patient, + see, + hour, + reaction, + injection	5
11	+ generalize, + minute, _ febrile seizure, + admit, temp, + second, + have, + episode, + follow + eye, + seizure, febrile, + hospital, + activity, + last	3
12	+ vaccination, vax, + do, + admit, + experience, + week, + time, + not, information, + dose, + post, + report, medical, + have, + receive	11
13	+ site, + injection site, + induration, + arm, + warm, + area, + itch, + pain, + injection, + red, warmth, + touch, + swell, erythema, + reaction	6
14	+ immunization, + swell, + local reaction, + leave erythema, cellulitis, dtap, local, + deltoid, + site, warmth, + give, + reaction, redness, + vaccine	4
15	Redress, + induration, + leave thigh, erythema. + site, + right thigh, + area, warmth, anterior, cm, + swell, + leg, upper, + red, + thigh	5

mendations were altered to include a pertussis vaccination one time under the age of 64 if that individual did not have one after the previously recommended 6 years of age. (Middleton, Zimmerman, & Mitchell, 2007) This added recommendation occurred with the development of an adolescent/adult vaccination that was previously unavailable.

In the National Inpatient Sample, there are 1303 inpatients with a diagnosis of pertussis out of a total number of 8 million inpatient events. Of that number, 1090, or 83% of those patients hospitalized were under one year of age. Approximately

175 of those patients have no co-morbidities; another 134 patients have an additional diagnosis of symptoms involving the respiratory system and asthma. The remaining patients also have the diagnoses of acute bronchitis, diseases of the esophagus, and pneumonia.

Of the 1303 patients, 11 died while in the hospital. Using the sample weights to generalize to the entire population, this would be the equivalent of 54 deaths nationally from pertussis and 6484 hospitalizations. All of the deaths were in patients under the age of 1 year; 10 of the deaths were in patients under the age of 3 months. Ap-

Table 6. Vaccine proportions in clusters

Cluster #	DTAP	FLU	HEP	HPV4	MMR	VARCEL
1	249 (10%)	1312 (21%)	483 (19%)	121 (5%)	281 (11%)	92 (4%)
2	3407 (91%)	119 (3%)	55 (1%)	3 (0%)	90 (2%)	75 (2%)
3	1181 (27%)	1726 (40%)	658 (15%)	269 (6%)	298 (7%)	224 (5%)
4	5308 (73%)	511 (7%)	686 (9%)	107 (1%)	388 (5%)	319 (4%)
5	354 (49%)	60 (8%)	118 (16%)	14 (2%)	153 (21%)	19 (3%)
6	2314 (48%)	1271 (27%)	291 (6%)	164 (3%)	227 (5%)	504 (11%)
7	1708 (32%)	625 (12%)	651 (12%)	124 (2%)	1438 (27%)	843 (16%)
8	302 (11%)	2182 (79%)	148 (5%)	53 (2%)	44 (2%)	32 (1%)
9	957 (24%)	996 (25%)	800 (20%)	786 (20%)	239 (6%)	180 (5%)
10	2212 (36%)	1622 (26%)	1281 (21%)	145 (2%)	506 (8%)	442 (7%)
11	651 (15%)	2128 (49%)	748 (17%)	295 (7%)	407 (9%)	106 (2%0
12	1125 (61%)	221 (12%)	148 (8%)	51 (3%)	248 (13%)	62 (3%)
13	1375 (34%)	1138 (29%)	689 (17%)	201 (5%)	345 (9%)	239 (6%)
14	6740 (68%)	1628 (16%)	429 (4%)	174 (2%)	252 (3%)	711 (7%)
15	1813 (45%)	959 (24%)	608 (15%)	222 (6%)	300 (7%)	121 (3%)
16	690 (21%)	501 (15%)	685 (21%)	0	335 (10%)	1033 (32%)
Total	30386 (44%)	16999 (25%)	8477 (12%)	2729 (4%)	5551 (8%)	5002 (7%)

proximately 60% of the hospitalizations were paid through private insurance with another 30% paid through Medicaid. Interestingly enough, 36% of the patients were in the top income quartile; only 16% were in the lowest income quartile. It indicates that more affluent patients are more likely to acquire the disease. These weights appear to over-count the number of deaths, reportedly at 12 per year, although other reports tend to validate the estimated number of hospitalizations. (Anonymous-MMWRpertussis, 2002)

In the VAERS reporting system, there were 32,000 reports concerning the use of the DTAP, or Diptheria, tetanus, and pertussis vaccination combination. The pertussis vaccine is almost always administered in combination with these other vaccines, so that it would be difficult to separate adverse effects for each one separately. However, it is not necessary to make such a separation since we are looking at the difference in risk of vaccination versus disease. Of the 32,000 reports on DTAP, 444 reported death and 482

reported life-threatening problems; 2279 were admitted to the hospital with 13,243 trips to the emergency room. Another 391 reported permanent disability. While the voluntary reporting may have questionable accuracy, we can use text analysis to investigate the reports to determine just how serious they were. Note that there is a higher ratio of deaths to hospitalizations for the voluntary reporting of vaccine adverse events compared to the ratio for the disease. It is feasible to assume that not all hospitalizations were reported, and it is not possible to assign weights to generalize to the population at large.

To investigate the reports in the VAERS system, we use text analysis, restricting attention to those patients serious enough to require hospital admission or who reported death. We want to investigate the description of symptoms to see if patterns exist in the data. We will first look at all of the admitted patients, and then separately, those who are identified as died or as having life threatening problems. Table 7 shows

Table 7. Text clusters of patients hospitalized after DTAP administration

Cluster Number	Descriptive Terms	Frequency
1	w/, sz, vax, p/vax, pt, devel, hosp, exp, adm, recv, + vomit, + diarrhea, + cry, + mom, + late, + reveal, + fever, + stool, + day	226
2	+ symptom, + rash, + cough, + fever, + develop, with, + admit, + summary, + reaction, + antibiotic, + discharge, dos, + state, + give, + day, + see, + immunization, on, + follow, + swell	478
3	+ reaction, upper, + thigh, + injection, + site, redness, erythema, + arm, + antibiotic, + red, cellulitis, + leg, + area, + warm, right, + swell, + leave, + pain, + discharge, + admit	243
4	Abdominal, + reveal, + surgery, air, bloody, + bloody stool, contrast, intussusceptions, dos, + bowel, reduction, + vomit, + reduce, d/c, + enema, + stool, barium, + pain, + record, + present	160
5	+ minute, + hour, + last, + activity, febrile, + seizure, + generalize, + episode, + eye, + fever, er, + start, + state, + dtap, + post, + have, + follow, + vaccination, + record, + day	424
6	+ hospitalize, + report, concomitant, additional information, unspecified, female, + vaccinate, male, + concern, additional, prevnar, + physician, information, + old, + include, + dose, + recover, + event, + month, + vaccine	281
7	+ breathe, + episode, + not, + pale, + back, + have, + call, + cry, + shoot, + eye, + hour, + minute, but, + give, + child, + do, + state, + up, in no	467

Table 8. Text clusters of patients with life threatening diagnoses after DTAP administration

Cluster Number	Descriptive Terms	Frequency
1	+ fever, vax, + have, + do, + vomit, + hospital, + day, + not, no	239
2	+ vomit, bloody, + enema, reduction, + bloody stoolo, intussusceptions, + reduce, dos, + stool	71
3	+ dose, information, + old, + vaccine, + month, + event, + give, medical, + patient, + receive	233
4	+ death, + cause, + report, + sid, crib, + state, as, + find, autopsy report, + infant	233
5	+ seizure, + have, + hour, + fever, er, with, + child, + day, + state, + hospital	195

the text clusters defined from the 2279 cases of hospitalization. Table 8 gives the text clusters for the patients with life-threatening concerns. They mostly include vomiting, diarrhea, bloody stool, and seizures. There appears to be little difference in the diagnoses, only in the severity.

It is also possible to investigate the age of the individual at death. Figure 20 gives the general age; Figure 21 gives the age restricted to children less than 1 year. While there were no deaths beyond the age of one for the disease, there are several reported deaths from the vaccine. Most of the deaths occur in the 2-4 month range when children are given the first and second dose of DTAP.

MMR

We also look at the MMR. The primary consideration concerning this vaccine is whether MMR is related to autism, and that cannot be studied using the VAERS system, so we also look at more immediate problems. Historical information indicates that death from any of the three MMR diseases was relatively small pre-vaccine. (O'Reilly, 2008) We perform a similar analysis using the National Inpatient Sample and the VAERS reporting system to investigate death and morbidity. The recommendation for vaccine is to administer it at 12-15 weeks, 4-6 years of age, and 11-12 years.

In the National Inpatient Sample, there is a reported 126 hospitalizations for measles, mumps,

Figure 20. Deaths by age after DTAP administration

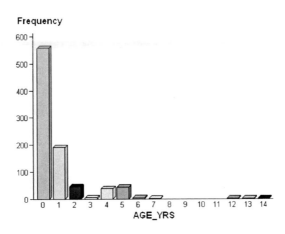

Figure 21. Deaths by age after DTAP administration restricted to less than one year of age

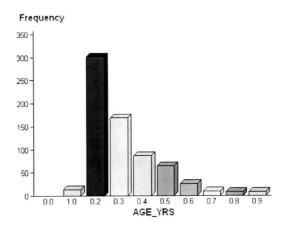

or rubella. Of that number, 2 resulted in death. Using the weights would define approximately 11 deaths nationally, and 630 cases total. Figure 22 has the age distribution of the reported cases.

Similarly, the VAERS system reported 30 deaths, 126 life-threatening conditions, 438 admitted to the hospital, and 191 with disabilities. A total of 4065 went to the emergency room. Therefore, the vaccine is a relatively benign. Of the deaths, 2/3 of them were at the age of one, timed at the first dose administration.

Of course, the most crucial problem was not mortality in this case, but in mothers passing along the infection to their newborns. In fact, the schedule was changed to include a booster at 11-12 years of age because young adults in their early twenty's had become the most susceptible to an infection of measles. As shown in Figure 22, that age remains susceptible.

HPV Vaccination

The HPV vaccine has just become available. Nevertheless, there are already 21 reported deaths immediately following vaccine administration. (Smith, 2008) In this case, there is the additional

Figure 22. Age distribution for MMR cases

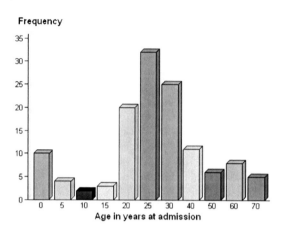

issue that HPV itself is rarely immediately life-threatening and is only life-threatening in later life with the potential onset of cervical cancer. In contrast, the vaccine is recommended for girls as young as 9 years of age. In the investigation of medical decision making, individuals are frequently surveyed on the question of whether it is better to endure 20 years of imperfect health versus the possibility of 10 years of perfect health followed by death. This is one of the primary questions in the administration of the HPV vaccine. Is it better to die at age 45 of cervical cancer, or to risk death at 13 from the HPV vaccine?

There is an additional question as well. Unlike the previous infectious diseases discussed, HPV is spread through sexual intercourse. Therefore, behavior can increase or decrease the risk of the disease. If an individual avoids sexual intercourse, there is virtually no risk of acquiring HPV, and no need of the vaccine. Such individuals have no risk from the disease, and no risk from the vaccine.

In the years 2006-2008 in the VAERS reporting system, there were 15 deaths, 97 life threatening conditions, 4511 visits to the emergency department that resulted in 261 hospitalizations. As a result of the vaccination, there were reports of 177 disabilities that were permanent and 1674 reports that the patients did not fully recover from the

vaccine. There were approximately 8400 reports related to the HPV vaccine.

Text analysis first found a total of 11 clusters. Several of the clusters were just identified as reporting symptoms. Therefore, the data were filtered to those reporting specific adverse effects and then re-clustered. Table 9 gives the remaining clusters.

The three different types of problems are clear from these clusters. Cluster #3 consists primarily of a rash; cluster #2 consists of more serious swelling at the injection site. Cluster #1 contains the most serious adverse events that include vomiting, fever, and pain. This cluster is almost comparable to the number of patients hospitalized. We can examine the relationship between the text clusters and the adverse events in the dataset. Table 10 shows the relationship between the two variables.

It appears that there is a much higher percentage of patients hospitalized in cluster #2 compared to cluster #1 even though cluster #1 seems to have more critical adverse events. Table 11 compares the life threatening events.

It appears again that patients in cluster #2 are more likely to be diagnosed with a life-threatening condition compared to the other two clusters of adverse effects. In addition, all of the reported deaths are related to cluster #2, suggesting that

Table 9. Text clusters for adverse events for HPV vaccine

Cluster Number	Descriptive Terms	Frequency
1	+ vomit, + fever, nausea, + headache, + hour, + experience, + symptom, + pain, + day, + vaccine	341
2	+ swell, pt, + leave, + arm, + pain, + feel, + give, in, + injection, + vaccine	777
3	+ year, + rash, + concern, first, + dose, information, + female, additional information, + request, additional	348

Table 10. Relationship of hospitalization to cluster

Table of _CLUSTER_ by Hospitalization			
Cluster ID	Hospitalization		Total
Frequency Row Pct Col Pct	N	Y	
1	330 96.77 23.55	11 3.23 16.92	341
2	724 93.18 51.68	53 6.82 81.54	777
3	347 99.71 24.77	1 0.29 1.54	348
Total	1401	65	1466

Table 11. Cluster by life threatening conditions

Table of _CLUSTER_ by Life-THREAT			
Cluster ID	Life-THREAT		Total
Frequency Row Pct Col Pct	N	Y	
1	340 99.71 23.66	1 0.29 3.45	341
2	750 96.53 52.19	27 3.47 93.10	777
3	347 99.71 24.15	1 0.29 3.45	348
Total	1437	29	1466

swelling at the injection site is a more crucial concern than the nausea and vomiting reported in cluster #1. In contrast, for 2005, in the National Inpatient Sample, there were 1363 diagnoses of HPV out of a total 8 million inpatient visits and 2660 inpatient visits for cervical cancer. Of that number, none of the patients with cervical cancer died in the hospital and 2 of the patients with HPV died.

There are some real competing risks concerning the decision to use the HPV vaccination. There is a small risk of death from the HPV vaccine when it is administered. However, when it occurs, that risk is small and occurs at a young age; death from cervical cancer occurs much later in life.

CURRENT AND FUTURE CHALLENGES FACING THE ORGANIZATION

The survey questionnaire covers a vast range of issues about an early adolescent student's eating habits, social behavior and lifestyle. These data have a tremendous scope to be helpful to provide rich research material for many interesting health studies that influence child health policies nationally and internationally.

A fraction of the data is used for the analysis to generate the predictive models to estimate the students' health with other independent variables. The factors that may affect the child's obesity are incorporated in the data analysis. Multiple models are developed and tested. Of them, Decision Tree is found to be the best fit for the estimation of the dependent variable. The study also gives us insights on the weight control behaviors that are most popular and least popular among the student community. The results indicate that the majority of the weight control measures are more successful with girls rather than boys, except for Exercising. Exercising, Eating more fruits and vegetables, drinking more water and eating less fat are shown to be the best methods to keep healthy weight. Using pills, Vomiting, Fasting and Smoking more are some of the least effective methods that helped the students keep their weight healthy.

The most effective weight control behaviors that helped the students have healthy weight are

Q36A - Exercise
Q36D - Eat Fewer Sweets
Q36H - Eat More Fruits/Veggies and
Q36I - Drink More Water

The least effective weight control behaviors that are observed are

Q36C - Fasting
Q36J - Restrict to 1 Food Group
Q36K - Vomiting
Q36L - Use Pills
Q36M - Smoke More
Q36N - Under Professional

Weight control behaviors that yielded mixed results for both boys and girls:

Q36E - Weight Control Behavior - Eat Less Fat
Q36F - Weight Control Behavior - Drink Fewer Soft Drinks
Q36B - Weight Control Behavior - Skip Meals
Q36G - Weight Control Behavior - Eat Less

Medical practice changes slowly, and its use of modern techniques of analysis also changes slowly. Much patient information still exists in paper records, making it very difficult to determine actual risk based upon evidence. Information is contained within separate systems and there is very little integration of this information. It also relies upon voluntary rather than mandatory reporting so that there are many unknowns concerning non-reported illnesses. In addition, it relies upon historical, pre-vaccine and often, pre-antibiotic estimates of risk from disease rather than to modify risk values in the present time. For this reason, outside organizations are starting to challenge the vaccine recommendations and a small group of individuals are refusing them altogether.

The study's findings can be helpful for the relevent health initiatives and these can be further extended to develop different strategies to address the problems relating to child health.

REFERENCES

Ait-Khaled, N., Enarson, D., Bissell, K., & Billo, N. (2007). Access to inhaled corticosteroids is key to improving quality of care for asthma in developing countries. *Allergy, 62*(3), 230–236. doi:10.1111/j.1398-9995.2007.01326.x

Anonymous-1985 recommendations. (1985). Diphtheria, tetanus, and pertussis: guidelines for vaccine prophylaxis and other preventive measures. Recommendation of the Immunization Practices Advisory Committee. Centers for Disease Control, Department of Health and Human Services. *Annals of Internal Medicine, 103*(6), 896-905.

Anonymous-asthma. (2007). Trends in asthma morbidity and mortality. Retrieved September, 2008, from http://www.lungusa.org/site/c.dvLUK9O0E/b.22884/k.7CE3/Asthma_Research__Studies.htm

Anonymous-attorney. (2008). *Gardasil Lawyers*. Retrieved 2008, from http://www.brownandcrouppen.com/gardasil-attorney.asp

Anonymous-Mayoasthma. (2008). Asthma. Retrieved September, 2008, from http://www.mayoclinic.com/health/asthma/DS00021/DSECTION=treatments-and-drugs

Anonymous-MEPS. (2007). Medical Expenditure Panel Survey [Electronic Version]. Retrieved December, 2007, from http://www.meps.ahrq.gov/mepsweb/.

Anonymous-MMWR. (2004, September 3). Suspension of rotavirus vaccine after reports of intussusception-United States, 1999. *MMWR*, 786–789.

Anonymous-MMWR. (2008). Syncope after vaccination-United States, January 2005-2007. *MMWR, 57*(17), 457–460.

Anonymous-MMWRpertussis. (2002). Pertussis-United States, 1997-2000. *MMWR, 51*(4), 73–76.

Anonymous-NIHasthma. (2008). What is Asthma? Retrieved September, 2008, from http://www.nhlbi.nih.gov/health/dci/Diseases/Asthma/Asthma_WhatIs.html

Anonymous-NIS. (2007). *Overview of the National Inpatient Sample*. Retrieved December, 2007, from http://www.hcup-us.ahrq.gov/nis-overview.jsp.

Anonymous-VAERS. (2008). Vaccine Adverse Event Reporting System. Retrieved September, 2008, from http://vaers.hhs.gov/

Austin, P. C., Alter, D. A., & Tu, J. V. (2003). The use of fixed- and random-effects models for classifying hospitals as mortality outliers: a monte carlos assessment. *Medical Decision Making, 23*, 526–539. doi:10.1177/0272989X03258443

Barlow, W. E., White, E., Ballard-Barbash, R., Vacek, P. M., Titus-Ernstoff, L., & Carney, P. A. (2006). Prospective breast cancer risk prediction model for women undergoing screening mammography. *Journal of the National Cancer Institute, 98*(17), 1204–1214.

Barrentt, B., & Wi. C.-E. A. (2002, March 11). Retrieved from http://www.here.research.med.va.gov/FAQ_AL.htm.

Berzuini, C., & Larizza, C. (1996). A unified approach for modeling longitudinal and failure time data, with application in medical monitoring. *IEEE Transactions on Pattern Analysis and Machine Intelligence, 16*(2), 109–123. doi:10.1109/34.481537

Bines, J. E. (2005). Rotavirus vaccines and intussusception risk. *Current Opinion in Gastroenterology, 21*(1), 20–25.

Brophy, J., & Erickson, L. (2004). *An Economic Analysis of Drug Eluting Coronary Stents A Quebec Perspective*. Québec, Canada: AETMIS.

Brown, R. (2001). Behavioral issues in asthma management. *Pediatric Pulmonology, 21*(Supplement), 26–30. doi:10.1002/ppul.2003

Bruin, J. S. d., Cocx, T. K., Kosters, W. A., Laros, J. F., & Kok, J. N. (2006). *Data mining approaches to criminal career analysis*. Paper presented at the Proceedings of the Sixth International Conference on Data Mining, Hong Kong.

Brus, T., Swinnen, G., Vanhoof, K., & Wets, G. (2004). Building an association rules framework to improve produce assortment decisions. *Data Mining and Knowledge Discovery, 8*, 7–23. doi:10.1023/B:DAMI.0000005256.79013.69

Cerrito, P., Badia, A., & Cerrito, J. C. (2005). *Data Mining Medication Prescriptions for a Representative National Sample*. Paper presented at the Pharmasug 2005, Phoenix, Arizona.

Cerrito, P., & Cerrito, J. C. (2006). Data and Text Mining the Electronic Medical Record to Improve Care and to Lower Costs [Electronic Version]. In *SUGI 31 Proceedings, 31*. Retrieved January, 2007, from http://www2.sas.com/proceedings/sugi31/077-31.pdf.

Cerrito, P. B. (2009). *Data Mining Healthcare and Clinical Databases*. Cary, NC: SAS Press.

Cerrito, P. B. (2009). *Text Mining Techniques for Healthcare Provider Quality Determination: Methods for Rank Comparisons*. Hershey, PA: IGI Global Publishing.

Cerrito, P. B., & Cerrito, J. C. (2006). *Data and text mining the electronic medical record to improve care and to lower costs*. Paper presented at the SUGI31, San Francisco.

CHi-Ming, C., Hsu-Sung, K., Shu-Hui, C., Hong-Jen, C., Der-Ming, L., Tabar, L., et al. (2005). Computer-aided disease prediction system: development of application software with SAS component language. *Journal of Evaluation in Clinical Practice, 11*(2), 139–159. doi:10.1111/j.1365-2753.2005.00514.x

Chipps, B., & Spahn, J. (2006). What are the determinates of asthma control? *The Journal of Asthma, 43*(8), 567–572. doi:10.1080/02770900600619782

Circulation, J. A. H. A. (n.d.). *Heart Association Statistics Committee and Stroke Statistics Subcommittee*. Retrieved from http://circ.ahajournals.org/cgi/reprint/113/6/e85.pdf.

Claus, E. B. (2001). Risk models used to counsel women for breast and ovarian cancer: a guide for clinicians. *Familial Cancer, 1*, 197–206. doi:10.1023/A:1021135807900

Conboy-Ellis, K. (2006). Asthma pathogenesis and management. *The Nurse Practitioner, 31*, 24–44. doi:10.1097/00006205-200611000-00006

Cox, J. L. A. (2005). Some limitations of a proposed linear model for antimicrobial risk management. *Risk Analysis, 25*(6), 1327–1332. doi:10.1111/j.1539-6924.2005.00703.x

David, J., Bakhai, C., Shi, A., Githiora, C., Lavelle, L., & Berezin, T. (2004). Cost-Effectiveness of Sirolimus-Eluting Stents for Treatment of Complex Coronary Stenoses. *ACC Current Journal Review, 13*(11), 55–56. doi:10.1016/j.accreview.2004.10.053

Eleuteri, A., Tagliaferri, R., Milano, L., Sansone, G., Agostino, D. D., Placido, S. D., et al. (2003). *Survival analysis and neural networks*. Paper presented at the 2003 Conference on Neural Networks, Portland, Oregon.

Fajadet, J. P. M., Hayashi, E. B., et al. (2002, March 18). *American College of Cardiology 51st Annual Scientific Session; Presentation #0032-1*. Retrieved from http://www.stjohns.com/doctorclark/AnswerPage.aspx?drclark_id=22

Foster, D. P., & Stine, R. A. (2004). Variable selection in data mining: building a predictive model for bankruptcy. *Journal of the American Statistical Association, 99*(466), 303–313. doi:10.1198/016214504000000287

Freedman, A. N., Seminara, D., Mitchell, H., Hartge, P., Colditz, G. A., & Ballard-Barbash, R. (2005). Cancer risk prediction models: a workshop on developmnet, evaluation, and application. *Journal of the National Cancer Institute, 97*(10), 715–723.

Gardner, P., Pickering, L., Orenstein, W., Gershon, A., & Nichol, K. (2002). Infectious diseases society of America. Guidelines for quality standards for immunization. *Clinical Infectious Diseases, 35*(5), 503–511. doi:10.1086/341965

Gaylor, D. W. (2005). Risk/benefit assessments of human diseases: optimum dose for intervention. *Risk Analysis, 25*(1), 161–168. doi:10.1111/j.0272-4332.2005.00575.x

Gillette, B. (2005, September). *Manage Health Care Executive, E. G. c. W. I. o. H. S. o. C. a. Q.* Retrieved from http://www.managedhealthcare-execytive.com/mhe/article.

Giudiei, P., & Passerone, G. (2002). Data mining of association structures to model consumer behaviour. *Computational Statistics & Data Analysis, 38,* 533–541. doi:10.1016/S0167-9473(01)00077-9

Giudier, P., & Passerone, G. (2002). Data mining of association structures to model consumer behavior. *Computational Statistics & Data Analysis, 38*(4), 533–541. doi:10.1016/S0167-9473(01)00077-9

Hand, D. J., & Bolton, R. J. (2004). Pattern discovery and detection: a unified statistical methodology. *Journal of Applied Statistics, 8,* 885–924. doi:10.1080/0266476042000270518

Hernandez, M. A., & Stolfo, S. J. (1998). Real-world data is dirty: data cleansing and the merge/purge problem. *Data Mining and Knowledge Discovery, 2,* 9–17. doi:10.1023/A:1009761603038

Hosking, J. R., Pednault, E. P., & Sudan, M. (1997). Statistical perspective on data mining. *Future Generation Computer Systems, 13*(2-3), 117–134. doi:10.1016/S0167-739X(97)00016-2

Iezzoni, L. I., Ash, A. S., Shwartz, M., Daley, J., Hughes, J. S., & Mackleman, Y. D. (1995). Predicting who dies depends on how severity is measured: implications for evaluating patient outcomes. *Annals of Internal Medicine, 123*(10), 763–770.

Jiang, T., & Tuxhilin, A. (2006). *Improving personalization solutions through optimal segmentation of customer bases.* Paper presented at the Proceedings of the Sixth International Conference on Data Mining, Hong Kong.

John, T. T., & Chen, P. (2006). Lognormal selection with applications to lifetime data. *IEEE Transactions on Reliability, 55*(1), 135–148. doi:10.1109/TR.2005.858098

Keim, D. A., Mansmann, F., Schneidewind, J., & Ziegler, H. (2006). Challenges in visual data analysis. *Information Visualization, 2006,* 9–16.

Kim, X., Back, Y., Rhee, D. W., & Kim, S.-H. (2005). *Analysis of breast cancer using data mining & statistical techniques.* Paper presented at the Proceedings of the Sixth International Conference on Software Engineering, Artificial Intelligence, Networking, and Parallel/Distributed Computing, Las Vegas, NV.

Lee, S. (1995). *Predicting atmospheric ozone using neural networks as compared to some statistical methods.* Paper presented at the Northcon 95. IEEE Technical Applications Conference and Workshops Northcon95, Portland, Oregon.

Linoff, G. S. (2004). *Survival Data Mining for Customer Insight. 2007.* Retrieved from www.intelligententerprise.com/showArticle.jhtml?articleID=26100528

Loebstein, R., Katzir, I., Vasterman-Landes, J., Halkin, H., & Lomnicky, Y. (2008). Database assessment of the effectiveness of brand versus generic rosiglitazone in patients with type 2 diabetes mellitus. *Medical Science Monitor, 14*(6), 323–326.

Loren, K. (n.d.). *Heart Disease: Number One Killer.* Retrieved from http://www.heart-disease-bypass-surgery.com/data/footnotes/f5.htm

Mannila, H. (1996). *Data mining: machine learning, statistics and databases.* Paper presented at the Eighth International Conference on Scientific and Statistical Database Systems, 1996. Proceedings, Stockholm.

Menon, R., Tong, L. H., Sathiyakeerthi, S., Brombacher, A., & Leong, C. (2004). The needs and benefits of applying textual data mining within the product development process. *Quality and Reliability Engineering International, 20,* 1–15. doi:10.1002/qre.536

Middleton, D. B., Zimmerman, R. K., & Mitchell, K. B. (2007). Vaccine schedules and procedures, 2007. *The Journal of Family Practice, 56*(2), 42–60.

Moches, T. A. (2005). *Text data mining applied to clustering with cost effective tools.* Paper presented at the IEEE International Conference on Systems, Mand, and Cybernetics, Waikoloa, HI.

Moses, J. W., & Leon, M. B. (n.d.). Lenox Hill Hospital and the Cardiovascular Research Foundation, U.S. SIRIUS Study: 1,058 Patients, Retrieved from http://www.investor.jnj.com/releaseDetail.cfm?ReleaseID=90711&year=2002

National HeartLung and Blood Institute. D. a. C. I. (n.d.). *Angioplasty.* Retrieved from http://www.nhlbi.nih.gov/health/dci/Diseases/Angioplasty/Angioplasty_WhatIs

O'Reilly, K. B. (2008). *Time to get tough? States increasingly offer ways to opt out of faccine mandates.* Retrieved September, 8, 2008, from http://www.ama-assn.org/amednews/2008/09/08/prsa0908.htm

O'Ryan, M., Lucero, Y., Pena, A., & Valenzuela, M. T. (2003). Two year review of intestinal intussusception in six large public hospitals of Santiago, Chili. *The Pediatric Infectious Disease Journal, 22*, 717–721.

Pazzani, M. J. (2000). Knowledge discovery from data? *IEEE Intelligent Systems,* (March/April): 10–13. doi:10.1109/5254.850821

Pear, R. (2007, August 19). Medicare Says It Won't Cover Hospital Errors. *New York Times.*

Pinna, G., Maestri, R., Capomolla, S., Febo, O., Mortara, A., & Riccardi, P. (2000). Determinant role of short-term heart rate variability in the prediction of mortality in patients with chronic heart failure. *IEEE Computers in Cardiology, 27*, 735–738.

Popescul, A., Lawrence, S., Ungar, L. H., & Pennock, D. M. (2003). *Statistical relational learning for document mining.* Paper presented at the Proceedings of the Third IEEE International Conference on Data Mining, Melbourne, FL.

Poses, R. M., McClish, D. K., Smith, W. R., Huber, E. C., Clomo, F. L., & Schmitt, B. P. (2000). Results of report cards for patients with congestive heart failure depend on the method used to adjust for severity. *Annals of Internal Medicine, 133*, 10–20.

Potts, W. (2000). *Survival Data Mining. 2007,* Retrieved from http://www.data-miners.com/resources/Will%20Survival.pdf

Ried, R., Kierk, N. D., Ambrosini, G., Berry, G., & Musk, A. (2006). The risk of lung cancer with increasing time since ceasing exposure to asbestos and quitting smoking. *Occupational and Environmental Medicine, 63*(8), 509–512. doi:10.1136/oem.2005.025379

Rotavirus, A.-M. (2008, April 18). Rotavirus vaccination coverage and adherence to the advisory committee on immunization practices (ACIP)-recommended vaccination schedule-United States, February 2006-May 2007. *MMWR*, 398–401.

Sabate, J. (1999). Nut consumption, vegetarian diets, ischemic heart disease risk, and all-cause mortality: evidence from epidemiologic studies. *The American Journal of Clinical Nutrition, 70*(Suppl), 500–503.

Sahoo, P. (2002). *Probability and Mathematical Statistics.* Louisville, KY: Department of Mathematics, University of Louisville.

Sargan, J. D. (2001). Model building and data mining. *Econometric Reviews, 20*(2), 159–170. doi:10.1081/ETC-100103820

Seker, H., Odetayo, M., Petrovic, D., Naguib, R., Bartoli, C., Alasio, L., et al. (2002). *An artificial neural network based feature evaluation index for the assessment of clinical factors in breast cancer survival analysis.* Paper presented at the IEEE Canadian Conference on Electrical & Computer Engineering, Winnipeg, Manitoba.

Shaw, B., & Marshall, A. H. (2006). Modeling the health care costs of geriatric inpatients. *IEEE Transactions on Information Technology in Biomedicine, 10*(3), 526–532. doi:10.1109/TITB.2005.863821

Siegrist, M., Keller, C., & Kiers, H. A. (2005). A new look at the psychometric paradigm of perception of hazards. *Risk Analysis, 25*(1), 211–222. doi:10.1111/j.0272-4332.2005.00580.x

Silverman, B. W. (1986). Density Estimation for Statistics and Data Analysis (Monographs on Statistics and Applied Probability. Boca Raton, FL: Chapman & Hall/CRC.

Simonsen, L., Viboud, C., Elixhauser, A., Taylor, R., & Kapikian, A. (2005). More on Rotashield and intussusception: the role of age at the time of vaccination. *The Journal of Infectious Diseases, 192*(Supple 1), 36–43. doi:10.1086/431512

Smith, P. J. (2008). Controversial HPV vaccine causing one death per month: FDA report. *LifeSiteNews.* Retrieved from http://www.lifesitenews.com/ldn/2008/jul/08070316.html

Sokol, L., Garcia, B., West, M., Rodriguez, J., & Johnson, K. (2001). *Precursory steps to mining HCFA health care claims.* Paper presented at the 34th Hawaii International Conference on System Sciences, Hawaii.

Tebbins, R. J. D., Pallansch, M. A., Kew, O. M., Caceres, V. M., Jafari, H., & Cochi, S. L. (2006). Risks of Paralytic disease due to wild or vaccine-derived poliovirus after eradication. *Risk Analysis, 26*(6), 1471–1505. doi:10.1111/j.1539-6924.2006.00827.x

Texas Heart Institute. (n.d.). *H. I. C., Coronary Artery Bypass, at St.Lukes'Episcopal Hospital.* Retrieved from http://texasheart.org/HIC/Topics/Proced/cab.cfm

Thomas, J. W. (1998). Research evidence on the validity of adjusted mortality rate as a measure of hospital quality of care. *Medical Care Research and Review, 55*(4), 371–404. doi:10.1177/107755879805500401

Thompson, K. M., & Tebbins, R. J. D. (2006). Retrospective cost-effectiveness analyses for polio vaccination in the United States. *Risk Analysis, 26*(6), 1423–1449. doi:10.1111/j.1539-6924.2006.00831.x

Tosh, P. K., Boyce, T., & Poland, G. A. (2008). Flu Myths: Dispelling the Myths Associated With Live Attenuated Influenza Vaccine. *Mayo Clinic Proceedings, 83*(1), 77–84. doi:10.4065/83.1.77

Tsanakas, A., & Desli, E. (2005). Measurement and pricing of risk in insurance markets. *Risk Analysis, 23*(6), 1653–1668. doi:10.1111/j.1539-6924.2005.00684.x

W. I. t. R. A. C. (n.d.). *Blue Cross Blue Shield of Texas.* Retrieved from http://www.bcbstx.com/provider/bluechoice_solutions_tool_raci.htm.

Wang, K., & Zhou, X. (2005). Mining customer value: from association rules to direct marketing. *Data Mining and Knowledge Discovery, 11*, 57–79. doi:10.1007/s10618-005-1355-x

Wong, K., Byoung-ju, C., Bui-Kyeong, H., Soo-Kyung, K., & Doheon, L. (2003). A taxonomy of dirty data. *Data Mining and Knowledge Discovery, 7*, 81–99. doi:10.1023/A:1021564703268

Wong, R. C.-W., & Fu, A. W.-C. (2005). Data mining for inventory item selection with cross-selling considerations. *Data Mining and Knowledge Discovery, 11*, 81–112. doi:10.1007/s10618-005-1359-6

Xie, H., Chaussalet, T. J., & Millard, P. H. (2006). A model-based approach to the analysis of patterns of length of stay in institutional long-term care. *IEEE Transactions on Information Technology in Biomedicine, 10*(3), 512–518. doi:10.1109/TITB.2005.863820

Yock, C. A., Boothroyd, D. B., Owens, D. K., Garber, A. M., & Hlatky, M. A. (2003, October 1). Cost-effectiveness of Bypass Surgery versus Stenting in Patients with Multivessele Coronary Artery Disease. *The American Journal of Medicine, 115*, 382–389. doi:10.1016/S0002-9343(03)00296-1

Yuhua, Li, D. M., Bandar, Z. A., O'Shea, J. D., & Crockett, K. (2006). Sentence similarity based on semantic nets and corpur statistics. *IEEE Transactions on Knowledge and Data Engineering, 18*(6), 1138–1148.

Zhu, X., Wu, X., & Chen, Q. (2006). Bridging local and global data cleansing: identifying class noise in large, distributed data datasets. *Data Mining and Knowledge Discovery, 12*(2-3), 275. doi:10.1007/s10618-005-0012-8

ADDITIONAL READING

Cerrito, P. B. (2007). *Introduction to Data Mining with Enterprise Miner*. Cary, NC: SAS Press.

Cerrito, P. B. (2009). *Data Mining Healthcare and Clinical Databases*. Cary, NC: SAS Press.

Evans, D., Cauchemez, S., Hayden, F. G., Evans, D., Cauchemez, S., & Hayden, F. G. (2009). "Prepandemic" immunization for novel influenza viruses, "swine flu" vaccine, guillain-barre syndrome, and the detection of rare severe adverse events. *The Journal of Infectious Diseases, 200*(3), 321–328. doi:10.1086/603560

Goldman, G. S. (2005). Cost-benefit analysis of universal varicella vaccination in the U.S. taking into account the closely related herpes-zoster epidemiology. *Vaccine, 23*(25), 3349–3355. doi:10.1016/j.vaccine.2003.10.042

Iskander, J., Pool, V., Zhou, W., & English-Bullard, R. (2006). Data mining in the US using the Vaccine Adverse Event Reporting System. *Drug Safety, 29*(5), 375–384. doi:10.2165/00002018-200629050-00002

Niu, M. T., Erwin, D. E., & Braun, M. M. (2001). Data mining in the US Vaccine Adverse Event Reporting System (VAERS): early detection of intussusception and other events after rotavirus vaccination. *Vaccine, 19*, 4627–4634. doi:10.1016/S0264-410X(01)00237-7

Smith, P. J. (2008). Controversial HPV vaccine causing one death per month: FDA report. *LifeSiteNews*. Retrieved from http://www.lifesitenews.com/ldn/2008/jul/08070316.html

Tosh, P. K., Boyce, T., & Poland, G. A. (2008). Flu Myths: Dispelling the Myths Associated With Live Attenuated Influenza Vaccine. *Mayo Clinic Proceedings, 83*(1), 77–84. doi:10.4065/83.1.77

Chapter 13
Healthcare Delivery in a Hospital Emergency Department

Joseph Twagilimana
University of Louisville, USA

ABSTRACT

The outcome of interest in this study is the length of stay (LOS) at a Hospital Emergency Department (ED). The Length of stay depends on several independent clinical factors such as treatments, patient demographic characteristics, hospital, as well as physicians and nurses. The present study attempts to identify these variables by analyzing clinical data provided by electronic medical records (EMR) from an emergency department. Three analysis methodologies were identified as appropriate for this task. First, data mining techniques were applied, and then generalized linear models and Time series followed. In spite of the fact that Data Mining and Statistics share the same objective, which is to extract useful information from data, they perform independently of each other. In this case, we show how the two methodologies can be integrated with potential benefits. We applied decision trees to select important variables and used these variables as input in the other models.

BACKGROUND

Medical data form a collection of observations about a patient. Among records on each patient are the patient identification (name and/or medical record), the parameters being observed, the values of the parameters, and the time of observation. Some parameters such as complaints, diagnoses, charges or treatments are in textual format. Some others such as age, blood pressure, and temperature are in numerical format. There are also pictures such as x-rays and CT scans. All of these characteristics make medical data analysis a challenging one. Krzysztof J. Cios and G. William Moore (2002) report the major points of the uniqueness of medical data:

• Heterogeneity or volume and complexity contained in the data. They can include Physician's interpretation (unstructured free-text English), sensitivity and specificity

DOI: 10.4018/978-1-61520-723-7.ch013

Copyright © 2010, IGI Global. Copying or distributing in print or electronic forms without written permission of IGI Global is prohibited.

analysis, poor mathematical characterization, and lack of canonical form (imprecision, lack of standard vocabulary).

- Ethical, legal, and social issues: Because of a fear of lawsuits directed against Physicians, unnecessary lab tests are ordered. This makes the analysis of the data difficult because there is no association or pattern with the patient's condition.

- Statistical Philosophy: Assumptions underlying Statistical methods such as normality and homogeneity of variance are constantly violated in medical data. Medical data are primarily patient care oriented rather than a research source, unless they are from designed experiments. The size of the patient sample is often too small for data mining techniques, which require a considerable amount of data for training/validation methodology. Medical data are highly noisy and often contain missing fields. Some data mining techniques such as neural networks do not handle missing data. There are also issues with clustering in large dimensional medical data. A major concern is how to incorporate medical domain knowledge into the mechanism of clustering. Without focus and at least partial human supervision, one may end up with results that do not make sense.

- Special status of medicine: Medicine has a special status in life. The outcomes of medical care can be life-or-death. Medicine is a necessity, not merely an optional luxury, pleasure, or convenience. Any medical data analysis must take into consideration that there is no room for errors. Any results must be accompanied by a certain confidence level to help decision makers make the right choices.

The ideas presented in the above paragraph were borrowed from the article written by Krzysztof J. Cios and G. William Moore (2002). We recommend this article to beginners in medical data analysis.

SETTING THE STAGE

The data to be analyzed were collected using the **Ibex Pulse Check, a** comprehensive and well-integrated emergency department information system (EDIS). **Ibex Pulse Check** is a fast-charting system that gives both emergency nurses and physicians the ability to view the medical record as it is being created (Pulse Chek, n.d.) The data were collected for a 3-month period in a hospital emergency department. It had originally 12 variables and 3345 observations. As any medical data, the datasets contain variables in text format (complaints, diagnosis, charges), numerical variables (age) and some other identifier such as patient name, Physician's initial, and Nurse's initial. Variables were recoded to maintain the privacy of patients, Physicians and Nurses. New variables were created as they were needed for the preprocessing and analysis phases of the study. A counter variable, **visits**, that counts the patients as they enter the emergency room, and a variable **count,** which accumulates the number of patients per hour were created. The variable **Time**, which specifies the hour interval time in which the patient was seen by the triage nurse, was created from the variable **triage.**

The variable, charges, which specifies the items for which the patient was charged, was used to create clusters of patients. It is believed that patients with similar symptoms and diagnoses are treated in a similar manner. Those clusters were created using the SAS Text Miner. Text mining can be used to group patients with similar complaints, diagnoses and charges in the same cluster. The new variable showing the clusters is labeled "CLUSTER'. The following table gives a summary description of the variables. The data have been de-identified according the HIPAA recommendations. Table 1 gives a brief description of the data.

Table 1. Description of the data

Variable name	Description
Gender	Male Female
Age	Age
Urgency	1-Emergent 2-urgent 3-Non-urgent
Complaint	How the patient describes his/her disease
Diagnosis	How the Physician describes the patient's clinical condition.
Medical Record	A fake record number of the file of the patient.
MD	Physician de-indentified: values MD1, MD2, MD3...
RN	Nurse de-indentified: Values RN1, RN2, RN3...
Triage	Date and time where the patient was triaged
Disposition	Tell if the patient was referred to a hospital or to nurse services, or sent home for self-care.
LOS	Length of stay from the triage time to exit. (in Minutes)
Charges	Items for which the patient was charged.
CLUSTER	Grouping of similar patients in regard to Charges
ClusDescription	Label of a cluster
ChargesCount	Count of a patient's charges

The variable of interest in this data set was LOS, the Length of stay from the triage time to the disposition or exit time.

The purpose of the analysis is to show how different methodologies can be combined and applied to the analysis of LOS (Length of stay) in order to identify variables that have a decisive impact on the length of stay at the Hospital emergency department, and use them for prediction purposes. Finding factors that have influence on length of stay and wisely managing them will benefit patients, the emergency department, and health insurance providers. By knowing which factors are predictive of prolonged LOS and therefore of ED overcrowding, hospitals can anticipate the likelihood of emergency departments heading towards critical-care divert situations. Possible divert status of the ED can be detected on time and avoided. This improvement can have a direct impact on the quality of care and can contribute to a significant reduction of healthcare costs, since prolonged LOS implies high costs.

An exploratory analysis of the data identified the variable LOS to be Log-normally distributed (Figure 1).

Figure 1 shows that the data are not normally distributed. We also ran a Bartlett's test of homogeneity of variance to find that the variance was not constant across patients' clusters. Because of the Non-normality and non-constant variance, classical linear models are invalid in analyzing these data. Only the Generalized mixed model can handle this case.

In preliminary analysis, it was also found that the crowding of the ED varies from time to time during the 24 hours (Figure 2), going from a peak between 8:00 and 16:00 to a trough between 0:00 to 6:00.

These observations suggest that the variable LOS is time stamped and that it can be analyzed using time series techniques (Figure 3). Because Triage can happen at any time as the patients enter the ED, instead of occurring at a regular time period, ordinary time series analysis techniques cannot be directly applied, and a transformation to regular Time series by defining accumulation intervals will be needed. Time series analysis will be used to forecast the LOS and the results will be compared to those obtained by the Generalized linear models. To our knowledge, analysis of LOS by time series techniques is innovative, and this was inspired by the fact that the variable LOS shares most of the common characteristics of time series or transactional data, namely being time stamped and exhibiting autocorrelations. Due to the challenging characteristics of medical data as discussed earlier, no one can pretend to have the best models unless he/she tried many and chose

Figure 1. The lognormal distribution seems to fit the variable LOS

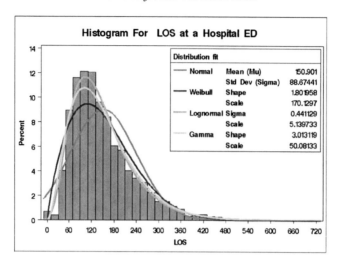

Figure 2. Variation in the number of visits by time of triage

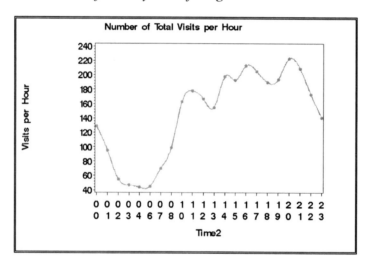

the best according to some criteria. In addition to statistical models such as the Generalized linear models and Time series models, we will perform the analysis of the data using data mining techniques and all the results will be compared.

CASE DESCRIPTION

The dataset contains variables in free-English text format (complaints, diagnosis, charges), numerical variables (age) and some other iden-

tifiers such as fake patient record, fake Physician's initial, fake Nurse's initial. Complaints, diagnosis, and charges constitute the highest source of information about the patient in the data. Unfortunately, they cannot be used in the analysis as they stand. A pretreatment of these variables is needed in order to be understandable by a machine. Patients who have similar symptoms and diagnoses should have similar charges, and can be grouped together according to these charges. We recall that charges means the items charged to the patient.

Figure 3. Variation in the average LOS by time of triage

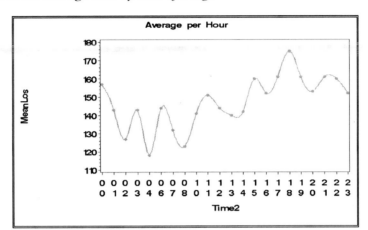

In order to group the patients, we performed a text analysis on the charges as defined into text strings. Some of the charges were described by groups of words. We used tokenization to prevent groups of words being separated, and therefore losing their meaning. We created one text string of charges for each patient, and parsed the text into different terms using the text mining node of the SAS Enterprise Miner Software. We then performed a clustering on these terms. The clusters that were obtained are in Table 2. Looking at the description of each cluster, and with the help of a pharmacist with domain expertise (Cerrito, 2005), we labeled each cluster. The label of each cluster corresponds to the main diagnoses that correspond to the charges in the list.

Table 2 shows the results of text analysis to define the clusters of patient diagnoses for those who enter the ED. While the patient conditions vary considerably, they can be grouped in a reasonable manner. Each cluster was given a label that can be used to identify the general patient condition defined by the cluster.

The SAS text mining tools add the clusters to the dataset where they can be used as any other categorical variable in the data. Clustered data exhibit correlations as the patients grouped together in a cluster are believed to have many similarities. That is why techniques that support correlated variables can be used when analyzing the data using statistical techniques.

Decision trees are powerful methods of predictive modeling for data mining purposes applied to classification problems. In such problems, the objective is to assign an observation to one of several pre-defined classes. In order to apply Decision Trees, the variable LOS (length of stay) was discretized into four categories (Figure 4).

Short: 0-2 hours
Medium: 2-3 hours
Long: 3-5 hours
Very Long: More than 5 hours

The Discretization in Figure 4 was inspired by the existing literature (Sollid, n.d., Practice Plan, n.d.) and the statistical measures of the variable LOS (Table 3). According to Leif Sollid (n.d.), in 2002-2003, the average wait to be seen by a physician in Emergency was 115 minutes, the average length of stay for patients who are treated and then discharged from Emergency was 4.03 hours (241 minutes), and the average length of stay in Emergency for patients who were admitted to an inpatient bed is 9.49 hours (569 minutes). Some other sources (Practice Plan, n.d., Shwartz, n.d.) mention an average length of stay of about 3 hours, with a goal of reducing it by an hour or

Table 2. Description of the charges clusters

#	Descriptive Terms	Freq	Percentage	Label
1	Crutch_training, ct-head_wo_contrast, + extremity_xray-ankle, injection_sq_ or_im_ther/pro/d, + strapping_ankle, + triage_simple, + splint_appl_(thigh/ ankle), shoulder_xray	688	21%	Ankle/Arm Injuries
2	+ cbc, extens_thpy_not_chemo_p/visit, ckmb_(ck_iso+total)_w/o_interp, ekg_(electrocardiogram), injectons_intravenous_th/pro/, + troponin_i, + speci- men_collection, bmp_(basic_panel)	1159	35%	URI (Upper Respira- tory infection)
3	koh_prep, + pregnancy_test_qualitative, wet_prep, + pelvic_exam_specimen_col- lection_points, + culture_blood, + urinalysis_clean_catch, + specimen_collection, extension_gc_dna_probe	241	7%	UTI (urinary tract infection)
4	+ spine_cervic-flexion/extension, + ct-spine_cervical-wo_contrast, injection_ sq_or_im_ther/pro/d, hip_xray-unilateral-two_view, + dc_instructions_simple, pelvis_xray-full_view, + triage_simple,	213	6%	Back Injury
5	+ eye_medication, visual_acuity, slit_lamp_e.r, + irrigation_one/both_eyes, tetanus_or_other_immunization, + dc_instructions_simple, + triage_simple, + oral_med_administration	104	3%	Eye trauma
6	tetanus_or_other_immunization, + dressing_complex, wound_cleansing/ir- rigation, laceration_tray, dermabond_adhesive, + dc_instructions_simple, + triage_simple, + extremity_xray-ankle	186	6%	Wound
7	+ dc_instructions_simple, injection_im_antibiotic, + oral_med_administration, rapid_strep_screen, + triage_simple, ear_med_administration, + mono_test, influenza_a_rapid_screen	209	6%	Infection
8	+ dc_instructions_simple, crutch_training, + splint_appl_(thigh/ankle), + extrem- ity_xray-ankle, + triage_simple, removal_cerumen_ear, + ct-spine_cervical- wo_contrast, + oral_med_administration	517	16%	Minor Injuries

Figure 4. Discretization of LOS

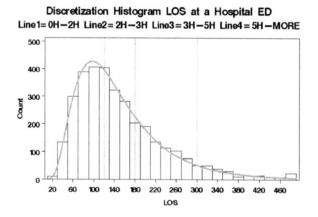

to less than 3 hours. In turn, the basic statistics measures of our data (Table 3) indicate an average of 2 hours and a half. The Discretization intervals are not uniquely determined, but the one used optimized predictions results.

After discretization, a Decision Tree was built using the SAS Enterprise Miner software. There are no specific rules of what the settings parameters should be to demonstrate a good fit, but some rules of thumb can be followed. Berry and Linoff

Table 3. Basic statistical measures of the variable LOS

Basic Statistical Measures			
Location		Variability	
Mean	151.4664	Std Deviation	85.35151
Median	130.0000	Variance	7285
Mode	108.0000	Range	458.00000

Table 4. Tree settings

Splitting criterion: Entropy Reduction Minimum number of observations in a leaf: 16 Observations required for a split search: 33 Maximum number of branches from a node: 2
Maximum depth of tree: 6 Splitting rules saved in each node: 5 Surrogate rules saved in each node: 6 Treatment missing as an acceptable value Model assessment measure: Misclassification Rate Subtree: Best assessment value Observations sufficient for split search: 1673 Maximum tries in an exhaustive split search: 5000 Do not use profit matrix during split search Do not use prior probability in split search

(1999) recommend setting the minimum number of observations in a leaf to be between 0.25 and 1 percent of the model set, and the observations required for a split search to not less than twice the minimum number of observations in a leaf. Following some of these recommendations and trying several settings, we came up with the optimal settings shown in Table 4.

The settings are self-explained except the *entropy reduction or information gain*. This measure tells us how well a given attribute classifies an observation according to the target.

The entropy for a probability distribution P is defined as

$$Entropy(P) = -\sum_{i} p_i(\log_2 p_i)$$

where p_i is the probability of event i These measures are automatically calculated by the software. The resulting tree is shown in Figure 5. The colors in the tree have the following mean-ings: dark represents the *short class*; the lighter color is for the *medium class*, and the very light and light are respectively for the classes *long* and *very long*.

From the top of the tree to the bottom, splitting variables are listed according to their importance in predicting the length of stay. The *number of charges* is ranked first followed by the *disposition*, the treating *Physician*, the *time* of *triage* and finally, the *nurse*. The particular relationships of each of these variables with LOS are illustrated in Figure 5.

In addition to the tree structure, the EM Decision Tree mining produces decision rules in the form of "*If ...Then*', some of which are listed below.

Rule1

```
IF Time of triage, IS ONE OF: 09:01 -
10:00 10:01 - 11:00
```

Figure 5. SAS enterprise miner decision tree

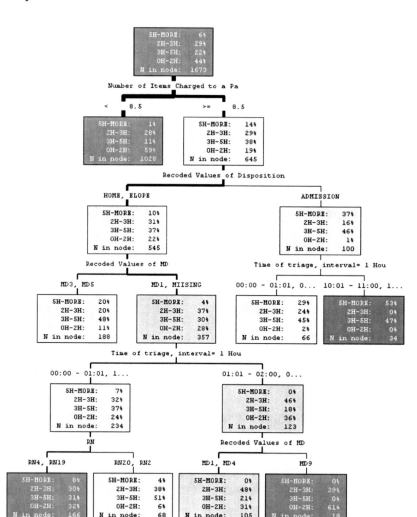

```
11:01 - 12:00 12:01 - 13:00 18:01 - 19:00
AND Disposition EQUALS ADMISSION
AND 8.5 <= Number of Items Charged to a
Patient
THEN
Long: 47.1%
Very Long: 52.9%
Medium: 0.0%
Short: 0.0%
N: 34
```

Rule1 says that if the visit of a patient arriving at the ED around noon or in the early evening results in a hospital admission, then that patient will have a long stay at the ED, probably waiting for a bed to be free, since in this rule, the patient has only a few charges (<= 8).

In the data set under study, there were 34 patients who fell in this category. In contrast, when the physician *MD9* is in the ED in the early morning (00:00 to 10:00), the patients' care is expedited (see Rule2 below).

Rule2

```
IF MD EQUALS MD9
AND Time of triage IS ONE OF: 01:01 -
02:00 02:01 - 03:00
```

Table 5. Confusion Matrix. table of target by output (assessed partition=VALIDATION)

target output					
Frequency|					
Percent						
Row Pct						
Col Pct |Short |Medium |Long |Very long| Total				
Short	341	24	16	1	382
	42.26	2.97	1.98	0.12	47.34
	89.27	6.28	4.19	0.26	
	58.19	39.34	10.88	7.69	
Medium	155	18	30	3	206
	19.21	2.23	3.72	0.37	25.53
	75.24	8.74	14.56	1.46	
	26.45	29.51	20.41	23.08	
Long	76	12	69	3	160
	9.42	1.49	8.55	0.37	19.83
	47.50	7.50	43.13	1.88	
	12.97	19.67	46.94	23.08	
Very Long	14	7	32	6	59
	1.73	0.87	3.97	0.74	7.31
	23.73	11.86	54.24	10.17	
	2.39	11.48	21.77	46.15	
Total	586	61	147	13	807
	72.61	7.56	18.22	1.61	100.00

```
03:01 - 04:00 04:01 - 05:00 05:01 - 06:00
06:01 - 07:00
07:01 - 08:00 09:01 - 10:00 12:01 - 13:00
16:01 - 17:00
22:01 - 23:00 23:01 - 00:00
AND Disposition IS ONE OF: HOME ELOPE
PHYSICIAN
AND 8.5 <= Number of Items Charged to a
Patient
THEN
Short: 61.1%
Medium: 38.9%
Long: 0.0%
Very Long: 0.0%
N: 18
```

The assessment criterion of the model was the *misclassification rate*. This rate was 0.47 for the training set, 0.46 for the validation set and 0.51 for the test set. A Table of target by output, called a confusion matrix (Table 5) is also a tool that helps in judging the accuracy of the model. The table indicates a good prediction for a length of stay of less than two hours, but performs badly in the medium LOS since 25.53% of the patients were actually observed in that class, but only 7.56% were predicted with a medium stay. Predictions in the long class are also satisfying, but again are poor for the very long class.

The confusion matrix is well visualized in a 3D graph, called the diagnostic chart (Figure 6). Globally, the diagnostic chart shows that the decision tree, in the absence of a better model, can serve as a basis for LOS predictions.

Decision trees have provided useful information through the decision rules, and have helped in identifying the most informative variables. These variables will serve as input for the Time series and the generalized linear models.

An analysis similar to the one done using Decision Trees was performed using an Artificial Neural Network. The architecture of the ANN used was the multilayer perceptron. The model selection criterion was set to the misclassification rate, and the training technique to Quasi-Newton. It had three input nodes, one for each category of variables: interval, ordinal and nominal. There

were also three hidden nodes with direct connections between them. To optimize the model, five preliminary runs were performed. The diagram in Figure 7 summarizes the ANN settings.

The neural network misclassification Rate was 0.42 on the training data, 0.43 on the validation data and 0.47 on the test data. These rates show a result slightly better than that of the decision tree. The confusion matrix (Table 6) also shows an improvement in the prediction. No LOS in the class "Very long" was classified as low as "Short" as was the case in the Decision Tree.

Again, the confusion matrix was graphically visualized by the diagnostic chart (Figure 8).

Many considerations must be taken into account when choosing an adequate accumulation interval. By choosing an accumulation interval of one hour, one may be able to predict LOS for each of the 24 hours of the day. With an accumulation interval of 4 hours, or 6 hours, one may be able to predict LOS for the 4 hours, or 6 hour periods. As shown in Figures 9, 10, 11, 12, and 13, a long accumulation interval tends to produce data that

Figure 6. Diagnostic chart for the decision tree model

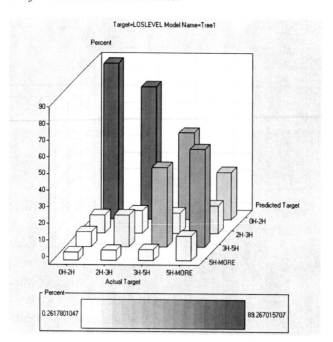

are more correlated than those produced by a short accumulation interval.

Time series have one or more variation components: Trend, Cyclic variation, Seasonal, and Irregular variation. A trend shows a shift variation in the level of the mean. A trend can be linear, having a constant rate of increase or decrease; or it can present a periodic variation (Figure 9 (a)). The trend main effect is in the increase or the decrease of the mean. If a time series oscillates

Figure 7. The ANN architecture and settings. There are three input nodes, one for each variable category: Interval, nominal and ordinal. The nodes H1, H2, and H3 are the hidden nodes and they are all interconnected. Finally, there is only one output node corresponding to the target LOSLEVEL

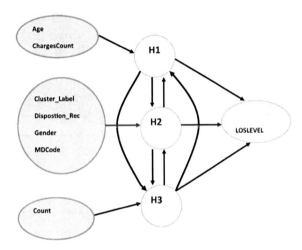

Figure 8. Diagnostic chart for the Neural Network model. None of the patients that spent less than two hours was predicted to spend more than five, which was the case with the decision tree

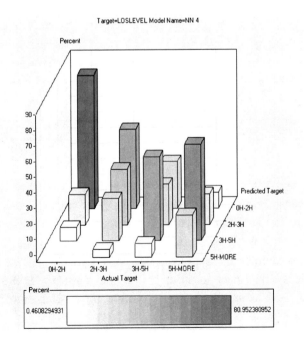

Table 6. Confusion Matrix. Table of target by output (assessed partition=VALIDATION)

Table of target by output				
target output				
Frequency|				
Percent					
Row Pct					
Col Pct |SHORT |MEDIUM |LONG |VERYLONG| Total				
---------+--------+--------+--------+--------+				
SHORT	289	53	15	0	357				
	36.22	6.64	1.88	0.00	44.74				
	80.95	14.85	4.20	0.00					
	66.44	32.32	8.38	0.00					
---------+--------+--------+--------+--------+				
MEDIUM	100	67	49	1	217				
	12.53	8.40	6.14	0.13	27.19				
	46.08	30.88	22.58	0.46					
	22.99	40.85	27.37	5.00					
---------+--------+--------+--------+--------+				
LONG	43	36	84	7	170				
	5.39	4.51	10.53	0.88	21.30				
	25.29	21.18	49.41	4.12					
	9.89	21.95	46.93	35.00					
---------+--------+--------+--------+--------+				
VERYLONG	3	8	31	12	54				
	0.38	1.00	3.88	1.50	6.77				
	5.56	14.81	57.41	22.22					
	0.69	4.88	17.32	60.00					
---------+--------+--------+--------+--------+				
Total 435 164 179 20 798				
54.51 20.55 22.43 2.51 100.00				

at regular intervals, we say that it has a cyclic component or a cyclic variation (Figure 9 (b)). *Seasonal variation* is cyclic variation that is controlled by seasonal factors. Water consumption has a seasonal high in summer and a low in winter. It happens that it is sometimes possible to disassociate trend and cyclic components. An Irregular component is an irregular fluctuation about the mean. The component can be additive or multiplicative. Decomposition of a time series into its components can be done automatically using statistics software packages. In this study, we have used the SAS software to decompose the time series LOS into its multiplicative compo-

Figure 9. Decomposition of the time series LOS into its components: The Trend-cycle (b), the Seasonal (c) and the irregular (d). The general trend shows that the LOS tends to decrease from January to March

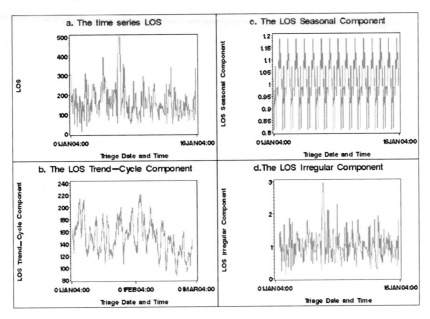

Figure 10. Seasonal component of LOS. This component shows a periodic variation of 24 hours. The LOS is short in morning (before noon) and increases in the afternoon hours

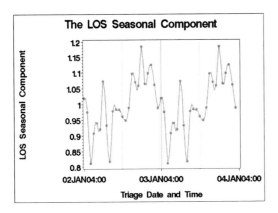

Figure 11. Linear Trend in the Time Series LOS. There is a global decrease in LOS from the month of January toward March, even if this trend is not strong

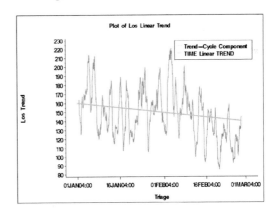

nents: the trend-cyclic component (Figure 9b), the seasonal component (Figure 9c) and the irregular component (Figure 9d).

In this study, we illustrate the time series method of LOS analysis using an accumulation interval of one hour.

Once the accumulation interval is found, the SAS high performance forecast procedure (PROC HPF) can be used to transform the transactional data into a multivariate time series. The proc HPF is very important as an automated forecasting procedure, especially in the following situations:

Figure 12. Marginal plots of the means of LOS by the most important predicting variables, revealed by the Decision Tree

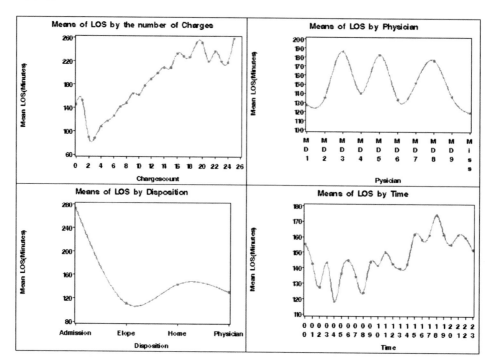

Figure 13. Correlogram of accumulated LOS for a 1 Hour, 4 Hours, 6 Hours and 8 Hours accumulation interval

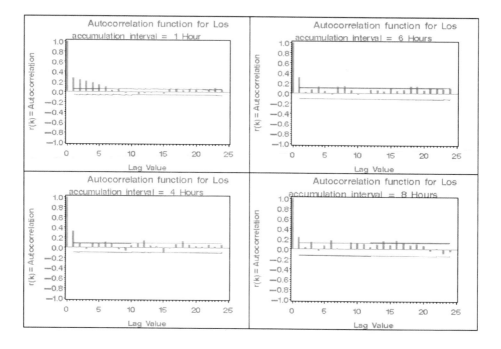

- A large number of forecasts must be generated.
- Frequent forecast updates are required.
- Time-stamped data must be converted to time series data.
- The forecasting model is not *a priori* known for each time series.
- Future values of the independent variables are needed to predict the dependent variable.

The big challenge with the HPF procedure is that it does not handle nominal variables. With medical data, the most important variables are nominal; for example, complaints, diagnoses, charges, and gender. Instead of leaving them out of the analysis, we recoded them using 0 and 1 dummy variables. As this may be a tedious task if there are several nominal variables with several classes, we recommend to a software developer that they incorporate an automatic dummy recoding into their statistics and data mining package. For example, the variable Cluster1 is a numerical binary variable with value 1 if the observation belongs to Cluster 1 and 0 otherwise. We did similar recoding for the variables, MD, RN, Disposition, Gender, Urgency, and Time, using SAS programming. Some other SAS procedures, such as proc GLM or Proc MIXED, perform automatically by recording nominal variables, but not PROC HPF.

When invoking the procedure HPF for accumulation purposes, no forecasts are needed and the option **lead** must be set to 0. The following code shows how the procedure was used:

```
proc sort data=sasuser.IbexFinal_Clus
out=Two;
By Triage;
Run;
proc hpf data=Two out=Three lead=0 ;
Id Triage interval=Hour6.
accumulate=Total;
forecast LOS Age visits ChargesCount;
```

```
forecast Cluster1 - Cluster8 MDCode1 -
MDCode8
RN_Code1 - RN_Code32 Disposition_Rec1 -
Disposition_Rec4
Time00 - Time23 Male Female Emergent Ur-
gent NonUrgent
/ Model=idm ;/*idm= intermittent time se-
ries */
run;
quit;
data sasuser.HPF2IbexFinal_Clus;
set Three ;
LOS=round(LOS/visits,1);
Age=round(Age/visits,1);
run;
Quit;
```

Accumulating the transactional variable, LOS, by one hour intervals leaves us with a time series with 25% missing values and many zeroes. Such time series are called intermittent time series. These time series are mainly constant valued except for relatively few occasions. With Intermittent series, it is often easier to predict when the series departs from the constant value and by how much from the next value. The HPF procedure uses special methods in handling these kind of data (SAS, n.d.). Intermittent models decompose the time series into two parts: the interval series and the size series. The interval series measure the number of time periods between departures. The size series measures the magnitude of the departures. This is specific to the procedure by using the option "*model=idm*" in the forecast statement.

In this analysis, the time series LOS components were identified. Only the irregular component was random. Using the SAS autoreg procedure, we predicted the irregular components and then recombined all the components to obtain the final predictions of LOS. A Plot of LOS versus its predictions is shown in Figure 14.

Generalized linear models were fit using the SAS procedure, Proc Glimmix (Glimmix, n.d.),

Figure 14. Plot of LOS versus its predictions. As this phenomenon was found with the Decision Tree and ANN, when the LOS becomes too long, it is hard to predict since the scatter points spread further from the 45 degree line

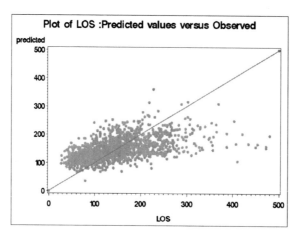

which is still an experimental procedure. The GLIMMIX procedure does not require that the response be normally distributed. It does not require a constant variability, nor does it require observations to be independent. The only requirements are that the response has a distribution that belongs to the exponential family and that the errors have a normal distribution with mean 0. Since errors come after fitting the model; it is required to check the distribution of the errors once the model has been fit.

The procedure can fit models with only fixed effects as well as models with random effects. As was discussed previously, there is no strict rule as to when to treat an effect as fixed or random. The only effects that are candidates to being fixed or random were the physician (MD) and the nurses (RN). We fitted two models, one considering MD and RN as fixed effects and another considering them as random. The code used is as follows:

```
goptions reset = all ctext = bl htext =
3pct ftext = swissb border;
ods html;
ods graphics on;
/*Fit fixed effect model*/
```

```
proc glimmix data=sasuser.IbexFinal_Clus;
class CLUSTER MDCode RN_Code Urgency Dis-
position_recoded Time gender;
MODEL LOS = chargesCount*chargesCount
CLUSTER*chargesCount MDCode|RN_Code Dis-
position_recoded Age Time Age Gender
Count|count / dist=LOGN link=identity
noint ;
nloptions technique=QUAnew;
Output Out=Glimmixout Pred=P
Resid=Residual;
run;
/*Transforming the output back to the
data scale*/
Data One;
set Glimmixout;
predicted=Exp(P);
N=_N_
run;
/* creating the 45 degree line*/
data Line;
set Two;
N=_N_;
If N LT 1600 then x=0;
else x=600;
If N LT 1600 then y=0;
else y=600;
```

Table 7. Fit statistics

Fit Statistics	
-2 Res Log Likelihood	3754.05
AIC (smaller is better)	4342.05
AICC (smaller is better)	4406.94
BIC (smaller is better)	6104.77
CAIC (smaller is better)	6398.77
HQIC (smaller is better)	4976.44
Pearson Chi-Square	468.14
Pearson Chi-Square / DF	0.16

```
run;
axis1 label=(a=90 r=0);
/* Ploting the actual values versus the
predicted*/
Proc GPlot Data=line;
plot predicted *Los=1 x*y=2/overlay
vref=100 200 300 400 500 href=100 200 300
400 500 lvref=20 lhref=20 vaxis=axis1;
symbol1 c=blue i=none v=dot w=2;
symbol2 c=red i=join v=none w=4;
Title1 BOLD C=BL H=18pt FONT=swissb
"Figa. Analysis of LOS by Proc Glimmix
Fixed Effect ";
Title2 BOLD C=BL H=18pt FONT=swissb "Ac-
tual vs Predicted Values of LOS";
Run;
Quit;
/*Checking the distribution of the re-
sidual*/
proc univariate data=One;
var Residual;
histogram Residual / vaxis=axis1
cbarline=black cfill=blue
normal(color=red w=4);
inset normal(mu std) /
pos = ne height = 3 header = 'Distribu-
tion fit' ;
axis1 label=(a=90 r=0);
Title1 BOLD C=BL H=18pt FONT=swissb
"Figc.Analysis of LOS by Proc Glimmix
Fixed Effects ";
```

```
Title2 BOLD C=BL H=18pt FONT=swissb "His-
togram For Residual";
run;
quit;
/*Fitting random effect model*/
proc glimmix data=sasuser.IbexFinal_Clus;
class CLUSTER MDCode RN_Code Urgency Dis-
position_recoded Time gender;
MODEL LOS = chargesCount*chargesCount
CLUSTER*chargesCount Disposition_recoded
Age Time Age Gender count|count
/ dist=LOGN link=identity noint;
random MDCode|RN_Code ;
nloptions technique=QUAnew;
Output Out=Glimmixout2 Pred=P
Resid=Residual;
run;
/* Putting the plots and the residual
plot in the same frame*/
proc greplay igout=work.gseg tc=sashelp.
templt
template=l2r2 nofs;
treplay 1:Gplot 2:Gplot1 3:univar 4:uni-
var1;
run;
ods graphics off;
ods html close;
```

The Table 7 shows the fit statistics of the models. Only the ratio of the Pearson chi-square by its degree of freedom is used to check the goodness of the model. All other fit statistics are good for comparing nested models. When the variability in the target variable is well modeled, the Pearson ratio is close to one. In our model, this value is rather too small. This means that the variability of the variable, LOS, is not well modeled through the given model. There may be various reasons for this lack of fit, but the main reason should be that although the variables included in the model have a significant influence on the response variable, there may be some other important predictors of LOS that were missed when collecting the data. This lack of fit can be seen in Figure 15.

In the Table 8, all the fixed effects have significant influence on LOS except the interaction, *Cluster*Gender,* and the variable, count. The interaction can be excluded from the model, but the predictor, *Count,* has to remain in the model since its interaction with Disposition is significant.

The GLIMMs model requires the residuals to be normally distributed with mean zero and some constant variance $\sigma2$ This requirement was checked using the SAS procedure, Proc Univariate. Figure 16 shows a distribution very close to a normal one, even if Table 9 does not agree with that assumption. This output shows that the hypothesis of normality of the residual is rejected.

Many of these tests have several limitations and their results cannot be trusted in this case.

In the case of the Kolmogorov-Smirnov, when location, scale, and shape parameters are estimated from the data, the critical region of the K-S test is no longer valid. It typically must be determined by simulation. (Fausett, 2004) The Anderson-Darling test is sensitive to the size of the data. With large datasets, small deviations from normality are detected as significant and small samples almost pass the normality test. The best way to evaluate how far the data deviate from Gaussian is to look at a graph and see if the distribution deviates considerably from a bell-shaped normal distribution (Sollid, n.d.). With these observations in mind, Figure 16 shows that the residuals are close to normally distributed, with mean 0 (Table 10).

The previous model assumes the variables, Physician and nurse, are fixed effects. However, the physicians and nurses considered are not the only ones treating at this Hospital. We want this study to be more general and not restricted to these specific physicians and nurses. If we want to extend the results of the analysis only for the medical personnel of the hospital, then we must treat the variable MD and RN as random effects. However, then we will need to apply a correction factor, since the population of Nurses and Doctors in a hospital is of finite size. If we decide not to limit the study to that hospital, then we can treat

Figure 15. Plot of predicted versus observed LOS. The predictions are good for Low values of LOS. For high values, the variation is uncontrollable

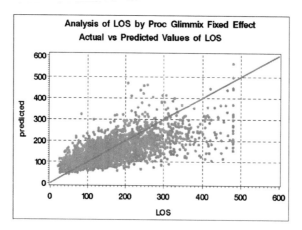

these variables without any constraint. The idea of a correction factor in a random effect is new and is not yet incorporated in the SAS software package. Due to this limitation, we have decided

to extend the study to any hospital that has a non-trauma emergency department.

The code for fitting with a mixed effect model is similar to the one used for fixed effects except

Table 8. Type iii tests of fixed effects

Type III Tests of Fixed Effects				
Effect	Num DF	Den DF	F Value	Pr > F
ChargesCo*ChargesCou	1	2983	82.17	<.0001
ChargesCount*CLUSTER	8	2983	55.67	<.0001
MDcode	9	2983	16.61	<.0001
RN_code	32	2983	2.13	0.0002
MDcode*RN_code	197	2983	1.70	<.0001
Disposition_recoded	3	2983	46.62	<.0001
Age	1	2983	23.71	<.0001
Time	23	2983	4.08	<.0001
Gender	1	2983	3.87	0.0494
COUNT	1	2983	20.00	<.0001
COUNT*COUNT	1	2983	9.82	0.0017

Figure 16. Distribution of residuals

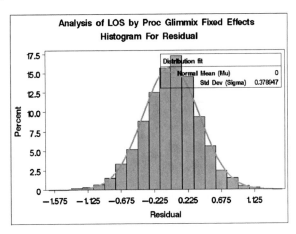

Table 9. The UNIVARIATE procedure: normality tests

Goodness-of-Fit Tests for Normal Distribution				
Test	Statistic		p Value	
Kolmogorov-Smirnov	D	0.02063671	Pr > D	<0.010
Cramer-von Mises	W-Sq	0.33638183	Pr > W-Sq	<0.005
Anderson-Darling	A-Sq	2.18214449	Pr > A-Sq	<0.005

Table 10. The UNIVARIATE procedure: fitted distribution for residual

Parameters for Normal Distribution		
Parameter	Symbol	Estimate
Mean	Mu	0
Std Dev	Sigma	0.378947

that this time, the variables MD and RN are moved from the Model statement to Random statement, as shown below.

```
proc glimmix data=sasuser.IbexFinal_Clus
plots=all;
class CLUSTER MDCode RN_Code Urgency Dis-
position_recoded Time gender;
MODEL LOS = chargesCount*chargesCount
CLUSTER*chargesCount
Age gender|CLUSTER Disposition_
recoded|count Time
/ dist=LOGN link=identity noint;
random MDCode|RN_Code ;
nloptions technique=QUAnew;
Output Out=Glimmixout2 Pred=P
Resid=Residual;
run;
```

The output of the fitting procedure is almost the same as the ones of the fixed effect except for the covariance parameter estimate (Table 11), which is not produced in the case of fixed effect.

The graphic of the fixed effect model and of the random effect model were put together in one frame (Figure 17) for easier comparison.

In this chapter, we have applied various techniques to analyze the Length of Stay at a Hospital Emergency Department. We also compare these techniques and show how they can be combined to produce better results.

In this study, we have applied two classes of techniques to perform the analysis of the dataset provided by electronic records in a Hospital Emergency Department (ED). One class was Data Mining techniques and the other was a class of

Statistical techniques. The Data mining techniques that we used include Text mining, Decision Trees, and Artificial Neural Network (ANN). The statistics techniques used were Generalized Linear Mixed Models (GLIMMs) and Time Series. All these techniques are incorporated in the statistical software package SAS (Statistical Analysis System).

The dataset contained interval, ordinal, nominal, and some other variables in an unstructured free-English format. Complaints, diagnosis, and charges were in the latter format, and as such they could not be included in several techniques for many reasons. Complaints and diagnoses had too many classes to be considered as nominal. In addition, the software distinguishes between capital and small letters so that identical instances such as *"Abdominal Pain"*, *"Abdominal pain"*, *"abdominal Pain"*, *"abdominal pain"*, *"abd pain"*, ... were considered different. The variable, charges, was simply too long to be understandable by any language machine. To include complaints, diagnosis, and charges in the analysis, we had to perform a text analysis, a data mining technique that analyzes text and groups together in one cluster by using related words. Text mining recognizes synonyms such as *headache* and *migraine*, the same words written with small or capital letters such as *"abdominal pain"* and *"Abdominal Pain"*, stemmed words such as *sleep* and *sleeping* as being from the same family. Hence, Text Analysis was applied to allow those variables to be used by other techniques.

In some complex systems, we need rules to understand the flow describing a course of action. Decision Trees, a data mining technique,

Table 11. The covariance parameter estimate

Covariance Parameter Estimates				
Cov Parm	Estimate	Standard Error	Z Value	Pr Z
MDcode	515.98	265.70	1.94	0.0261
RN_code	53.5450	48.8095	1.10	0.1363
MDcode*RN_code	275.21	68.4231	4.02	<.0001
Residual	3877.23	100.93	38.42	<.0001

Figure 17. Predictions and residual plot of the fixed effect and random effect models

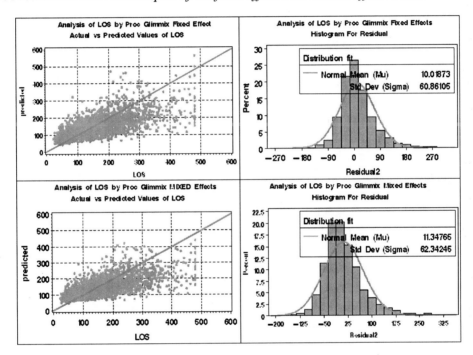

generates these rules. Each distinct path through the decision tree node produces distinct rules. These rules are often easier to understand than the tree itself.

Although the software generates those rules, we can generate them ourselves by tracing each path in the decision tree, from the root node to leaf nodes, recording the test outcomes as antecedents and the leaf-node classification as the consequent. Decision trees deliver an unparalleled understanding of the system through those decision rules. In addition, Decision Trees were used as a variable selection technique. In fact, in a Decision Tree, the splitting variables are ranked from the root node to a leaf node according to their importance. This way, when applying linear or generalized linear models after a decision tree, one would include higher powers of the variables ranked first in the tree. We have done that with the variable *chargescount* and both *chargescount* and *chargescount*chargescount* were highly significant.

Decision trees are efficient in analyzing ordinal and nominal variables. Artificial Neural network models can be applied to both nominal and interval variables. We applied ANN to discretized LOS

Table 12. Fit statistics of decision tree and ANN

	Training	Validation	Test
DECISION TREES			
Misclassification Rate	0.45	0.47	0.47
Root Average Squared Error	0.38	0.38	0.39
ANN			
Misclassification Rate	0.43	0.42	0.47
Root Average Squared Error	0.37	0.37	0.38

using the same inputs as those used for the decision trees, and ANN performed better than the Decision Trees judging by the misclassification rate as shown in Table 12.

The misclassification rate is a simple measure of how well the classifier is performing. Unfortunately, neural networks do not generate decision rules. Therefore, using both models will provide a good classification result and a good understanding of the system that generates the data.

Among the Statistical techniques that were used for the analysis of the dataset, the Generalized Linear Models (GLIM), the Generalized Linear Mixed Models (GLIMM), and the Time Series Models provided insight into the data. Treating MDCode and RN_code as fixed underestimates the variance and as a consequence, the model can predict values that lie outside of the range of the actual (Figure 18).

The system of Emergency Departments in the United States are organized almost the same, and we believe that the chosen hospital is representative of many others. Therefore, we may treat physicians and nurses as a sample from the population of Physicians and nurses in the whole country, and consider the factors MDCode and RN_Code as random effects. Figure 19 shows the improvement made to the model. No more predicted values lie outside of the range of the actual values.

Globally, the mixed model produced betters predictions. We also compared the Glimmix procedure, the time series procedure, Proc Autoreg, that fits Time series models, and the Artificial Neural Network. From Figures 20 and 21, we conclude that the time series models applied to the accumulated data performed better than the Glimmix procedure when applied to the same data,

Figure 18. Plot of Actual VS predicted values of LOS for a fixed effect Model

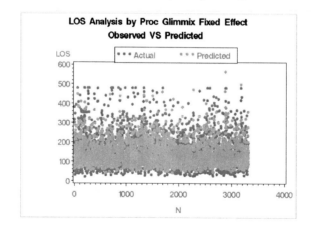

Figure 19. Plot of actual values vs predicted values with the mixed model

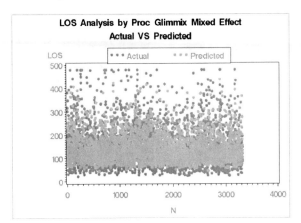

and that both perform better than the Artificial Neural Network.

However, all of this analysis must be used to make decisions to improve patient care. Therefore, we also look to the issue of scheduling throughout the day in order to optimize the use of personnel.

The analysis of electronic data from a Hospital Emergency Department (ED) using the HPF procedure showed that the crowding of the ED varies from time to time during the 24 hours (see Figure 22 and Table 13), going from a peak between 8:00 and 16:00 to a trough between 0:00 to 6:00, and day to day with a peak on the weekend

Figure 20. Comparison predictions of Glimmix procedure, Time series models (Proc Autoreg) and Artificial Neural Network

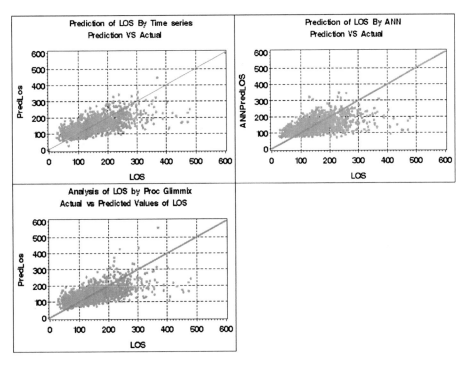

Figure 21. Comparison of Residual of Glimmix procedure, Time series models (Proc Autoreg) and Artificial Neural Network

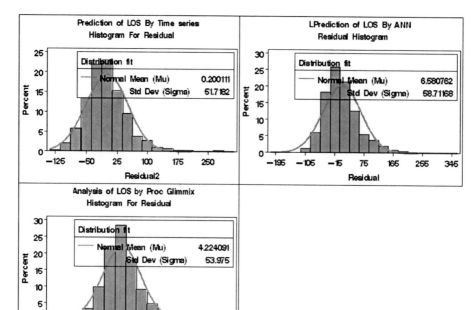

Figure 22. Boxplot showing the variation of the number of patients in the ED for a period of 24 Hours. This figure shows that the ED is more crowded in the afternoon, with a high variation between 12:00 and 18:00

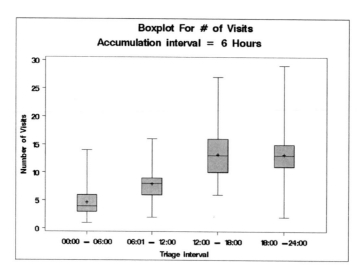

Table 13. Variation in the number of visits and in the LOS in the ED for all patients for a period of three months

Triage Time	LOS			
	# Patients	MeanLOS	Min	Max
00:00 - 01:01	121	161	35	648
01:01 - 02:00	94	143	34	392
02:01 - 03:00	48	131	33	472
03:01 - 04:00	46	144	36	380
04:01 - 05:00	41	124	40	348
05:01 - 06:00	30	138	45	434
06:01 - 07:00	42	147	44	331
07:01 - 08:00	67	137	31	495
08:01 - 09:00	94	127	26	285
09:01 - 10:00	121	146	22	580
10:01 - 11:00	160	142	29	533
11:01 - 12:00	173	153	32	552
12:01 - 13:00	157	145	39	655
13:01 - 14:00	151	142	49	686
14:01 - 15:00	190	144	32	567
15:01 - 16:00	184	163	15	482
16:01 - 17:00	193	159	30	454
17:01 - 18:00	198	164	38	653
18:01 - 19:00	181	174	32	521
19:01 - 20:00	178	165	29	465
20:01 - 21:00	212	154	36	419
21:01 - 22:00	195	162	32	552
22:01 - 23:00	159	161	37	728
23:01 - 00:00	130	151	31	496

(Table 14). We can show that the scheduling of the medical personnel can be done efficiently allowing for a reduction in the patient "Length of Stay" (LOS).

From the dataset under analysis, it has been found that the scheduling basis is one Physician with two or sometimes three nurses from 6:00 AM to 6:00 PM and one Physician from 6:00 PM to 6:00 AM. From Figure 21, it is clear that from 00:00 to 06:00, there are few visits, whereas there are a large number of visits between 12:00 and 18:00. This means that the

actual scheduling is inadequate as it does not take care of the time varying character of the number of visits at the ED. Figure 23 shows that the variable, LOS, is strongly associated with the variable visits.

In order to include independent variables in (auto) regression models where future values of the independent variable are needed to predict the dependent variable, the HPF procedure can be extended by the AUTOREG procedure. The user can let the HPF automatically select the forecast model, or he/she can provide one if known. A

299

Table 14. Variation of the number of patients by the day of the week

Visits: Day of the week	Triage Time				Total
	00:00 - 06:00	06:01 - 12:00	12:01 - 18:00	18:00 - 24:00	
FRIDAY	46	104	132	139	421
MONDAY	43	104	171	182	500
SATURDAY	77	102	199	165	543
SUNDAY	58	91	172	152	473
THURSDAY	61	101	155	163	480
TUESDAY	54	84	131	142	411
WEDNESDAY	62	94	158	178	492

Figure 23. Variation of the number of visits by the time of visit. The number of visits and the Average LOS attain a global maximum between 16:00 and 20:00

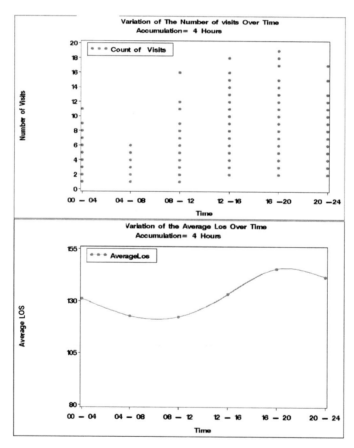

transformation of the independent variable is also possible with the HPF procedure.

In our study, we produced the LOS forecast for a week including the variable, visits, as an independent variable and invoking the log transformation to ensure a normal distribution of the data (Figure 24). The code used looks like this:

Figure 24. Forecast of LOS by extending the HPF procedure to include the independent variable visits using Proc Autoreg. The R-square=78%, which means that 78% of the variation in LOS is explained by the crowding of the Emergency Department alone

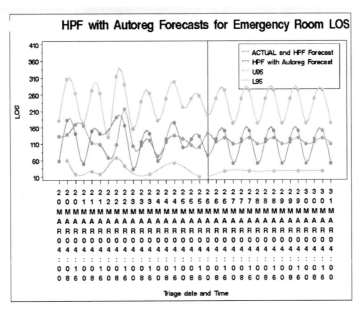

```
goptions reset = all ctext = black htext
= 2.5pct ftext = swissb border;
proc hpf data=sasuser.Hpf6day
out=nextweek lead=24;
id datetime interval=hour6.
accumulate=none;
forecast los / transform=log;
forecast visits ;
run;
proc autoreg data= nextweek;
model los = visits /noint;
output out=sasuser.LosForecast p=Forecast
UCL=U95 LCL=L95;
run;
quit;
Title BOLD C=BL H=22pt FONT=swissb 'Fig-
ure 5: HPF with Autoreg
Forecasts for Emergency Room LOS';
symbol1 c=blue i=spline w=2 v=dot ;
symbol2 c=red i=spline w=2 v=dot ;
symbol3 c=magenta i=spline w=2 v=dot ;
symbol4 c=green i=spline w=2 v=dot ;
axis1 offset=(1 cm)
label=('Triage date and Time') minor=none
order=('20mar04:00:00:00'dt
to'31MAR04:00:00:00'dt by Hour8.);
axis2 label=(angle=90 'LOS')
order=(10 to 410 by 50);
legend1 across=1
cborder=black
position=(top inside right)
offset=(-2,0)
value=(tick=1 'ACTUAL and HPF Forecast'
tick=2 'HPF with Autoreg Forecast'
tick=3 'U95'
tick=4 'L95')
shape=symbol(2,.25)
mode=share
label=none;
proc gplot data=sasuser.
LosForecast(firstobs=181 obs=273);
plot Los * datetime = 1
forecast*datetime=2 (U95 L95)*datetime=4
/ overlay
href='26MAR04:00:00:00'dt
chref=maroon
```

```
vaxis=axis2
vminor=1
haxis=axis1
legend=legend1;
run;
quit;
```

There are many analyses of medical data, but most have been done without consideration of the fact that medical data are time-stamped as shown in Tables 13 and 14. The scheduling of medical personnel does not utilize statistical analysis that examines the time varying character of the number of visits in the Hospital Emergency Department and length of treatment needed for each patient. Figures 21 and 23 show that the LOS and the number of visits at the ED are generally high during the second half of the day (between 12:00 and 24:00). Therefore, more medical personnel should be scheduled for those hours; otherwise, there will be considerable crowding in the ED, resulting in significant increases in the average LOS causing the ED to go to a divert or bypass status.

The number of visits to the ED is an important factor for the LOS, as by itself, it explains 78% of the variation in LOS. It has to be taken into consideration when scheduling the medical personnel. The actual scheduling as shown in Table 14, is based on only one physician for every 12-hour shift with the support of only two nurses (rarely, three nurses are scheduled).

CURRENT AND FUTURE CHALLENGES FACING THE ORGANIZATION

This study has attempted to model the Length of Stay at a Hospital Emergency department, using Data mining techniques and statistical Techniques. Each model can be applied alone, or the information from one model can be used in the other models. The Figure 25 shows a hierarchy of how these models can be integrated. Text mining

is done prior to any other method. Then Decision Trees models can be built to selection variables and produce decision rules that help understand the system. Using the variables identified by the Decision Trees, Neural Network, generalized Linear models, and Time series models can be built.

In the case of Time series or transactional data, a decomposition of the time series into its components can be done first, and the Artificial Neural Network, the Generalized Linear Model (Glimmix procedure), and the autoregression (Autoreg procedure) can be applied to predict the irregular component. Results of each model can be recombined with the other components to produce the final predictions.

Some models, such as Decision Trees, are descriptive and should not be missing in any analysis since they help understand the data. Descriptive models are expected to identify factors that contribute the most to the variation of the target variable. In the case of the Length of Stay at a Hospital Emergency Department, the variables that contribute the most to the variation of the LOS variable are the number of items (exams, specimen collections) charged to the patients, the type of diagnosis (identified in the data by CLUSTER),

Figure 25. Flow of integration of analysis models

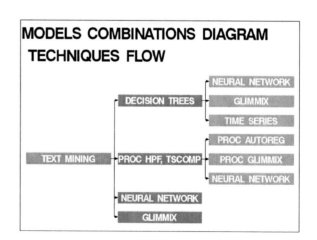

the treating physician, the time of presentation at the ED, and the nurses. These variables are not the only ones available. However, these variables contribute about 50% of the variation of LOS, according to the misclassification rates. Other factors still need to be identified. We think that some of these factors can be organizational. We have found that despite the fact that the number of patients at the ED varies by the time of the day, only one Physician and mainly 2 nurses are scheduled for a period of 12 hours. Also, the policy of shift change should be reviewed since we have an increase of the LOS at the shift change time of 3:00 PM and 6:00 PM.

In the future, we plan on continuing our investigation, trying to identify more factors that are linked to the long length of stay at the ED.

REFERENCES

Berry, M. J. A., & Linoff, G. (1999). *Mastering Data Mining: The Art and Science of Customer Relationship Management.* New York: John Wiley & Sons, Inc.

Cerrito, J. C. & Pharm (Personal Communication, October, 2005).

Faculty Practice Plan boosts emergency room operations.(1999). Retrieved 2007, from http:// record.wustl.edu/archive/1999/09-09-99/articles/ practice.html

Fausett, L. (n.d.). *Fundamentals of Neural Networks: Architectures, Algorithms, and Applications.* Englewood Cliffs, NJ: Prentice Hall.

Friedman, J., Hastie, T. & Tibshirani, R. (n.d.). *The Elements of Statistical Learning: Data Mining, Inference and Prediction.* New York: Springer Verlag.

Krzysztof, J., Cios, G., & Moore, W. (2002). Uniqueness of Medical Data Mining. *Artificial Intelligence in Medicine, 26*(1), 1–24. doi:10.1016/ S0933-3657(02)00049-0

Sahai, H., & Ageel, M. I. (2000). *The Analysis of variance: Fixed, Random and mixed models,* library of Boston: Birkhausser

SAS 9.1.3 (n.d.). High-Performance Forecasting, User's Guide, Third Edition. Retrieved 2007, from http://support.sas.com/documentation/ onlinedoc/91pdf/sasdoc_913/hp_ug_9209.pdf

Schwartz, M. (2007). *Wanted: Emergency Care Just For Kids.* Retrieved from http://www.lpfch. org/fundraising/news/spring03/emergency.html

Sengupta, D., & Jammalamadaka, S. R. (2003). *Linear Models: An Integrated Approach.* Washington, DC: World Scientific Publishing Co.

Sollid, L. (2007). *The Evolution Of Emergency Room Medecine: Today's patients often need a high level of medical care,* Calgary Health Region's hospital Emergency Departments. Retrieved from http://www.calgaryhealthregion.ca/newslink/ er_pack052103/evol_er052103.html

The Glimmix Procedure. (2005, November). Retrieved 2007, from http://support.sas.com/rnd/ app/papers/glimmix.pdf

Verbeke, G. (1997). *Linear Mixed Models in Practice: A SAS-Oriented Approach.* New York: Springer Verlag.

ADDITIONAL READING

Berry, M. J. A., & Linoff, G. S. (2004). *Data Mining Techniques* (2nd ed.). New York: Wiley Publishing.

Friedman, J., Hastie, T. & Tibshirani, R. (2009, February)*The Elements of Statistical Learning: Data Mining, Inference and Prediction.* New York: Springer Verlag.

Kantardzic, M. (2003). *Data Mining: Concepts, Models, Methods, and Algorithms.* New York: Wiley-Interscience.

Maddala, G. S., & Kim, I.-M. (1998). *Unit Roots, Contegration and Structural Change*. Cambridge, UK: Cambridge University Press.

Sahai, H., & Ageel, M. I. (2000). *The Analysis of variance: Fixed, Random and mixed models*. Boston: Birkhausser.

Sengupta, D., & Jammalamadaka, S. R. (2003). *Linear Models: An Integrated Approach*. Washington, DC: World Scientific Publishing.

Verbeke, G. (1997). *Linear Mixed Models in Practice: A SAS-Oriented Approach*. New York: Springer Verlag.

Chapter 14
Utilization of the Emergency Department

David Nfodjo
University of Louisville, USA

ABSTRACT

The primary role of the Emergency Department (ED) is to treat the seriously injured and seriously sick patients. However, because of federal regulations requiring the ED to treat all who enter, EDs have become the providers of a large number of unscheduled, non-urgent care patients. The role of the ED has changed considerably in recent years to treat those without insurance, and without primary care physicians. The main purpose of this study is to investigate the use of the hospital ED for non-urgent care in relationship to socio-economic status and payer type. This study will identify the socio-economic factors related to the utilization of the emergency department for health care. The study will identify for the purpose of shifting patients that use the Ed as primary care to a nearby clinic. The clinic is within a mile of the ED. It is a Nurse-managed health center that provides free care.

BACKGROUND

The primary role of the Emergency Department (ED) is to treat the seriously injured and seriously sick patients. However, because of federal regulations requiring the ED to treat all who enter, the EDs have become the providers for a large number of unscheduled, non-urgent care patients. The role of the ED has changed considerably in recent years to treat those without insurance, and without primary care physicians.

Many patients choose to go into the ED instead of using a primary healthcare provider. The National Center for Health Statistics states that most patients who go to the ED do not need urgent care. In 1996, a record fifty percent of the 90 million visits to the ED were deemed unnecessary. These unnecessary visits translated, in terms of dollars and cents, to a mean of 40.5 million people paying up to three times as much for routine care as they would have paid at a physician's office or clinic. Many of the patients who visit the ED are uninsured and without the means to pay, creating a financial burden

DOI: 10.4018/978-1-61520-723-7.ch014

Copyright © 2010, IGI Global. Copying or distributing in print or electronic forms without written permission of IGI Global is prohibited.

on EDs across the United States (US). Also, if a patient goes to the ED with a skin rash or a sprain or other non-urgent problem, insurance may not cover it. These non-urgent visits create economic and financial burdens on both the patient and the ED. The number of EDs in the US has been cut by 14%, but the number of visits has increased to about 114 million, according to the Centers for Disease Control (CDC). (CDC, 1996)

Health care policymakers need to investigate some, if not all of the characteristics of the most frequent users of the ED. It was reported that in 2003, 20.9 percent of all children made one or more visits to the ER (ED). The Urban Institutes' 1997 and 1999 data showed that the most frequent users of the ER are more likely to be publicly insured and to have worse health conditions compared to others. (Urban, 1999)

Previous studies have shown the inappropriateness of the use of the ED by non-urgent patients. However, these studies have different estimates of non-urgent care that ranges from 5 percent to 82 percent (CDC, 2003). In general, many insurance payers consider a primary care setting to be more cost-effective, and there are many suggestions presented in an attempt to decrease the burden on the ED. There is also a general concern that non-urgent patients delay care to the seriously injured or ill by crowding the ED. The Centers for Disease Control and Prevention have reported that in 2003, visits to the ED reached a record high of nearly 114 million, but the number of EDs decreased by 12% from 1993 to 2003. The number of visits increased 26% during this time period when the United States population increased by 12.3%. The report indicated that Medicare patients were 4 times as likely (81 visits per 100 people) to seek treatment from the ED than those with private insurance (22 visits per 100 people). This information is based on data from the 2003 National Hospital Ambulatory Medical Care Survey (NHAMCS) Emergency Department Summary, which is a national probability-based sample survey of visits to US ER. (CDC, 2003)

EDs in the US are more crowded than ever. EDs do not operate on a first come, first served basis. The ED uses a triage method to classify patients; providers assign patients into categories based upon the severity of the medical need. The most severe are seen first regardless of the time of arrival. The last thing a patient wants to do is to sit for long hours in the waiting room. Overall, patients spend an average of 3.2 hours in the ED. The average wait time is 46.5 minutes. A recent government report indicated that overcrowding is occurring in most EDs, along with an increase in the number of people who leave the ED before seeing a doctor because they get tired of waiting (called elopement). One of the reasons for overcrowding is that many patients choose the ED because of a lack of a primary provider. Those without primary providers tend to use the ED for the treatment of everything from a fractured toe to a cough. Use of the ED for such minor problems helps create the overcrowding. An urgent condition is defined as one that does not pose an immediate threat but does require prompt medical attention; non-urgent are those who do not require prompt attention.

Reports have questioned the ability of the ED to handle the widespread overcrowding. (Gao, 2002). Reports have indicated that more than 90% of large hospitals are operating at or over their capacity. Overcrowding not only causes delays in both diagnosis and treatment, but is a risk to the critically ill. When the ED is overcrowded, the average wait time is 5.8 hours. With overcrowding, there is not enough staff to give the severely ill the undivided attention they require, so there is an increased risk of medical errors. Errors have been linked to overcrowding as the quality of patient care is compromised, since the medical staff is constantly under pressure by the needs of all the patients (Jcrinc, 2004).

When EDs are overcrowded, ambulances carrying the severely injured or ill are sometimes diverted to more distant sites. In many urban areas, there is as much as a 20% to 50% diversion rate of medical vehicles. Overcrowded EDs will not be ready if there were a natural disaster or a terrorist act as we saw on September 11th, 2001.

Previous reports have blamed a large amount of overcrowding on non-urgent patients, but while there is a vague concept that non-urgent conditions do not require immediate attention, no standardized consensus definition of non-urgent exists. There are several different suggestions on how to handle the non-urgent patient population; however, reports have shown that the rate of hospitalization has increased for patients who were identified as needing non-urgent care and initially turned away by the ED (Nursing center, 2004). Because of these concerns, EDs are more inclined to accept all patients who enter. In addition to these concerns, the Health Care Financing Administration (HCFA) strictly enforces the Emergency Medical Treatment and Labor Act (EMTALA), which makes the ED the only guaranteed access to health care for all uninsured Americans.

The NHAMCS reports that visit rates were higher in the Northeast (44.4 visits per 100 persons) and the South (44.0) with a higher proportion of visits occurring in the south than in the other three regions. It was also reported that the majority of patients arrived at the ED between 8 am and 10 pm. Medicaid patients have been identified as the greatest users of the ED. There is a general notion that the non-urgent users delay care. The idea that the ED is being used inappropriately by non-urgent care is not a new one. There have been a number of retrospective studies that have had dramatically different results of non-urgent patients in the ED. The range is from 5% to 82%. Some have suggested re-directing or shifting the non-urgent care to reduce cost and overcrowding. However, while the non-urgent demand is the reason for overcrowding in the waiting room, that demand is not the reason for overcrowding in the treatment area. Reports have indicated that the total number of ED visits has a poor correlation with ED overcrowding (Hschange, 2004).

There is no easy solution to the problem of overcrowding. Some EDs have constructed an observational unit, and this has been shown to decrease the wait time by 40% while also reducing the overcrowding problem. Studies have been done to determine who waits the longest in the ED. It is no secret that prolonged waiting times in the ED are negatively associated with patient satisfaction and an increased risk of patients leaving without medical attention (called elopement). Current initiatives are not adequate to tackle the problem of overcrowding and wait times. To help reduce the overcrowding in the ED, the Saint Mary's hospital, a subsidiary of Barnes Jewish Hospital, has offered a non-urgent care facility adjacent to their traditional ED (BJC, 2001). The Athens regional will soon begin construction of a new express care facility adjacent to the ED to treat non-urgent patients. The University Hospital in Louisville has created a similar facility.

The main purpose of this study is to investigate the use of the hospital ED for non-urgent care in relationship to the socio-economic status and payer type, and to compare those patients to patients who utilize a no-cost clinic to see if there are differences in the patient populations. The specific aims are listed below.

1. To determine the nature of the patient population of the area within 5 and 10-miles of the local, free clinic located only one mile from the Hospital's ED. Patient location will be compared to socio-economic data available in ESRI's Tapestry database. The clinic is a Nurse-managed health center. The clinic improves community health through neighborhood-based primary health care services that are accessible, acceptable and affordable.

2. To determine if a shift from the ED to the Clinic will decrease costs while simultaneously increasing the quality of care. Socioeconomic status is strongly associated

with risk of disease and mortality. This study will examine the Socio-economic factors related to utilization of the emergency department for health care.

Another purpose of this project is to examine whether recommended follow up for non-urgent care can be redirected to the clinic, which is located about 1.5 miles from the hospital. The transfer will ensure more and better management of patient care for non-urgent needs, so that the ED can focus on more urgent patients. In this study, we use data mining techniques such as cluster analysis to cluster patients based on certain attributes and characteristics. Cluster analysis is used to discover the socio-economic reasons that affect the utilization of the ED. Linear models and classification methods are used to determine the grouping, and predictive modeling will be used to examine resource utilization.

Traditional statistical techniques for identifying non urgent care utilizations of the ED include Chi-square, the Bonferroni multiple comparison test, means and proportions, correlation, ordinary least squares, and multiple linear regression analysis with the method of choice for most researchers being multiple logistic regression. The weaknesses of these techniques include the inability to model nonlinear relationships between inputs and targets, and the inability to model effectively large volumes of data. These techniques also require distribution assumptions.

One study used proportions and means in comparing non-urgent care utilization of the ED in two different hospitals. Subjects were interviewed before and after their ED visit. Four expert judgments were used to define non urgent and urgent patients. The findings reported that the young and the socially fragile with no source of regular income accounted for a third of the visits out of 12,000 visits per year. Their results indicated a need for a structure providing primary care both inside and outside of normal working hours. A second study analyzed their data on parents

taking their children to the ED. This study used a non-parametric statistic (Chi-square). Parents of subjects were given a 53-item questionnaire to answer. Eighty-two percent of parents were found to have overstated or were unsure of the seriousness of their child's illness. A total of 114 parents filled out the questionnaire during a two week period in 1992. Their results suggested the need for more community primary care services. The results of a third study, using multiple logistic regression on 541 patients who participated in a survey questionnaire, indicated that age and sex were significant factors for the utilization of the ED. Two expert judgments were used to define non urgent and urgent patients. They suggested a further evaluation of the use of primary care. (Nfodjo, 2006)

The analysis here differs from that in previous studies in that the actual clinical data are used instead of relying on patient surveys. This will allow decision makers to gain more insight into the nature of the patients they deal with. It will help target the clustered patients before they go to the ER. The idea is to help shift the non urgent care patients to the nearby clinic. Using the same techniques and strategies for all patients is ineffective and very expensive. This research will help the hospital reduce cost by identifying ways to shift the non urgent care patients to the clinic.

SETTING THE STAGE

Geographic Information Systems (GIS) is a simple, but powerful concept that is used to solve real-world problems from tracking delivery trucks to modeling global atmospheric circulation. For many GIS users, the end result is best when it is displayed in a map or graph format. GIS can perform a variety of analyses, including mapping, data management, geographic analysis, and data editing. By mapping objects, we can see patterns and easily locate where things are. GIS maps also help monitor the occurrence of events in a geographic location. By mapping, we can gain insight into the behavior of objects. Our future needs may be adjusted accordingly to this behavior. Maps allow us to see relationships, patterns or trends that may not be possible to see with charts or spreadsheets.

GIS provides methods to input geographic (coordinates) and tabular (attributes) data. It also provides utilities for finding specific geographic features based on location, or on an attribute value. GIS is used to answer questions regarding the interaction of spatial relationships between multiple datasets. There are many tools in GIS for visualizing geographic features. Results can be displayed in a variety of formats such as maps, graphs and reports. The *vector* and *raster* forms are the two data models for the storage of Geographic data. The raster data type is made up of rows and columns of cells. A single value is stored in each cell. These values can be discrete or continuous. The vector data model represents geographic features using lines (series of points) and polygons (areas) to represent objects. Vector features respect spatial integrity through the application of topological rules. Vectors represent the features by their x, y (Cartesian) coordinate system. The raster assigns values to cells that cover coordinate locations instead of just representing features by their x, y coordinates.

The advantage of a vector over a raster is that it requires less storage space. Raster datasets record a value to represent each point in the area covered. However, overlay implementations, which are the combination of two separate points, lines, or polygons to create a new output, are more difficult in vector data. While raster data appear as blocky in appearance, vector data display a vector graphic that is used to generate traditional maps.

A GIS query can be used to determine the location that satisfies a condition of interest. It can also be used to determine what type of characteristic is associated with a particular area. Three common types of geographic analyses exist in GIS: the proximity, the overlay, and the Network analysis.

The proximity analysis is used to determine how many objects are within a certain distance of a second object or objects; for example, determining the location and number of houses that lie within a certain distance of a hospital, or determining what proportion of liquor stores are within 500 meters of a school. The overlay combines the features of two layers to create a new layer. This new layer can be analyzed to determine the area of overlap. These overlays are similar to a Venn diagram. The network is used to examine how linear features are connected, and how easily resources can flow through them.

The accuracy of the data can affect the results of any query or analysis that is performed in GIS. Since the purpose of GIS is to analyze and visualize relationships among objects, it is important to depict the real world as accurately as possible. All locations on the earth are referenced to the data. Two maps can have different coordinate values for the same location on the earth's surface if two different data points are used. Checking the data as well as the projected coordinate system of a dataset is vital for matching different data sources in the same coordinate space.

A map projection is a method of converting the earth's three-dimensional surface to a two-dimensional surface. All projections use mathematical formulas that convert data from a geographic location to represent a location on a flat surface. The conversions may cause distortion. The shape, area, distance or direction of a spatial property may be distorted. Care must be employed in choosing a projection since the spatial properties are used to make decisions. When a Peter's projection is chosen, for example, an accurate area calculation is achieved at the expense of inaccurate shape; a Mercator projection maintains the true direction, but gives inaccurate area and distance; and a Robinson projection is a compromise of all the properties. Any chosen projection has little effect on a large scale map, but significantly affects a small-scale map. The other types of projections are Equal area, Conformal, Equidistant and Azimuthal.

The Equal area maintains the area of a map. The map of the United States generally uses the Albers Equal Area Canonic projection. The Conformal map maintains shape for small areas and is very useful for weather maps and navigation charts. The Equidistant map preserves distance. Since no projection can maintain distance from all points to all other points, distance can be held true from one point or from a few points to all other points. The Azimuthal map preserves direction from one point to all the other points. This can be combined with the Equal area, Conformal, and Equidistant projections as in the Lambert Equal Area Azimuthal or the Azimuthal Equidistant projections. The most pleasing visually and most used projection for general mapping is the Robinson projection, which is neither equal area nor conformal.

GIS can be used to map objects where they are. This capability allows people to see where features lie, and the distributions of these features. The distributions of features allow us to see patterns in the features. GIS also allows us to map quantities. This gives us an additional level of information such as pointing to where the most and least of a quantity exist spatially.

GIS has been used by district attorneys to monitor drug-related arrests, and also to find out if an arrest is within 1000 feet of a school in order to stiffen the penalties. It has also been used extensively by public health officials to map the number of physicians per 1000 people in each census tract to see which areas are inadequately served and which are not. Catalog companies have used it to target the concentration of young families with high income in order to market their products.

For some businesses such as insurance companies, geography is an essential key in understanding customers. Many factors affect profit, and GIS helps insurance companies in a variety of ways. It provides the tools needed to segment customers into geographical location so that exposure to losses can be managed successfully

Another important facet often overlooked is the impact of GIS technology on financial institutions. These mathematical models provide an almost personal profile of customers. Aspects such as purchasing habits, financial behavior, and perceived need for additional products and services can all be studied comprehensively. These institutions can then target aggressively their best prospects by precision and promotional marketing while efficiently distributing their advertising resources, which can lead to huge cost savings while at the same time fulfilling mandatory compliance requirements.

Table 1. Segment Codes

L1: High Society	U1: Principal Urban Centers I
L2: Upscale Avenues	U2: Principal Urban Centers II
L3: Metropolis	U3: Metro Cities I
L4: Solo Acts	U4: Metro Cities II
L5: Senior Styles	U5: Urban Outskirts I
L6: Scholars and Patriots	U6: Urban Outskirts II
L7: High hopes	U7: Suburban Periphery I
L8: Global Roots	U8: Suburban Periphery II
L9: Family Portrait	U9: Small Towns
L10: Traditional Living	U10: Rural I
L11: Factories and Farms	U11: Rural II
L12: American	

Tapestry is an ESRI segmentation system that classifies United States (US) neighborhoods by using proven methodology. Neighborhoods are grouped by similarities in their characteristics. The segmentation provides an accurate, detailed description of US neighborhoods. The residential areas of the US are divided into 65 segments based on more than 60 attributes or demographic variables such as occupation, age, income, education and behavior characteristics. These 65 are organized into 12 life mode and 11 urbanization summary groups with similar consumer and demographic patterns, and similar levels of densities respectively. Tapestry, the combination of traditional statistical segments analysis methodology and the ESRI data mining techniques was used to produce this segmentation of the US neighborhoods.

The twelve life mode summary groups are based on life styles while the eleven urbanization summary groups are based on geographic features along with income.

The Life mode summary groups are defined as shown in Table 1.

We display the zip code map of the County in Figure 1, and Figure 2 gives a zip code map detailing the segment code for the life mode summary group. The map of the urbanization summary group is displayed in Figure 3.

Life Mode Group: L1 High Society

This group represents about 12% of the population and is employed in the high paying professional and managerial positions. The median house hold income is almost twice the national median at $94,000 and their median home values approach $300,000. It is also a prolific group with a 2% annual growth each year.

Life Mode Group: L2 Upscale Avenues

This group is just as educated as the previous one with incomes well above the national median at

Figure 1. A zip code map of the county of interest

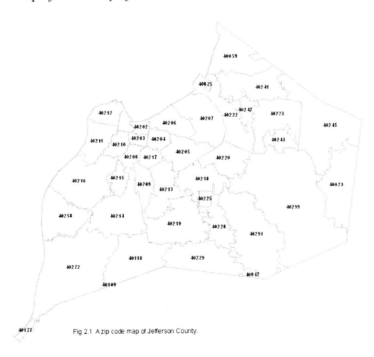

Fig 2.1 A zip code map of Jefferson County.

Figure 2. A zip code map detailing the segment codes for the life mode summary group

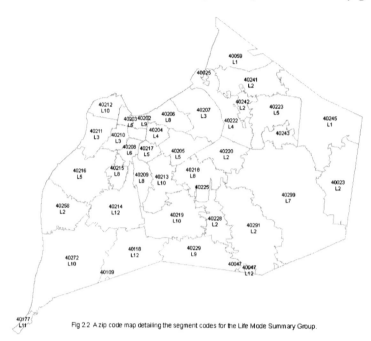

Fig 2.2 A zip code map detailing the segment codes for the Life Mode Summary Group.

Figure 3. A zip code map detailing the segment codes for the urbanization summary group

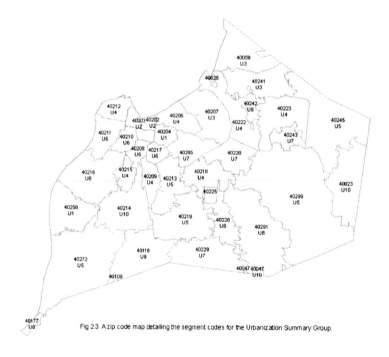

Fig 2.3 A zip code map detailing the segment codes for the Urbanization Summary Group.

$65,000. They choose various suburban home types and some even rent, depending on distinct individual preferences.

Life Mode Group: L3 Metropolis

This group lives in older homes built earlier than 1940. They reside in smaller cities and commute to service related jobs. This group has diversity in age with married couples with children and single family homes.

Life Mode Group: L4 Solo Acts

These are educated, established singles with at least a college degree. Their income is based on experience ranging from about $40,000 to $87,000 and they migrate mainly to the large cities. They tend to live in start-up homes in densely populated neighborhoods.

Life Mode Group: L5 Senior Styles

The median income in this group is from retirement savings or earnings from social security. As a result, their housing selections depend entirely on their income. Some stay in their homes, others in retirement communities, and yet others move to more agreeable climate areas.

Life Mode Group: L6 Scholars and Patriots

This group is transient, comprised mostly of college students and military serviceman and as a result, home ownership is limited. Residence is usually in town homes, multi-housing on a temporary basis during either active duty or until a college degree is earned.

Life Mode Group: L7 High Hopes

Less than half own homes and the households are a mix of married couples, single-parent families and singles, on average less than 35 years old. They have a college education and have a net worth of about $80,000.

Life Mode Group: L8 Global Roots

The households are younger and more ethnically diverse, with a strong Hispanic background. Their modest income allows them to rent in multi-unit dwellings. Most are recent immigrants to the States; they strive for the American dream of better jobs and homes for their families.

Life Mode Group: L9 Family Portrait

This group is young, ethnically diverse and many own single-family homes. Families generally have a large household size. Youth, family and children characterize this group.

Life Mode Group: L10 Traditional Living

This group is hard-working and well settled. They live modestly in established neighborhoods. Characteristically, these communities have families completing child-rearing, and the youth migrate to other places in search of better jobs. The dominant homes in these communities are single-family homes

Life Mode Group: L11 Factories and Farms

This segment has a median household income of $37,000 from factory or agricultural based jobs. The households are made up of married couples with or without children and most own their own homes in these rural American communities

Life Mode Group: L12 American Quilt

This segment lives in small rural areas and towns. Mobile homes and single family homes are typical for this group of people who consist

313

mainly of skilled laborers in the manufacturing and construction sectors.

Urbanization Group: U1
Principal Urban Centers I

These urbanites reside in high rises in the big cities and metropolises, and tend to consist of younger singles. They prefer high density apartments and public transport to ownership of homes and cars. They have professional jobs, are ethnically diverse and rely on modern conveniences.

Urbanization Group: U2
Principal Urban Centers II

These live in gateway cities and aspire to find affordable housing. As a result, they reside in the row houses, duplexes and low density areas. Families are more common than the previous group, and so is family based entertainment.

Urbanization Group: U3 Metro Cities I

This group combines suburban living with city life and as a result, lives in densely populated upscale neighborhoods. They are the well-educated and wealthiest with a median home value at nearly twice the national average and income in excess of 75% of the national average. Households are composed of married couples with or without children.

Urbanization Group: U4 Metro Cities II

This group is basically that of households in transition. The majority of households rent in multi-unit dwellings and a few, especially retirees, in starter households own homes. The younger population is still mobile, changing jobs and getting into college. They are economically conscious but utilize urban conveniences such as fast foods.

Urbanization Group: U5
Urban Outskirts I

This segment resides in higher density suburban areas in close proximity to metro entertainment and employment. This convenience appeals to this much younger group whose median income per household is at the national average. The houses include rental apartments and single family homes in which they undertake home improvement.

Urbanization Group: U6
Urban Outskirts II

The population is still younger, but they reside in older homes that can be single family or multi-unit dwellings built before 1960. They still live in high density suburban areas, but they have lower incomes and tend to have less extravagant tastes. Typically, the households are diverse, ranging from single parents to shared student households.

Urbanization Group: U7
Suburban Periphery I

The households are low density away from the centers of city living. Families are mainly made up of married couples, some with children, some without; and they have two cars and utilize technology extensively for shopping, investments.

Urbanization Group: U8
Suburban Periphery II

These live in older houses that are single family homes or military quarters and have a short commute to work. Mixed households are typical with some being single and others being married families with children. However, median net incomes and home values are lower then the national average, and yet the median age is higher at 40 and has a higher population of older adults.

Urbanization Group: U9 Small Towns

These are close knit communities away from city life, with a modest living and median salaries. They can afford typically single family or mobile homes. Even though most are retired, those employed work in the construction, manufacturing and retail industries. The communities are established but still experience immigration of younger generations. They are economically conservative related to their modest income median of $3,000.

Urbanization Group: U10 Rural I

These are hardworking adults with a median age of 40 who have left the cities to own large houses with huge acreage in non-farming rural settlements. Their children have usually left the nest and as a result, they spend much of their time in home remodeling and outdoor leisure such as hunting and fishing. The income median is higher than $50,000.

Urbanization Group: U11 Rural II

This segment is located in the low density rural areas whose employment comes from mining or manufacturing, mainly farming. The majority of the population consists of home owners at a median age of 38 years, and their lives are centered on family and home. Their lifestyles are more practical than the rest of the segments.

CASE DESCRIPTION

Data for the following selected zip codes were analyzed. These were carefully selected not only because they are the surrounding neighbors of zip code 40203, the home of the local clinic, but also the majority of visits come from them. In other words, roughly 83% of all the county visits came from these areas. As stated previously, these zip codes are within 5-10 miles of the Clinic. 15,274

out of the 18,390 visits are from these zip codes (Table 2).

Table 3 lists the frequency of visits for the 19 zip codes and Table 4 lists the corresponding tapestry names for each zip code. In each of the selected 19 zip codes, Private pay dominated all the financial classes. Overall, 8351 out of the 15,274 (55%) had no insurance, and so had to pay themselves. This is followed by Medicaid and Medicare. There were 4594 out of the 15,274 (30%) with such a method of payment. Only 2011 (13%) had insurance and 318 (2%) left before treatment or after registration. The use of Medicare and Medicaid was the second dominant method of payment except for zip codes 40258, 40220, 40205, 40207 and 40209 where Insurance dominated Medicaid and Medicare. There was no difference when the data were segmented into patients with and without a primary care physician.

Patient's gender is illustrated in Figure 4 where M stands for males and F for females. A total of 42.71% of the visits were from females and 57.29% are from males.

Figure 5 illustrates the final class for patients' with (1) and without (0) Primary Care Physicians (PCP). It is clear from the figure that private pay, Medicare and Medicaid are the dominant financial classes. The number of visits that resulted in leaving before treatment is greater with patients without PCP. The bar graph tells us that private pay together with Medicaid and Medicare is the most used form of payment for this Zip code for both patients with and without PCP.

The four payment types are

Table 2.

40212	40209	40258	40203
40211	40207	40220	40218
40210	40213	40202	40217
40208	40214	40206	40216
40217	40215	40204	

Table 3. Zip code frequency count

Zip_Code	Frequency	Percent	Cumulative Frequency
40203	2856	18.7	2856
40211	1630	10.67	4486
40212	1413	9.25	5899
40202	1392	9.11	7291
40210	1260	8.25	8551
40214	846	5.54	9397
40206	830	5.43	10227
40216	796	5.21	11023
40215	760	4.98	11783
40218	710	4.65	12493
40208	700	4.58	13193
40204	521	3.41	13714
40213	345	2.26	14059
40217	344	2.25	14403
40258	290	1.9	14693
40220	256	1.68	14949
40205	156	1.02	15105
40207	142	0.93	15247
40209	27	0.18	15274

Table 4. Zip codes with its tapestry names

Zip	Tapestry Code	Tapestry Name
40220	13	In Style
40205	14	Prosperous Empty Nesters
40258	17	Green Acres
40207	22	Metropolitans
40204	23	Trendsetters
40216	29	Rustbelt Retirees
40213	32	Rustbelt traditions
40212	34	Family foundations
40214	41	Crossroads
40206	52	Inner City Tenants
40218	52	Inner City Tenants
40208	55	College Towns
40217	57	Simple Living
40209	60	City Dimensions
40215	60	City Dimensions
40210	62	Modest Income Homes
40211	62	Modest Income Homes
40202	64	City Commons
40203	65	Social Security Set

Figure 4. Distribution of sex

PERCENT of Sex

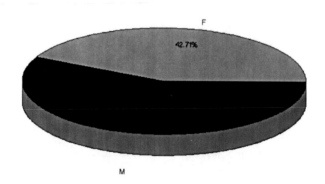

F
42.71%

M

Figure 5. Financial class statuses of patients with and without PCP

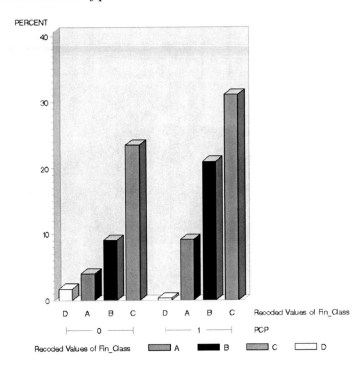

A=Private Insurance
B=Medicaid/Medicare
C=Private Pay
D=Left on Own Accord

This pie chart as in Figure 6 illustrates the four financial classes. We see that 54.67% of the visits resulted in private pay. These patients did not have insurance. A total of 30.08% used either Medicare or Medicaid. Only 13.7% of the visits resulted in some form of insurance.

Figure 7 combines all the visits of patients with and without PCP. This figure represents the financial class of all the visits from this zip code. It is clear here that codes B and C dominate all others in this region. We state again for clarity that C stands for different types of private pay, B for Medicaid and Medicare, A for insurance and D for the patients that left before treatment.

Figure 8 represents the disposition of patients. Code A indicates that most visits resulted in a discharge to patients' residence. All others com-

bined still are fewer compared to the discharge to private residence.

A=Discharged
B=Transferred
C=Left on Own Accord (LOA)
D=Admitted

This is followed by visits resulting in leaving (Code C) the ED before either being evaluated, or right after evaluation. Admissions follows code C closely while a few are transferred to other facilities (Code B).

Figure 9 indicates that there are no significant differences as to the disposition of patients when the data were segmented into visits with and without a PCP (Primary Care Physician). For those with PCP, admission is higher compared to leaving without treatment. The opposite is true for those without a PCP.

Figure 10 tells the same story for both visits with and without a PCP during triage. We have

Figure 6. Financial class distributions

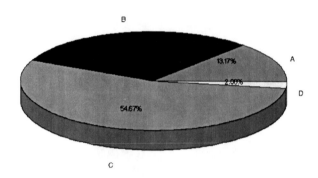

FREQUENCY of Fin_Class_recoded

Figure 7. Financial class distributions of all visits

Figure 8 Distribution of patients' disposition status

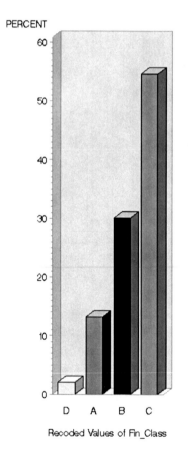

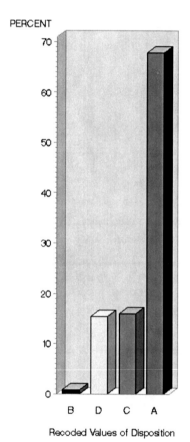

Figure 9. Disposition status of patients with and without PCP (Primary Care Physicians)

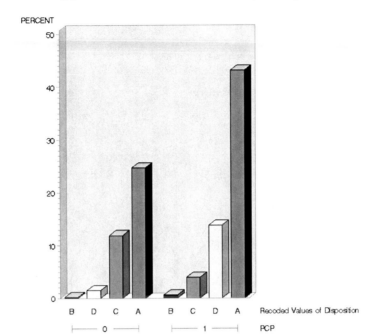

Figure 10. Distribution of triage acuity of patients with and without PCP

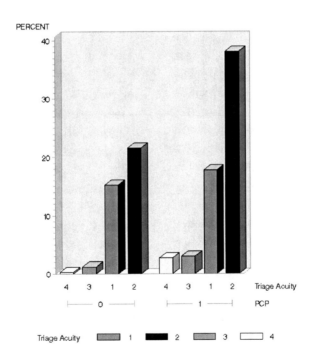

identical distributions from lowest to highest, 4<3<1<2. Most people are seen within 2 and 4 hour time intervals.

Figure 11 re-emphasizes Figure 10. We see that only a handful of visits were actually triaged a code of 3 or 4, seen within 15 minutes and seen immediately, respectively.

1=Non-urgent
2=Urgent
3=Emergent
4=Life-threatening

The next section is dedicated to table summaries where Tables 3 and 4 display patient disposition by triage acuity. These tables may help give us an insight into whether the triage system is a good predictor of disposition. A serious problem will arise when a patient is triaged with a code of 1 or 2 (to be seen within 2 or 4 hours respectively), and the resulting disposition is a transfer to the morgue. Table 5 is set up for all patients.

Out of a total of 15,274 patients visits that we see in Table 5, 9133 were triaged 2 (to be seen within 2 hours), 5044 were triaged 1 (to be seen within 4 hours), 643 were triaged a 3 (to be seen within 15 minutes) and 454 were triaged 4 (to be seen immediately). A total of 14,177 (9133+5044), which is 93% were deemed non-urgent while 1097 (7%) were triaged as urgent. A record number of 10,369 (68%) visits resulted in a discharge to a private home. This makes sense since only 472 (5%) of the 10,369 were triaged as urgent.

Of great interest and a test of the triage system is the 33 patients that were transferred to the morgue. 8 (24%) of these were triaged as non urgent and 25 (76%) as urgent. Of the 33, seven were triaged a code of 1, 1 a code 2, and 25 a code of 4. Another test of the triage system is that of the 261 visits that resulted in an admission to a critical care unit, 122 (47%) were initially triaged as non-urgent while 53% were triaged as urgent. Additionally, of the 150 admitted to the operat-

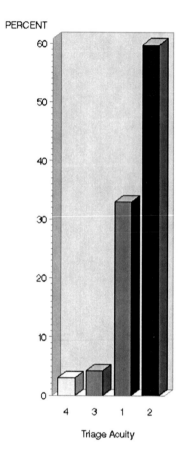

Figure 11. Triage acuity distributions for all visits

ing room, 87 were triaged as non-urgent, which is more than half of the admissions.

From Table 6, we have a total of 128 transfers to other facilities, 2347 resulted in admissions, and 2430 left on their own accord without treatment. The triage for these 2430 was appropriate since 2372 (1508+864) of these were deemed as non-urgent. Of concern is that out of the 2347 admissions, 1817 (1496+321) were triaged as non-urgent while only 530 were triaged as urgent.

The neural network misclassification rate was 0.08 on the training data, 0.15 on the validation data set and 0.16 on the test. This presented a slightly better rate than that of a decision tree when compared. The misclassification rate for the decision tree was 0.17 for the training set and 0.16

Table 5. Disposition by triage acuity

DISPOSITION	TRIAGE ACUITY				TOTAL
	2	1	3	4	
1	6066	3831	349	123	10369
3A	1191	257	162	114	1724
7B	805	478	18	0	1301
7A	456	335	20	1	812
3C	105	17	42	97	261
3B	121	14	22	26	182
7	130	23	10	3	166
3F	59	28	4	59	150
7C	117	28	6	0	150
2	51	15	5	0	71
6	1	7	0	25	33
3D	19	5	1	2	27
4	9	5	3	4	21
5	2	1	0	0	3
3E	1	943	1	0	2
TOTAL	9133	5044	643	454	15274

Table 6. Display of aggregated disposition by triage acuity

DISPOSITION	TRIAGE ACUITY				TOTAL
	2	1	3	4	
A	6066	3381	349	123	10369
C	1508	864	54	4	2430
D	1496	321	232	298	2347
B	63	28	8	29	128
	9133	5044	643	454	15274

for the validation set. We list the 3 clusters that were produced below and the cluster rule.

Cluster

```
ID Variable Value 1 Value 2 Value 3 Value
4
1 SEX F (%27.93) M (%72.07)
1 TRIAGE_ACUITY 1 (%50.80) 2 (%49.20)
1 PCP 0 (%60.24) 1 (%39.76)
1 FIN_CLASS A (%2.78) B (%8.55) C
(%85.49) D (%3.18)
1 DISPOSITION A (%70.08) B (%0.80) C
(%25.94) D (%3.18)
2 SEX F (%61.55) M (%38.45)
2 TRIAGE_ACUITY 1 (%17.09) 2 (%80.60) 3
(%2.31)
2 PCP 0 (%14.20) 1 (%85.80)
2 FIN_CLASS A (%22.75) B (%54.04) C
(%22.63) D (%0.58)
2 DISPOSITION A (%68.71) B (%0.69) C
(%7.85) D (%22.75)
```

3 SEX F (%28.13) M (%71.88)

3 TRIAGE_ACUITY 3 (%53.13) 4 (%46.88)

3 PCP 0 (%25.00) 1 (%75.00)

3 FIN_CLASS A (%21.88) B (%21.09) C
(%56.25) D (%0.78)

3 DISPOSITION A (%44.53) B (%4.69) C
(%6.25) D (%44.53)

Cluster 1: Male, non-urgent, No PCP, Private
pay, Discharged

Cluster 2: Female, non-urgent, PCP,
Medicaid/Medicare, Discharged

Cluster 3: Male, urgent, PCP, Private pay,
Admitted/discharged.

The cluster tree rule for our model is listed as
follows. These are the 'rules' that were used to
assign the clusters

IF Sex EQUALS M

AND Triage Acuity IS ONE OF: 3 4

THEN

NODE: 7

N: 92

1: 0.0%

2: 0.0%

3: 100.0%

IF PCP EQUALS 1

AND Recoded Values of Fin_Class IS ONE

OF: B A

AND Triage Acuity IS ONE OF: 1 2

THEN

NODE: 9

N: 526

1: 0.8%

2: 99.2%

3: 0.0%

IF PCP EQUALS 0

AND Recoded Values of Fin_Class IS ONE

OF: C D

AND Triage Acuity IS ONE OF: 1 2

THEN

NODE: 11

N: 496

1: 100.0%

2: 0.0%

3: 0.0%

IF Triage Acuity EQUALS 4

AND Sex EQUALS F

THEN

NODE: 13

N: 18

1: 0.0%

2: 0.0%

3: 100.0%

IF Triage Acuity EQUALS 1

AND PCP EQUALS 0

AND Recoded Values of Fin_Class IS ONE

OF: B A

THEN

NODE: 14

N: 83

1: 100.0%

2: 0.0%

3: 0.0%

IF Recoded Values of Fin_Class IS ONE OF:

C D

AND Triage Acuity EQUALS 3

AND Sex EQUALS F

THEN

NODE: 21

N: 12

1: 0.0%

2: 0.0%

3: 100.0%

IF Recoded Values of Disposition IS ONE

OF: A D B

AND Triage Acuity EQUALS 2

AND PCP EQUALS 0

AND Recoded Values of Fin_Class IS ONE

OF: B A

THEN

NODE: 23

N: 102

1: 0.0%

2: 100.0%

3: 0.0%

IF Triage Acuity EQUALS 1

AND Sex EQUALS F
AND PCP EQUALS 1
AND Recoded Values of Fin_Class IS ONE
OF: C D
THEN
NODE: 26
N: 76
1: 98.7%
2: 1.3%
3: 0.0%
IF Recoded Values of Disposition IS ONE
OF: A C B
AND Sex EQUALS M
AND PCP EQUALS 1
AND Recoded Values of Fin_Class IS ONE
OF: C D
AND Triage Acuity IS ONE OF: 1 2
THEN
NODE: 29
N: 298
1: 99.3%
2: 0.7%
3: 0.0%
IF PCP EQUALS 0
AND Recoded Values of Fin_Class IS ONE
OF: B A
AND Triage Acuity EQUALS 3
AND Sex EQUALS F
THEN
NODE: 30
N: 6
1: 0.0%
2: 0.0%
3: 100.0%
IF PCP EQUALS 1
AND Recoded Values of Fin_Class IS ONE
OF: B A
AND Triage Acuity EQUALS 3
AND Sex EQUALS F
THEN
NODE: 31
N: 20
1: 0.0%
2: 100.0%

3: 0.0%
IF Sex EQUALS F
AND Recoded Values of Disposition EQUALS
C
AND Triage Acuity EQUALS 2
AND PCP EQUALS 0
AND Recoded Values of Fin_Class IS ONE
OF: B A
THEN
NODE: 32
N: 21
1: 0.0%
2: 100.0%
3: 0.0%
IF Sex EQUALS M
AND Recoded Values of Disposition EQUALS
C
AND Triage Acuity EQUALS 2
AND PCP EQUALS 0
AND Recoded Values of Fin_Class IS ONE
OF: B A
THEN
NODE: 33
N: 27
1: 100.0%
2: 0.0%
3: 0.0%
IF Recoded Values of Disposition EQUALS C
AND Triage Acuity EQUALS 2
AND Sex EQUALS F
AND PCP EQUALS 1
AND Recoded Values of Fin_Class IS ONE
OF: C D
THEN
NODE: 34
N: 16
1: 87.5%
2: 12.5%
3: 0.0%
IF Recoded Values of Disposition IS ONE
OF: A D B
AND Triage Acuity EQUALS 2
AND Sex EQUALS F
AND PCP EQUALS 1

AND Recoded Values of Fin_Class IS ONE
OF: C D

THEN

NODE: 35

N: 154

1: 0.0%

2: 100.0%

3: 0.0%

IF Triage Acuity EQUALS 1

AND Recoded Values of Disposition EQUALS
D

AND Sex EQUALS M

AND PCP EQUALS 1

AND Recoded Values of Fin_Class IS ONE
OF: C D

THEN

NODE: 36

N: 11

1: 100.0%

2: 0.0%

3: 0.0%

IF Triage Acuity EQUALS 2

AND Recoded Values of Disposition EQUALS
D

AND Sex EQUALS M

AND PCP EQUALS 1

AND Recoded Values of Fin_Class IS ONE
OF: C D

THEN

NODE: 37

N: 42

1: 0.0%

2: 100.0%

3: 0.0%

Similarly, the predictive model rules for the disposition of patients are listed as follows.

IF Triage Acuity EQUALS 4

AND PCP EQUALS 1

THEN

NODE: 5

N: 163

C: 0.6%

A: 26.4%

D: 63.2%

B: 9.8%

IF Recoded Values of Fin_Class EQUALS D

AND PCP EQUALS 0

THEN

NODE: 7

N: 106

C: 99.1%

A: 0.0%

D: 0.0%

B: 0.9%

IF Recoded Values of Fin_Class EQUALS D

AND Triage Acuity IS ONE OF: 1 2 3

AND PCP EQUALS 1

THEN

NODE: 9

N: 21

C: 95.2%

A: 0.0%

D: 0.0%

B: 4.8%

IF Triage Acuity IS ONE OF: 1 2 3

AND Recoded Values of Fin_Class IS ONE
OF: C B A

AND PCP EQUALS 0

THEN

NODE: 10

N: 2216

C: 27.9%

A: 68.3%

D: 3.2%

B: 0.6%

IF Triage Acuity EQUALS 4

AND Recoded Values of Fin_Class IS ONE
OF: C B A

AND PCP EQUALS 0

THEN

NODE: 11

N: 17

C: 0.0%

A: 29.4%

D: 70.6%

B: 0.0%

```
IF Triage Acuity EQUALS 1
AND Recoded Values of Fin_Class IS ONE
OF: C B A
AND PCP EQUALS 1
THEN
NODE: 12
N: 1119
C: 5.8%
A: 82.6%
D: 10.7%
B: 0.9%
IF Recoded Values of Fin_Class IS ONE OF:
C A
AND Triage Acuity IS ONE OF: 2 3
AND PCP EQUALS 1
THEN
NODE: 16
N: 1571
C: 6.6%
A: 73.0%
D: 19.7%
B: 0.7%
IF Triage Acuity EQUALS 2
AND Recoded Values of Fin_Class EQUALS B
AND PCP EQUALS 1
THEN
NODE: 24
N: 830
C: 7.3%
A: 61.1%
D: 30.7%
B: 0.8%
IF Triage Acuity EQUALS 3
AND Recoded Values of Fin_Class EQUALS B
AND PCP EQUALS 1
THEN
NODE: 25
N: 67
C: 4.5%
A: 37.3%
D: 55.2%
B: 3.0%
```

The implication of these rules is that triage for males differ from triage for females. A non-urgent female is likely to be triaged a code 2 (to be seen in 2 hrs) while the male is likely to be triaged a code of 1 (to be seen in 4 hours). Also, non-urgent visits with insurance or patients who are considered as private pay are more likely to be discharged than those on Medicare/Medicaid.

CURRENT AND FUTURE CHALLENGES FACING THE ORGANIZATION

We recognize some of the limitations of this study. In the course of the study, we realized that race and age would have been helpful in explaining some of utilization of the ED. We also note that the outpatient ED visits could have been for urgent cases but did not result in admissions or a transfer; our assumption was that if a patient were triaged a code of 1 or 2, and eventually discharged to private residence, then that patient was non-urgent to begin with. To help reduce the use of the ED for non-urgent patients, policy makers may target the cluster groups that we have listed in the preceding sections.

This group of people can be targeted and thus shifted to the local clinic. This shift will not only decrease cost for the ER, but reduce the number of visits. This may reduce the overcrowding and waiting times while simultaneously increasing the quality of care. If the ED eliminates these unnecessary visits, nurses and physicians can then focus on urgent patients.

A suggestion on how to shift patients from the ED to the Clinic, (which is left to the policy makers and may be beyond the scope of this study) is to have patients call in to the ED before their visit. We realized during our cross-reference that patients of the Harambee Clinic do not go to the ED for any care, and vice-versa. Our model is based on the 2004 data, and we plan to use 2005 data to test the model. Age and race will also be needed in the 2004 data for further studies of the utilization of the ED.

REFERENCES

Barnes Jewish Hospital. (n.d.). Retrieved 2007, from http://www.bjc.org

Center for Studying Health System Change. (2004). Retrieved 2007, from http://www.hschange.com/CONTENT/799/

Centers for Disease Control. (1996). Retrieved from http://www.cdc.gov/nchs/products/pubs/pubd/series/sr13/150-141/sr13_150.htm

Centers for Disease Control. (2003). Retrieved 2007, from http://www.cdc.gov/nchs/products/pubs/pubd/ad/300-291/ad293.htm

Centers for Disease Control. (n.d.). Retrieved 2007, from http://www.cdc.gov/nchs/about/major/ahcd/ahcd1.htm

Government Accounting Office. (2002). Retrieved 2007, from www.gao.gov/new.items/d03460.pdf, www.gao.gov/new.items/d03769t.pdf

Joint Commission on Healthcare Quality. (2004). Retrieved 2007, from www.jcrinc.com/generic.asp?durki=9649

Nursing Center. com. (2004). Retrieved 2007, from http://www.nursingcenter.com/prodev/ce_article.asp?tid=512689

Urban Institute. (2002). Retrieved 2007, from http://www.urban.org/publications/1000728.html

ADDITIONAL READING

Afifi, A., Clark, V. A., & May, S. (2004). *Computer-Aided Multivariate Analysis*. New York: Chapman and Hall.

Arabie, P., Hubert, L. J., & De Soete, G. (1999). *Clustering and Classification*. Washington, DC: World Scientific.

Berry, M. J. A., & Linoff, G. (1999). *Mastering Data Mining: The Art and Science of Customer Relationship Management.* New York: John Wiley & Sons, Inc.

Bishop, C. M. (1995). *Neural Networks for Pattern Recognition.* Oxford, UK: Oxford University Press.

Chester, D. L. (1990). Why two Hidden Layers are Better then One. *IJCNN, 90*(1), 265–268.

Flury, B., & Riedwyl, H. (1988). *Multivariate Statistics: A Practical Approach*. New York: Chapman and Hall.

Mirkin, B. (1996). *Nonconvex Optimization and its Applications: Mathematical Classification and Clustering*. Boston: Kluwer Academic Publishers.

Nirmal, K. B. (1996). *Neural Network Fundamentals with Graphs, Algorithms and Applications*. New York: Mcgraw-Hill.

Romesburg, C. (2004). *Cluster Analysis For Researchers*. Raleigh: North Carolina. Lulu Press.

Chapter 15
Physician Prescribing Practices

Mussie Tesfamicael
University of Lousiville, USA

ABSTRACT

The purpose of this project is to develop time series models to investigate prescribing practices and patient usage of medications with respect to the severity of the patient condition. The cost of medications is rising from year to year; some medications are prescribed more often compared to others even if they have similar properties. It would be of interest to pharmaceutical companies to know the reason for this. In this case, we predict the cost of medications, private insurance payments, Medicaid payments, Medicare payments, the quantity of medications, total payment and to study why the cost is rising in one medication compared to others. We investigate how much patients are spending on average for their prescriptions of medications, taking the inflation rate into account as a time-dependent regressor. Both forecasts, the one that incorporates the inflation rates and the one that does not are compared.

BACKGROUND

There are over 100 antibiotics in the market, but the majority of them come from only a few types of drugs. The main classes of antibiotics are Penicillin, such as penicillin and Amoxicillin, Cephalosporin such as Cephalexin (Keflex), Macrolides such as erythromycin, Clarithromycin and Azithromycin (Zithromax), Fluoroquinolones, such as ciprofloxacin (Cipro), Levoflaxacin (Levaquin), and Tetracycline such as Tetracycline and Doxycycline

(Vibramycin). In this project, we will study the cost analysis of these antibiotics in relation to time. (Mol, et. al., 2005)

Antibiotics are among the most frequently prescribed medications. Antibiotics cure disease by killing or injuring bacteria. The first discovered antibiotic was penicillin, which was discovered from a mold culture. Today, over 100 different antibiotics are available to doctors to cure minor discomforts as well as life-threatening infections.

Antibiotics only treat bacterial infection, although they are used in a wide variety of illnesses. Antibiotics do not cure viral infections such as the

DOI: 10.4018/978-1-61520-723-7.ch015

Copyright © 2010, IGI Global. Copying or distributing in print or electronic forms without written permission of IGI Global is prohibited.

common cold; nor can they treat fungal infections. (Mol, et.al., 2005) Most antibiotics have two names, a brand name created by the drug company that manufactures the drug and a generic name based on the chemical composition of the drug. The main purpose of this study is to develop time series models to forecast the cost of medications and to classify patient usage of medications with respect to patient conditions using text-mining clustering. We will also study on average how much patients are spending on medications.

SETTING THE STAGE

The purpose of this study is to examine the use of time series forecasting and data mining tools to investigate the prescription of medications. The specific objective is to examine the relationship between the total payments, private insurance payments, Medicare payments, Medicaid payments, number of prescriptions and quantity of prescriptions for different antibiotics. Currently, there are no methods available to forecast medication prescription costs, so we have adopted several methods that will help health care providers and hospitals to know about the prescription of the antibiotics prescribed. The payment made for each antibiotic is based upon an average cost and total cost that will include the cost of the antibiotics and insurance payments. It will be beneficial to show health care providers the trends of these medications in terms of the cost analysis. It is also beneficial to make comparisons between several antibiotics in terms of the number of prescriptions and to do further study as to why one medication is prescribed more often than others.

We developed time series models that will be used to forecast the prescription practices of the antibiotics. We used exponential models to develop forecasting for antibiotics on which cost increases exponentially. We also developed an autoregressive integrated moving average model for non-stationary data on which the series has no

constant mean and variance through time. We developed Generalized Autoregressive Conditional Heteroskedastic Models for volatile variance, and we also incorporated the inflation rate as a model dynamic regressor to see the effect on model forecast. We finally used text mining and clustering to classify the ICD-9 codes into six clusters and make comparisons within each cluster, by plotting the data using kernel density estimation.

In this study, we use medications listed in the Medical Expenditure Panel Survey. The Medical Expenditure Panel Survey provides actual reimbursement information from private insurers, government agencies, and payments by patients. It provides summaries of all contact with the healthcare industry for a cohort of patients. (J. W. Cohen, et al., 1996; S. B. Cohen & Cohen, 2002; Newacheck, et al., 2004) With this information, studies have examined the specific costs of chronic diseases such as asthma, diabetes, and congestive heart failure. (Chan, et al., 2002; S. B. Cohen, Buchmueller, Cohen, & Buchmueller, 2006; Guevara, et al., 2003; Halpern, Yabroff, Halpern, & Yabroff, 2008; Law, et al., 2003; McGarry, Schoeni, McGarry, & Schoeni, 2005; Miller, et al., 2005; Newacheck, Kim, Newacheck, & Kim, 2005) However, because many patients have co-morbidities, it is extremely difficult to isolate the treatment for one particular chronic disease.

CASE DESCRIPTION

We begin with an exponential smoothing model building to forecast the prescription of medications for the antibiotics dataset. Exponential smoothing models are characterized by giving heavier weights to recent events and lower weights to past events. Before we build a model for the prescription of medications, we set the fit period and evaluation period. The fit period is the period on which the model fits the data while the evaluation period is the period where we evaluate the model we built. We used a holdout sample of 20% of the total

Figure 1. Prediction error plots: private insurance payment

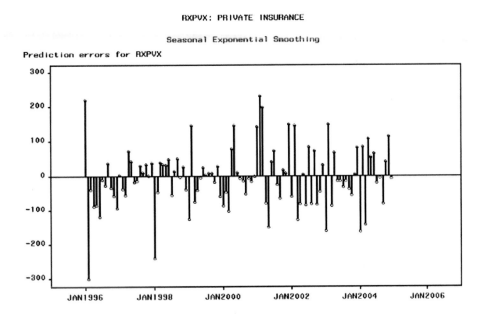

data set. By holdout sample, we mean that we use 80% of the data to build a model and we use the remaining 20% to forecast for future values. For a better fit, it is better if a holdout sample is chosen.

As an example, we will build a model fit for the antibiotic, Amoxicillin. The private insurance payments made for the prescription of Amoxicillin will be forecast. Here, we are building a time series model to study the prescription practice of Amoxicillin. Plotting the forecasted private insurance payments vs. time gives the structure of the data, and gives a clue as to what kind of model might be appropriate for the dataset. The plot of private insurance payments versus time. Figure 4 shows how the series data grow or decay exponentially with a seasonal nature; as a result, we used exponential models. We fitted a model of exponential smoothing models and we chose the one with the smallest root mean square error (RMSE). Statistically speaking, the model with the smallest error is considered the best. We begin the analysis of the private insurance payment with Amoxicillin. The prediction error plots for

private insurance payments made for Amoxicillin are given in Figure 1, while Figure 2 describes the autocorrelation plots (autocorrelation, partial autocorrelation and inverse autocorrelation). Figure 3 describes a white noise plot and Figure 4 describes the forecast plot.

The residuals do not appear to be white noise, with visual evidence of higher variability at the beginning of the time range. Figure 1 is the residual error plot for private insurance payments for the antibiotic, Amoxicillin. The autocorrelation plot, Figure 2, is within the bounds of two standard deviation errors, an indication that the residuals are white noise. The partial autocorrelation plots also reveal that the correlations are within 2 standard errors, an indication that the residuals are white noise.

We did also check white noise, unit root test and seasonal unit root tests that are given in figure 3. The white noise test indicates failure to reject a null hypothesis of white noise for alternative lags up to 24. The unit root tests indicate a rejection of a null hypothesis of a unit root for all polynomials up to lag 5, and the seasonal root tests indicate

Figure 2. Prediction error autocorrelation plots: private insurance payments

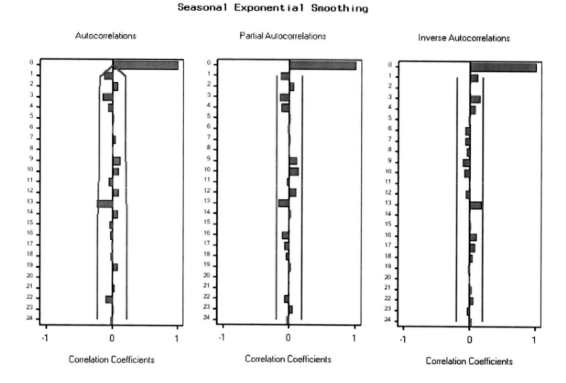

rejection of a null hypothesis of a seasonal unit root up to lag 5.

We chose the best model for the private insurance payment made for the antibiotic, Amoxicillin, based on the smallest root mean square error (RMSE). We fitted an exponential smoothing model, a simple exponential smoothing model, double (brown) exponential smoothing model, linear (holt) exponential smoothing model and damped trend exponential smoothing model. From Table 1, we selected the best model of fit for the private insurance payments made for the antibiotic, Amoxicillin.

We can see that the seasonal exponential smoothing model is selected as a model of forecast, with the smallest RMSE. The seasonal exponential smoothing model has also the smallest mean square error (MSE), mean absolute percent error (MAPE), mean absolute error (MAE) and Pearson correlation (R^2) time series.

Even though we used the RMSE for model selection in Table 1, it is advisable to use MAPE for error interpretation since the RMSE value tends to be larger when compared to the MAPE. The MAPE in Table 1 indicates that many cases have a percent error less than 32%. The model estimate parameter of private insurance payment for the antibiotic, Amoxicillin is given in Table 2.

The smoothed seasonal factor one is for January. The exponential smoothing model detects a seasonal difference decrease of $105.18 (99.94191-205.12659=105.18468) for February compared to January for private insurance payments made. On the other hand, the smoothed seasonal factor eleven indicates November; the exponential smoothing model detects a seasonal difference in-

Figure 3. Prediction error white noise: private insurance payments

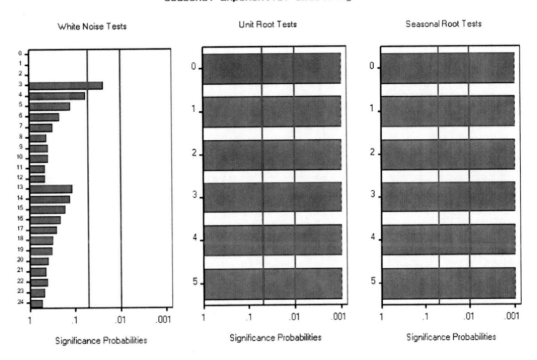

Figure 4. Forecast for private insurance payments: Amoxicillin

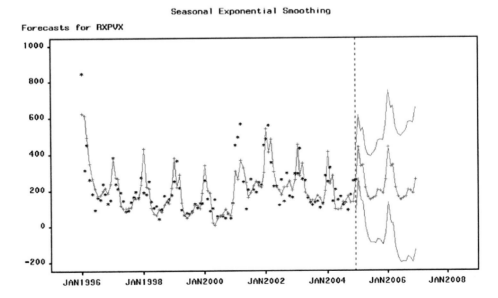

Table 1. Exponential models and statistics of fit

Time series model	MSE	RMSE	MAPE	MAE	R²
Seasonal exponential smoothing model	6916.4	83.1649	32.594	69.004	0.406
Simple exponential smoothing model	8344.5	91.348	34.519	72.565	0.2840
Double(brown) exponential smoothing model	10797.5	103.911	35.754	76.145	0.073
Linear Holt exponential smoothing model	8338.7	91.316	34.388	72.597	0.284
Damped trend exponential smoothing model	8599.2	92.732	34.664	73.141	0.262
Winters additive model	6898.6	83.058	32.513	68.925	0.408
Winters multiplicative model	12111.1	110.051	32.484	74.254	-0.040

Table 2. Parameter estimates of private insurance payment: Amoxicillin

Model Parameter	Estimates	Std. Error	T	Prob>|T|
LEVEL Smoothing weight	0.4230	0.0661	6.3971	<0.001
Seasonal Smoothing Weight	0.0010	0.1107	0.0090	0.9928
Residual Variance	7826			
Smoothed Level	339.3064			
Smoothed Seasonal Factor 1	205.1266			
Smoothed Seasonal Factor 2	99.9419			
Smoothed Seasonal Factor 3	106.0882			
Smoothed Seasonal Factor 4	-17.9435			
Smoothed Seasonal Factor 5	-67.4995			
Smoothed Seasonal Factor 6	-86.7825			
Smoothed Seasonal Factor 7	-77.4002			
Smoothed Seasonal Factor 8	-69.2203			
Smoothed Seasonal Factor 9	-33.8578			
Smoothed Seasonal Factor 10	-35.2863			
Smoothed Seasonal Factor 11	-49.4234			
Smoothed Seasonal Factor 12	26.1430			

crease of \$75.56 (26.14302-(-49.42344)=75.566) for December compared to November for private insurance payments made.

We have shown so far that forecast values for private insurance payments of Amoxicillin were fit by the exponential smoothing model. The seasonal exponential model has multiple steps ahead prediction, and Table 2 gives up to a smoothed seasonal factor level 12; this is an indication that seasonal data forecast over a longer time period will be more accurate than forecasts over a short period of time. Here, we are analyzing the private insurance payments made that were obtained by summing daily expenses paid for a period of every month.

The forecast plot for private insurance payments made for Amoxicillin shows seasonality with a period of approximately 12 months, which supports the model chosen. Figure 4 reveals that predicted and actual private insurance payments are very close to each other, making the residual term very small.

Figure 5. Prediction error plots: total payments: Amoxicillin

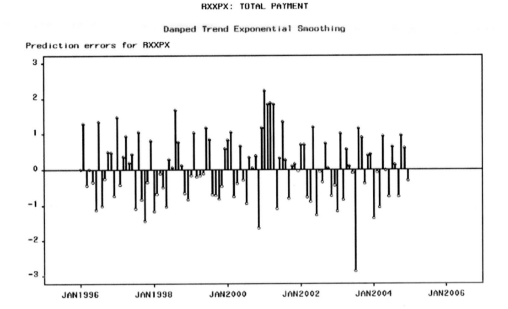

The predicted plot for private insurance payment for the antibiotic, Amoxicillin, also indicates that the values are higher around January and lower around June; this event repeats at approximately 12 months. We observe that the predicted series is very close to the actual series, which is an indication that the model that we built fits the data well. We have used the historical data to build what the private insurance payment will be in the future. One has to be cautious in forecasting for a longer period; in the future, the forecast might not be as accurate as we expect. For this reason, we forecast what the private insurance payments might be for the next two years, i.e. for the years 2005-2006.

We have also investigated on average how much patients are spending on prescriptions. At this time, we predict the total payments made on medications instead of private insurance payments made.

The residuals do not appear to be white noise, with visual evidence of higher variability at the middle and at the end of the time range. Figure 5 is the residual error for total insurance payment for the antibiotic, Amoxicillin.

The autocorrelation plot, Figure 6, is within the bounds of 2 standard deviation errors, an indication that the residuals are white noise. The partial autocorrelation plots also reveal that the correlations are within 2 standard errors, an indication that the residuals are white noise.

We also checked white noise, unit root test and seasonal unit root tests, which are given in Figure 7. The white noise test indicates failure to reject a null hypothesis of white noise for alternative lags up to 24. The unit root tests indicate a rejection of a null hypothesis of a unit root for all polynomials up to lag 4, and the seasonal root tests indicate rejection of a null hypothesis of a seasonal unit root up to lag 5.

We chose the best model for the total payment made for the antibiotic, Amoxicillin, based on the smallest root mean square error (RMSE). It should be noted that here we are investigating how much patients on average are paying for the antibiotic, Amoxicillin. We fitted a seasonal exponential

Figure 6. Prediction error autocorrelation plots: total payments

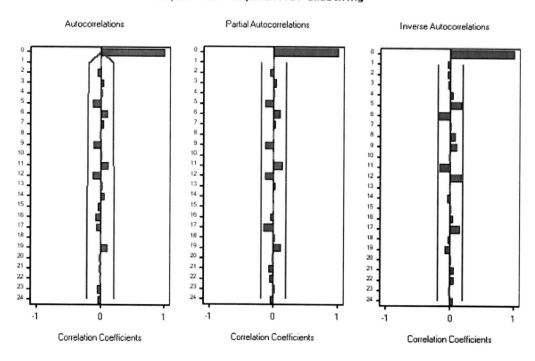

Figure 7. Prediction error white noise: total payments: Amoxicillin

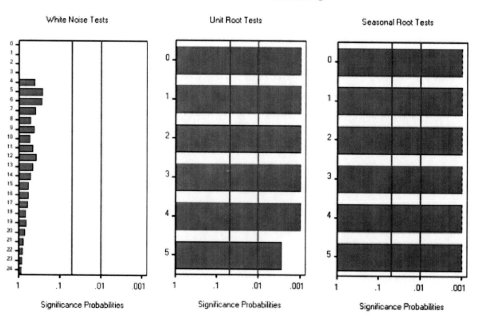

smoothing model, simple exponential smoothing model, double (brown) exponential smoothing model, linear (holt) exponential smoothing model and damped trend exponential smoothing model. From Table 3, we selected the best model of fit for the total payments made for the antibiotic, Amoxicillin. We can see that the damped trend exponential smoothing model is selected as a model forecast, with the smallest RMSE. The damped trend exponential smoothing model has also the smallest mean square error (MSE), mean absolute percent error (MAPE), mean absolute error (MAE) and Pearson correlation (R^2) time series.

Even though we used RMSE for model selection in Table 3 as mentioned in the previous paragraph, it is advisable to use MAPE for error interpretation because the RMSE value tends to be larger when compared to the MAPE. The MAPE in Table 3 indicates that many cases have a percent error less than 27%. The model estimate parameter of total payment for the antibiotic, Amoxicillin, is given in Table 4.

The t-test p-value in Table 4 may be questionable due to the fact that the trend smoothing weight falls on the boundary of zero estimation bounds.

The forecast plot for total payments made for Amoxicillin shows a slightly increasing trend from January, 2001 up to June, 2002 with damping seasonality. Figure 8 reveals that predicted and actual total payments made are very close to each other, making the residual term very small.

The predicted plot for total payment for the antibiotic, Amoxicillin, also indicates that the values are higher around January and lower around June; this event repeats at approximately 6 months. We also observe that the predicted series is very close to the actual series, which is an indication that the model is a good fit. We used the historical data to build what the total payment will be in the future.

Table 3. Exponential models and statistics of fit

Time series model	MSE	RMSE	MAPE	MAE	R²
simple exponential smoothing model	0.4943	0.7031	27.4015	0.5496	-0.094
Double(brown) exponential smoothing model	0.5244	0.7242	28.2752	0.5817	-0.160
Seasonal exponential model	0.5145	0.7173	28.4545	0.5672	-0.138
Linear Holt exponential smoothing model	0.4968	0.7049	27.8328	0.5549	-0.099
Damped trend exponential smoothing model	0.4943	0.7030	27.4014	0.5495	-0.094
Winters additive model	0.5207	0.72163	28.84722	0.5726	-0.152
Winters multiplicative model	0.5257	0.72506	29.10547	0.5694	-0.163

Table 4. Parameter estimates of total payment on average: Amoxicillin

Model Parameter	Estimate	Std. Error	T	Prob >|T|
Level smoothing weight	0.24354	0.0722	3.3717	0.0019
Trend smoothing weight	0.07557	0.1038	0.7280	0.4717
Damping smoothing weight	0.99106	0.1746	5.56775	<0.001
Residual variance	0.81101			
Smoothed level	12.12410			
Smoothed trend	0.12634			

Figure 8. Forecast for total payments: Amoxicillin

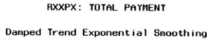

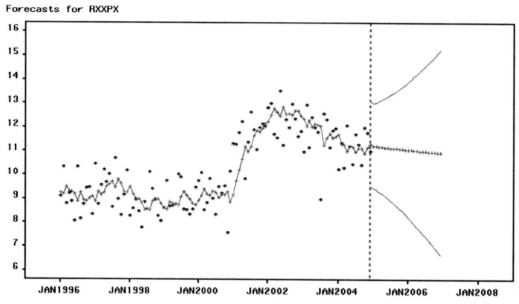

Erythromycin Results

In this section of the analysis, we will talk about autoregressive models (AR), moving average models (MA), autoregressive moving average models (ARMA) and autoregressive integrated moving average models (ARIMA). We will build models for the antibiotic, Erythromycin. We use this example in contrast to the use of Amoxicillin in the previous section because the optimal model is ARIMA in contrast to exponential smoothing.

We showed previously that an autoregressive process of order p is a linear function of p past values plus an error term. We have shown in the previous section that if an autoregressive model does not have a constant mean and variance through the sequence of time, there is a need for differencing.

As a result, an autoregressive integrated moving average (ARIMA) model is introduced to solve the problem of non-stationarity. What an ARIMA

model does is to take the difference of the series of data to make the series stationary.

As a start for the analysis of the antibiotic, Erythromycin, we plotted the total payment against the start date of medications; this plot is given in Figure 9. We will fit an autoregressive model of order p, i.e., AR(p). Based on the smallest MAPE, we will select p. As a result, the AR(p) model that fits the data well will be selected. We will analyze the fit of the data by checking autocorrelation plots, white noise and stationarity test, and the forecasted plot.

Figure 9 differs from that of Figure 4 for Amoxicillin in the previous section in that there is variability in the payments made from January, 1997 through January, 1998, but for the case of Amoxicillin, there is seasonal variability with exponential increasing in the payments made.

We first investigated whether the series of data is generated from white noise; to do this, we plotted the total payments made versus the

Figure 9. Plot of total payments vs. start date: Erythromycin

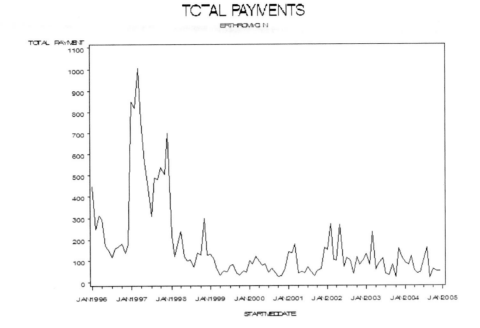

start date of medication, given in figure 9. Visual inspection shows the series is not generated from white noise, but visual inspection is not enough to conclude whether the series is generated from a white noise or not. As a result, we will check the residual plot, autocorrelation plot, white noise stationarity test and see how the model built fits the data.

The residual plot given in Figure 10 does not appear to be white noise, even though there is some variability at the beginning of the series. Figure 10 is the residual error for total payments made for the antibiotic, Erythromycin. Figure 10 differs from that of Figure 5 in the previous section in that the residual is smaller and less variable in the distribution of the error terms.

The autocorrelation plot, Figure 11, is within the bounds of two standard deviation errors, an indication that the residuals are white noise, even though at lag twelve, the inverse autocorrelation is non-significant; that is, outside the bound of two standard deviation errors. The partial auto-correlation plots also reveal that the correlations

are within two standard errors, an indication that the residuals are white noise.

Figure 11 differs from that of Figure 6 for Amoxicillin since all lags are not significant while the inverse autocorrelation function value at lag 12 is marginally significant. We also checked white noise, unit root test and seasonal unit root tests, which are given in Figure 12. The white noise test indicates failure to reject a null hypothesis of white noise for alternative lags up to 24. The unit root tests indicate a rejection of a null hypothesis of a unit root for all polynomials up to lag 5, and the seasonal root tests indicate rejection of a null hypothesis of a seasonal unit root up to lag 5.

Figure 12 differs from that of Figure 7 for Amoxicillin in that the unit root tests indicate a rejection of a null hypothesis of a unit root for all polynomials up to lag 5 while in figure 7, the unit root tests indicate a rejection of a null hypothesis of a unit root for all polynomials up to lag 4.

We chose the best model for the total payment made for the antibiotic, Erythromycin, based on

Figure 10. Prediction error plots: total payments: Erythromycin

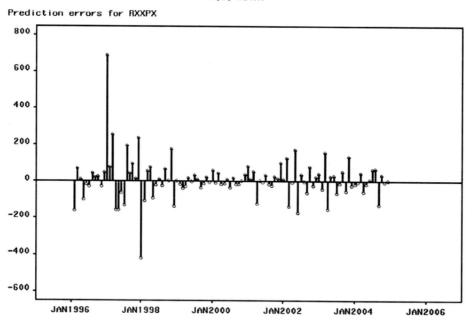

Figure 11. Prediction error autocorrelation plots: total payments

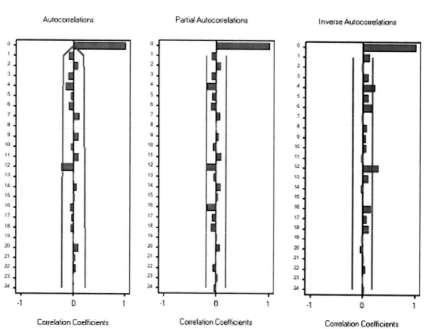

Figure 12. Prediction error white noise: total payments: Erythromycin

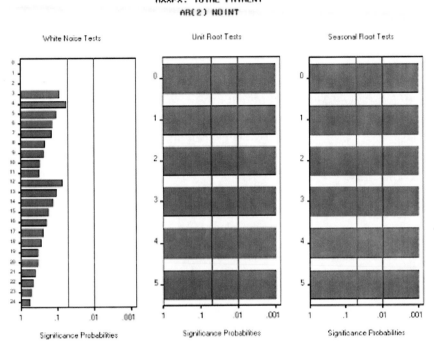

Table 5. Autoregressive models and statistics of fit

Time series model	MSE	RMSE	MAPE	MAE	R²	AIC	SBIC
AR(1)	6487.7	80.546	28.985	59.98	-0.738	317.996	319.579
AR(2)	6075	77.942	27.45	57.758	-0.627	317.629	320.797
AR(3)	6694.1	81.817	32.856	63.131	-0.793	325.123	331.457
AR(4)	7152.7	84.574	33.784	65.089	-0.916	327.509	333.843
AR(5)	6505.7	80.658	34.765	61.600	-0.743	326.096	334.013

the smallest root mean square error (RMSE). It should be noted that here we are investigating how much patients are paying in total for the antibiotic, Erythromycin. The autoregressive order two, *AR(2)* was a perfect fit for the data and the parameter estimates of the model are given in Table 5. We can see that the *AR(2)* model is selected as a model of forecast, with the smallest RMSE. The MAPE in Table 5 indicates that many cases have a percent error less than 27%.

We have mentioned in the analysis of the antibiotic, Amoxicillin, that the RMSE was very large when compared to the MAPE; but for the antibiotic, Erythromycin, the RMSE value is not that big as we can see from Table 5. For error interpretation, the MAPE is better, and from Table 5, the MAPE indicates that many cases have a percent error less than 27%. The model estimate parameter of total payment for the antibiotic, Erythromycin is given in Table 6.

Even though the parameter estimate for autoregressive lag 2 in table 6 is non-significant, an autoregressive model of order 2, *AR(2)* was perfectly fit to the data.

Table 6. Parameter estimates of total payment: Erythromycin

Model Parameter	Estimate	Std. Error	T	Prob >|T|
Autoregressive, Lag 1	0.8536	0.118	7.213	<.0001
Autoregressive, Lag 2	0.0629	0.118	0.531	0.598
Model Variance	15839			

Figure 13. Forecast for total payments: Erythromycin

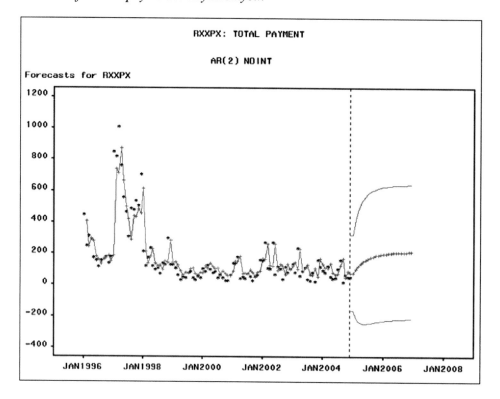

The forecast plot for total payments made for Erythromycin shows a slightly decreasing trend starting January, 1998 and peaks starting January, 2005. In contrast, the forecast for Amoxicillin shown in Figure 8 is exponentially increasing through the range of time. Figure 13 reveals that predicted and actual total payments made are very close to each other, except for values between June, 1997 and January, 1998; there is a small difference between the actual and forecasted values.

The predicted plot for total payment for the antibiotic, Erythromycin, also indicates that the values are higher around January and lower around June; this event repeats at approximately 6 months, and is similar to that for Amoxicillin. We also observe that the predicted series is very close to the actual series, which is an indication that the model is a good fit. So far from our analysis examples, the cost analysis of antibiotics has a seasonal nature. By seasonal nature, we mean that an event happens repeatedly; for example, if the event happens every six months, we say it has six-month seasonality.

High Performance Forecasting

In this section, we will use the High Performance Forecasting procedure to forecast prescriptions of antibiotics. The High Performance Forecasting analyzes time series (observations that are equally spaced at a specific time interval, for our case, month), or transactional data (observations that are not equally spaced with respect to a particular time interval as in our original antibiotic dataset). We will also plot the forecast series for several antibiotics in the same plot; in that case, comparisons can be made very easily. The historical series and forecasted series for several antibiotics can be drawn in the same plot, so that comparisons can be made and further studies can be performed on the nature of the trend of the forecast. In this section, we will identify and forecast series components such as the actual, predicted, lower confidence interval, upper confidence limit, prediction error, trend, seasonality and error (irregular). Trend usually refers to a deterministic function of time, which means the deterministic component exhibits no random variation and can be forecast perfectly, while a stochastic component is subject to random variation and can never be predicted perfectly except for chance occurrence.

Seasonality refers to the repetitive behavior at known seasonal periods, for instance, six months for antibiotics prescription. The High Performance Forecasting splits the current value of observation into trend, seasonal and error Components. In contrast to the previous section on time series forecasting, high performance forecasting can be used to forecast several variables by group, determines the best model from a list of models using the technique HPF DIAGNOSE and HPF ENGINE and can be used to forecast for a database with a large number of observations.

In this analysis section, we will use the antibiotic, Cipro, as an example to show and forecast the variables of interest (such as total payment, private insurance payment, quantity, amount of prescription, Medicare and Medicaid). Cipro is a commonly prescribed antibiotic, and the dataset we have shows a tremendous number of observations. Figure 14 gives the plot of total payment, private insurance payment, Medicare payment and Medicare against the start date of medication. From this plot, we can visually inspect how much difference really occurs between total payment, private insurance payment, Medicare payment and Medicare payments and give ideas as to what to expect when we make the forecast for these variables. We have used SAS CODE 1 to create the Cipro dataset and plot the Figure 14.

SAS Code 1. SAS codes for model forecasting and plotting: Cipro

```
Data cipro; set diser.disertation;
where RXNAME IN ('CIPRO');
RUN;
PROC SORT DATA=cipro;
by RXNAME STARTMEDDATE;
run;
Proc hpf data=cipro out=cipro lead=0;
id startmeddate interval=month
accumulate=total;
forecast RXMDX RXMRX RXPVX RXXPX /
model=none;
run;
title1 'Cipro Variables';
axis2 label=(a=-90 r=90 "PAYMENT");
SYMBOL1 INTERPOL=JOIN HEIGHT=10pt
VALUE=NONE CV=BLUE LINE=1 WIDTH=2;
SYMBOL2 INTERPOL=JOIN HEIGHT=10pt
VALUE=NONE CV=GREEN LINE=1 WIDTH=2;
SYMBOL3 INTERPOL=JOIN HEIGHT=10pt
VALUE=NONE CV=RED LINE=1 WIDTH=2;
SYMBOL4 INTERPOL=JOIN HEIGHT=10pt
VALUE=NONE CV=CYAN LINE=1 WIDTH=2;
Legend1 FRAME;
Axis1 STYLE=1 WIDTH=1 MINOR=NONE;
PROC GPLOT DATA=CIPRO;
PLOT RXMDX*STARTMEDDATE
RXMRX*STARTMEDDATE RXPVX*STARTMEDDATE
RXXPX*STARTMEDDATE /OVERLAY HAXIS=AXIS1
```

Figure 14. Cipro variables plot vs. start date of medication

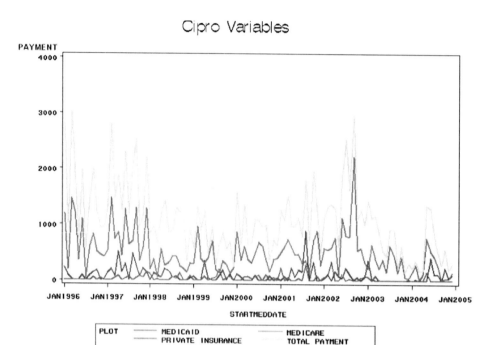

```
VAXIS=AXIS2
HAXIS='01JAN1996'D TO '01JAN2005'D BY
YEAR;
FRAME LEGEND=LEGEND1;
RUN;
```

We have used SAS CODE 1 to accumulate the daily observations into an accumulated sum of monthly values, and then plotted each variable of interest (Medicaid, Medicare, Private Insurance and Total Payment) against the start medication date. Figure 14 gives a starting point to see the relationships between these variables, and we can easily see that the Total Payment made surpasses Medicaid, Medicare and Private Insurance payments. On the other hand, the Medicare payment made for Cipro is smaller when compared to the Medicaid for almost every time point. As we can see from Figure 14, the plot for insurance payment fluctuates randomly; this might indicate that the data for Cipro is non- stationary. As a result, an

ARIMA model is one of the choices as a model prediction.

Also from Figure 14, we can see that between April, 2002 and July, 2002, there is a sudden increase in the insurance payment made for Cipro. We can think of this as a level shift or an event that happened at that moment of time that makes the increase, or that a particular observation could just be an outlier. The model that we will build automatically detects whether a particular observation is an outlier or not. The dataset, Cipro, has 1674 daily observations obtained from the means procedure given in Table 7. Cipro is a commonly prescribed antibiotic, and we have a reasonable number of observations for model building and forecasting; as a result, we will use it as an example to build a model for prediction. The Proc Means SAS procedure given in SAS CODE 2 was used to analyze the distribution of the observations. Once we have an idea of how the observations are linked, we can select a model based on the

Table 7. The means procedure for private insurance

MEDICATION NAME	N Obs	Sum	Minimum	Maximum	STDV
AMOXICILLIN	20457	44292.52	0.00	111.88	4.61
AMPICILLIN	1038	1693.86	0.00	54.60	3.52
AZITHROMYCIN	377	1985.20	0.00	262.27	18.45
CEFACLOR	597	14392.84	0.00	187.05	30.07
CEFADROXIL	239	5741.64	0.00	181.00	28.61
CEFUROXIME	28	2039.83	0.00	156.80	41.52
CEPHALEXIN	4788	41841.26	0.00	124.10	13.69
CIPRO	1674	53009.37	0.00	323.45	44.45
CLARITHROMYCIN	156	4785.03	0.00	87.38	35.39
CLINDAMYCIN	403	4597.68	0.00	123.40	16.53
CLOTRIMAZOLE	647	2210.43	0.00	142.11	14.63
DICLOXACILLIN	487	1277.08	0.00	49.24	8.06
DOXYCYCLINE	1054	8482.74	0.00	121.12	14.96
ERYTHROMYCIN	2226	5077.73	0.00	62.16	5.60
KEFLEX	1490	27802.95	0.00	115.78	29.37
SULFAMETHOXAZOLE	113	561.46	0.00	19.00	8.10
TEQUIN	408	11831.47	0.00	174.75	33.81
TETRACYCLINE	477	1395.82	0.00	97.48	10.21
TOBRAMYCIN	839	4003.18	0.00	44.69	5.16
VANCOMYCIN	73	703.34	0.00	262.60	34.17

number of observations, maximum, minimum and standard deviation of the antibiotics dataset.

SAS CODE 2. The Means Procedure

```
Proc means data=Diser.Disertation sum
nway min max std maxdec=2;
class RXNAME;
VAR RXPVX;
```

From the means procedure given in Table 7, we selected the antibiotic, Cipro, to investigate the private insurance payments made. As the main purpose of this case study is to build model forecasts for antibiotics, building model forecasts for Cipro's private insurance payment would be an ideal situation.

We will first build several models using the PROC HPFDIAGNOSE statement shown in SAS

CODE 3, and put the models into the model repository (warehouse). We then utilize the models built in HPFDIAGNOSE to the dataset using HPFENGINE. These methods select the best model using the criterion specified; for our case, we selected RMSE as an error of model selection. The model repository is a collection of a set of models to use to forecast the antibiotic, Cipro. The HPFDIAGNOSE procedure builds a model based on MODELREPOSITORY, and models specified are ARIMAX (autoregressive moving integrated moving average model), ESM (exponential smoothing model) and UCM (unobserved components model). The HPFENGINE procedure selects the models based on the smallest RMSE, and plots several graphs such as forecast, residual, autocorrelation plot etc.

We have built a model to forecast the private insurance payment made for the antibiotic, CIPRO.

The parameter estimates given in Table 7 indicate that there is an outlier on September, 2002; we have visually estimated the range of points where an outlier might happen as discussed previously. The plot of private insurance payments versus the start medication date given in figure 14 gives a starting point to show how the data behave through time. We can see that there is fluctuation of the data points across different time points, which we suspect indicates non-stationarity. For this reason, an ARIMA model would be a typical model of choice. We built a predictive model using the SAS CODE 9 for private insurance payments made for the antibiotic, Cipro.

The component in the parameter estimate given in Table 8 suggests that the event in September, 2002 resulted in an increase of $1700.40 in the payment of private insurance for the antibiotic, Cipro. We also have significant AR(1) and AR(2) parameters that indicate the model is well built. The parameter, AR1_1, of the component, RX-PVX (Private Insurance payment), represents an autoregressive process of order 1 with a difference of one, while AR1_2 is an autoregressive process of order 2 of difference one. The parameter, AO01SEP2002D, represents an additive outlier at September, 2002 and the scale indicates that the increase occurred due to the additive outlier.

SAS CODE 3. Building Private Insurance model for Cipro

```
PROC HPFDIAGNOSE DATA=CIPRO
OUTEST=CIPROSTATE CRITERION=RMSE
BASENAME= AMXESM PRINT=SHORT
```

```
MODELREPOSITORY=SASUSER.ANTIBIOTICSMOD-
ELS;
ID STARTMEDDATE INTERVAL=MONTH;
FORECAST RXPVX ;
ARIMAX PERROR=(12:24) P=(0:12) Q=(0:12)
CRITERION=SBC METHOD=MINIC;
ESM; UCM;
RU ODS RTF;
ODS GRAPHICS ON;
PROC HPFENGINE DATA=CIPRO
MODELREPOSITORY=SASUSER.ANTIBIOTICSMODELS
INEST=CIPROSTATE
GLOBALSELECTION=TSSELECT
PRINT=(SELECT ESTIMATES) LEAD=24
```

The HPFDIAGNOSE procedure builds models from the selected list (ARIMAX, ESM and UCM); the MODELREPOSITORY is a warehouse for the model built and the model estimates are put in the OUTEST=dataset. The HPFENGINE procedure builds the best model from the MODELREPOSITORY, which also uses some models from GLOBALSELEC-TION= where the new models built are stored in MODELREPOSITORY=SASUSER.ANTIBI-OTICS. The statements, OUTFOR= OUTEST= and OUTSTAT=, put the values of the forecast, estimates and statistics respectively in a dataset.

The PERROR= specifies the range of the AR order for obtaining the series, P=specifies the AR order, Q= specifies the range of the MA order, CRITERION=SBC specifies that the Swartz Bayesian Criterion is selected and the METHOD=MINIC specifies that the Minimum Information Criterion is selected. We have selected

Table 8. Parameter estimates of private insurance payment: Cipro

Component	Parameter	Estimate	Standard Error	T Value	Apporx Pr>|t|
RXPVX	AR1_1	-0.52158	0.09584	-5.44	,.0001
RXPVX	AR1_2	-0.26791	0.09718	-2.76	0.0069
AO01SEP2002D	SCALE	1700.4	351.03913	4.84	<.0001

the best model for Cipro private insurance payment from the listed models in SAS CODE 3. The SAS CODE 3 selects the best model of forecast based on the smallest RMSE, and from Table 9, we see that an ARIMA model with autoregressive order two and difference of one is chosen as the predictive model. The models AMXESM50, AMXESM 51 and AMXESM 52 are the models that were selected from the list of models in the model repository.

We have also investigated the prediction error for the normal curve and kernel density estimation for private insurance payments. Figure 15 reveals that the normal curve fitting is closer to the kernel density estimation (for unknown distribution).

The occurrence of the outlier on September, 2002 caused the gap between the two fits.

We have also investigated the prediction error for autocorrelation plot, partial autocorrelation plot and inverse autocorrelation plot. Each observation in a time series is correlated with previous prescriptions made, so it is important to analyze the autocorrelation function plots.

The error prediction for the autocorrelation function (Figure 16) and partial autocorrelation function (Figure 17) for the ARIMA model built shows that the correlations are within the bound of two standard errors; this reveals that the models are fitting the data well. As a consequence, we might adopt the ARIMA model as a model forecasting

Table 9. Model selection private insurance payment: Cipro

Model Selection Criterion = RMSE			
Model	**Statistic**	**Selected**	**Label**
AMXESM50	398.24401	Yes	ARIMA: RXPVX ~ P = (1,2) D = (1) NOINT
AMXESM51	428.92004	No	Simple Exponential Smoothing
AMXESM52	511.79995	No	UCM: RXPVX = LEVEL + ERROR

Figure 15. Prediction error for insurance payment

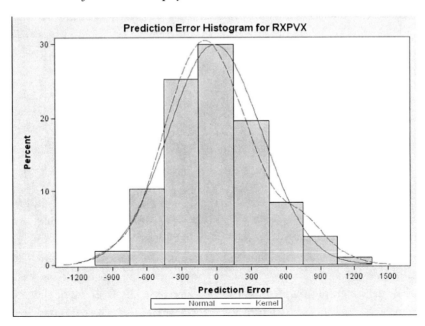

Figure 16. ACF plot of private insurance payment of Cipro

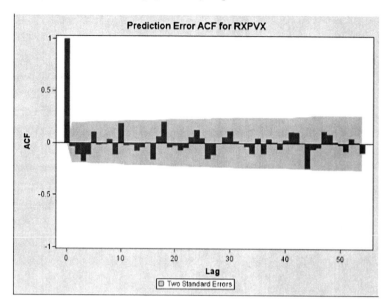

Figure 17. PACF plot of private insurance payment of Cipro

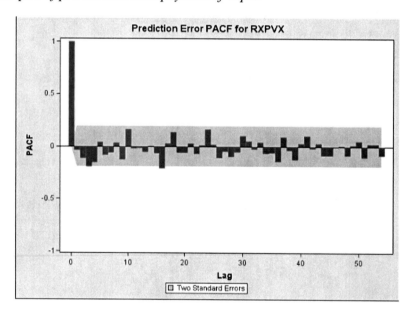

for the private insurance payment of the antibiotic, Cipro. The autocorrelation function plot and partial autocorrelation plot are also associated with the forecast model plot. The more the lags are outside the bounds of confidence, the more the model and forecast diverge. We also investigated the predictive model for private insurance payments for Cipro.

The points in Figure 18 represent the monthly private insurance payments for the antibiotic, Cipro and the thick blue line is the predictive model that was built. Most of the observations, with very few exceptions, lie within the 95% confidence band. There is a fairly constant increase in Private Insurance payments until the middle of

Figure 18. Model and forecast for private insurance payment of Cipro

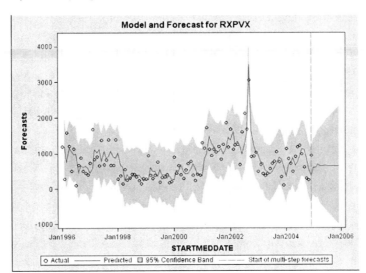

Figure 19. Stationarity component private insurance for Cipro

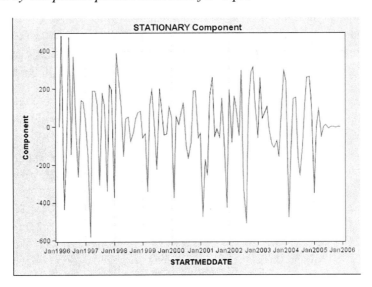

January, 2001; then there is a sudden increase in September, 2002. As mentioned earlier, in time series forecasting, we use the historical data to predict or forecast what tomorrow's value will be based on today's value.

The fact of the matter is that we chose to forecast for two years (year 2005 and year 2006) to get a better fit of the data; otherwise, we could forecast for the next 50 years and so forth. However, forecasting for a very long period of time gives a poorer fit; the reason is that there might be some other covariates that will occur in the near future that influence the forecast method used at the present time.

Figure 19 is the stationary component of the model that was built, and we can see that after differencing the data, which was done by the ARIMA procedure given in SAS CODE 3, the series is stationary.

Figure 20 is obtained by plotting each data point of the series forecast and connecting them by a line. This plot also reveals that in September, 2002, there is a sudden increase, which we define as an outlier. Figure 21 plots the outlier or event obtained through the model that was built. Outliers or events can be taken as single data points that we call point interventions in a time series. We will consider the data point of September, 2002 as a single data point; in other words, we will construct a dummy variable, and see if this can improve the forecast plot.

The payments made for all the antibiotics in our dataset were calculated without taking inflation rate as a factor. From an economic standpoint, inflation rate is important to consider when determining the price of items at a given period of time. As the inflation rate increases, the price of commodities increases as well and vice versa. Therefore, we introduced the inflation rate as a dynamic regressor and compared the model error with the one without a dynamic regressor.

The difference between the regressor variable and dynamic regressor is that the latter uses past values of the predictor series, so that it will help us to model effects that take place gradually. We added inflation rate to the dataset of Amoxicillin and investigated whether considering inflation rate as a dynamic regressor improves the model forecast.

The new model, which includes a dynamic regressor (Figure 22), fits the data much better than ARIMA (2, 1, 0) without a dynamic regressor (Figure 18). The predicted private insurance payment for the years 2005-2006 was constantly decreasing when a dynamic regressor was introduced. One possible reason is that the inflation rate affects the payments made for private insurance, and also the inflation rate was increasing through the time period. The root mean square error was dropped from 559 to 430, which is an indication that introducing the dynamic regressor improved the model forecast. The plot of inflation rates from 1996-2004 is given in Figure 23.

Figure 20. Y component of private insurance for Cipro

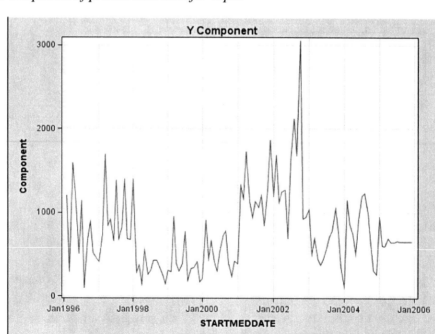

Heteroskedasticity and GARCH Models

In this section, we discuss approaches to dealing with heteroskedasticity. The ordinary regression model is used when the errors have the same variance throughout the time points; in such a scenario, the data are called Homoscedastic. On the other hand, if the errors have non-constant variances, then the data are called Heteroskedastic. Erroneously using ordinary least-squares regression for Heteroscedastic data causes the ordinary least squares estimate to be inefficient. As a consequence, we look for models that account

Figure 21. Outlier: private insurance for Cipro

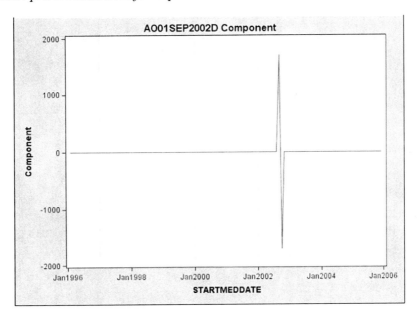

Figure 22. Forecasting plot of Cipro using inflation as dynamic regressor

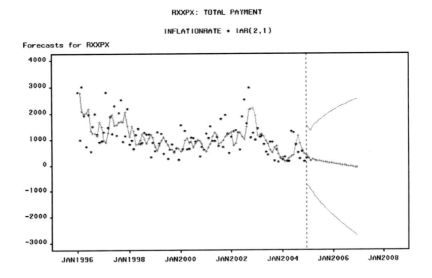

Figure 23. Inflation rates as a dynamic regressor

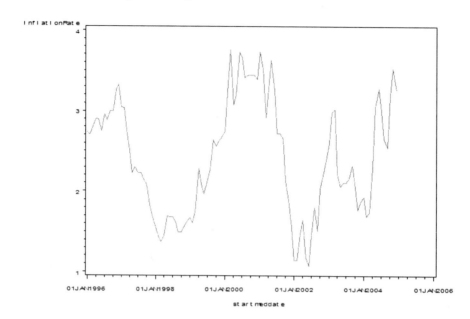

for the changing variances that make efficient use of the data.

The weighted regression method is a good method if the error variance at different time points is known, but if the error variance at different time points is not known, we must estimate it from the data by modeling the changing error variance. The generalized autoregressive conditional heteroskedasticity (GARCH) will be used to model for the heteroskedasticity errors. The analysis of the antibiotic, Erythromycin given in the previous section of this section reveals that there is higher variability in the beginning of the series that is given in Figure 9. A GARCH model is a weighted average of past squared residuals that has a declining weight on which recent observations are given larger weight than distant, past observations. Even if the series of time points given in Figure 9 looks Heteroskedastic, we need to test it statistically.

SAS CODE 4. SAS code to test heteroskedasticity

```
Ods html;
Proc autoreg data=hpfertro;
model RXXPX = STARTMEDDATE / nlag=12
archtest dwprob noint;
output out=out out=RXXPXresid;
```

We used SAS CODE 4 to test for heteroskedasticity, by regressing Private Insurance payments on start medication date and we used the ARCHTEST option to test for Heteroscedastic ordinary least squares residuals (Table 10). We used the DWPROB option to test for autocorrelation.

The Q statistic tests for changes in variance across time using lag windows ranging from 1 through 12 (Table 11). The p-values for the test statistics are significant and strongly indicate heteroskedasticity, with $p < 0.0001$ for all lag windows. The Lagrange multiplier (LM) tests also indicate heteroskedasticity. Both Q statistics and the Lagrange multiplier help to determine the order of the ARCH model needed for modeling the heteroskedasticity, on which the changing variance is assumed to follow an autoregressive conditional heteroskedasticity model.

350

Table 10. Ordinary least squares estimates

Ordinary Least Squares Estimates			
SSE	4030688.02	DFE	107
MSE	37670	Root MSE	194.08756
SBC	1448.12303	AIC	1445.4409
Regress R-Square	0.4108	Total R-Square	0.4108
Durbin-Watson	0.3475		

Table 11. Q and LM tests for ARCH disturbances

Q and LM Tests for ARCH Disturbances				
Order	Q	Pr > Q	LM	Pr > LM
1	50.0071	<.0001	48.7292	<.0001
2	77.6249	<.0001	49.1592	<.0001
3	80.8958	<.0001	56.3419	<.0001
4	81.1530	<.0001	56.4903	<.0001
5	81.3417	<.0001	59.5441	<.0001
6	82.0714	<.0001	59.5462	<.0001
7	84.4500	<.0001	59.5559	<.0001
8	88.7266	<.0001	60.2213	<.0001
9	95.2285	<.0001	60.9780	<.0001
10	96.1345	<.0001	66.4472	<.0001
11	96.4317	<.0001	66.6586	<.0001
12	97.0906	<.0001	67.2222	<.0001

Ordinary Least Squares Estimates

The parameter estimates given in Table 12 are also significant, an indication that the data have a Heteroskedastic property. Once we checked for heteroskedasticity of the data, then we used a generalized autoregressive conditional heteroskedasticity model (GARCH) that takes care of the Heteroskedasticity of the data. SAS CODE 5 was used to build a GARCH model and test the parameter estimates.

SAS Code 5. SAS code to build GARCH model for Private Insurance of Cipro

```
ods html;
Proc autoreg data=hpfertro;
model RXXPX = STARTMEDDATE / nlag=12
garch=(q=1,p=1) maxit=500 noint;
output out=out cev=vhat;
```

SAS CODE 5 was used to build GARCH (1, 1), by going back 12 lags into the past. This code will test how many autoregressive orders are needed for the Heteroskedastic variable, Private insurance payments, made for the antibiotic, Erythromycin. We fitted an AR(12) and GARCH(1,1) model for the Private Insurance Payment series regressed on start medication date. The AR(12) specifies an autoregressive error of order 12, while GARCH(1,1) specifies a conditional variance

Table 12. Parameter estimate

Variable	DF	Estimate	Standard Error	t Value	Approx Pr > |t|
STARTMEDDATE	1	0.0109	0.001261	8.64	<.0001

Table 13. GARCH estimates

GARCH Estimates			
SSE	1263311.36	Observations	108
MSE	11697	Uncond Var	14945.1458
Log Likelihood	-655.97225	Total R-Square	0.8153
SBC	1382.17648	AIC	1341.94451
Normality Test	1918.0137	Pr > ChiSq	<.0001

model (Table 13). SAS CODE 5 will compute the estimated conditional error variance at each time period in the variable, VHAT (estimated conditional error variance series) and output the dataset named OUT.

The normality test is significant ($p < 0.0001$), which is consistent with the hypothesis that the residuals from the GARCH model, $\varepsilon_t / \sqrt{k_t}$, are normally distributed. The parameter estimate is significant. The parameter estimates given in Table 14 include rows for the GARCH parameters. ARCH0 represents the estimate for the parameter ω, ARCH1 represents α_1, and GARCH1 represents δ_1. The parameter estimates for the autoregressive errors are significant up to lag 1; as a result, we adopt AR(1). Also, the GARCH1 parameter estimate is significant. The model for Erythromycin Private Insurance is therefore built with AR(1) + GARCH(1,1) on which the heteroskedasticity nature of the data is controlled. As we have discussed in the beginning of this section, an AR(2) was the best model predicted with a negative correlation of $R^2=-0.627$.

The autoregressive order of lag one is the only one significant, so we do not need lags of up to 12. The estimate of the mean term in the Hetereskedastic process is 0.0850, which is not significant, but the estimate of the coefficient of the square of error terms 0.2103 is significant. The estimate of error variance at lag 1 is 0.7376, which is significant at a 5% level of significance.

We also investigated the average Medicare and Medicaid payments made for the prescriptions of antibiotics. The term, Medicaid, is referred to as the amount of support in terms of healthcare given to low income people. A family is in the category of low income if the percentage of income of the household is less than 15,000. (Cerrito, Badia, Cerrito, 2005) Medicaid only consists of a very small portion of the total payment made; that means the majority cost is paid by the patient. The government pays only a small portion of the total payment. We have built a model of prediction for both Medicare and Medicaid payments made for the antibiotic, Cephalexin. Cephalexin is a commonly prescribed antibiotic. A model of forecast was built for the Medicaid payment of Cephalexin; a double (brown) exponential smoothing model was built. The Medicaid payment was increasing through the years 1996 up to 2004, and the forecasted Medicaid payment for the years 2005 and 2006 was increasing as well; this means the government was paying more money

Table 14. GARCH parameter estimates

Variable	DF	Estimate	Standard Error	t Value	Approx Pr > |t|
STARTMEDDATE	1	0.0185	0.005313	3.48	0.0005
AR1	1	-0.5830	0.2065	-2.82	0.0047
AR2	1	-0.3273	0.2008	-1.63	0.1030
AR3	1	0.0545	0.2386	0.23	0.8195
AR4	1	0.1816	0.2391	0.76	0.4474
AR5	1	-0.0956	0.2075	-0.46	0.6448
AR6	1	-0.0242	0.2607	-0.09	0.9260
AR7	1	-0.1437	0.2584	-0.56	0.5782
AR8	1	0.0351	0.3917	0.09	0.9286
AR9	1	0.0115	0.3367	0.03	0.9726
AR10	1	0.0312	0.2624	0.12	0.9055
AR11	1	-0.0825	0.2040	-0.40	0.6858
AR12	1	-0.004789	0.1342	-0.04	0.9715
ARCH0	1	0.0850	0.0757	1.12	0.2614
ARCH1	1	0.2103	0.0847	2.48	0.0130
GARCH1	1	0.7376	0.0960	7.68	<.0001

for Medicaid than the previous years. One has to keep in mind that this increase in payment is due to cost increase; insurance payments increase overall due to total payment increase.

We also investigated the average Medicare payments made for the prescription of Cephalexin. The term, Medicare, is referred to as the amount of support in terms of healthcare given to the American elderly people of age 65 or more. People with disabilities are also eligible for Medicare payments. Figure 25 indicates that on average, the government pays a maximum of less than three dollars for the prescription of Cephalexin. The data for Medicare payments has many missing observations, but in order to maintain the series of the data, we set missing values to zero; that is why a mean model was built as a model of prediction. As we can observe from figure 24, the model built did not capture most of the data, the reason being that the data have two observations of zero at November, 2004 and December, 2004. Statistically speaking, when we have as many observations missing, it is ideal to consider the mean as a model of prediction.

Comparing Medicaid payment (Figure 24) and Medicare payment (Figure 25), we see that Medicaid payments are three times as large as Medicare payments; further studies can be made if the number of low income people are three times as many as elderly or disabled people.

We finally built a model of forecast for the remaining antibiotics for the total payment made. As we have seen earlier in this section using the Means procedure, we found out that Amoxicillin was the most prescribed with 20,457 transactions while Cefuroxime was the least prescribed with only 28 transactions. The model forecast for all antibiotics was built using SAS CODE 6.

SAS CODE 6. For all antibiotics model building

```
Proc sort data=diser.disertation;
by RXNAME STARTMEDDATE ; RUN;
PROC HPF DATA=diser.disertation
```

Figure 24. Model forecast for Medicaid payment: Cephalexin

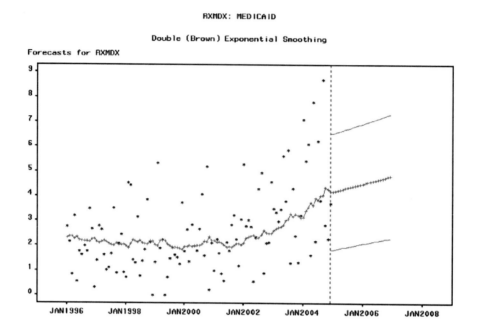

Figure 25. Model forecast for Medicare payment: Cephalexin

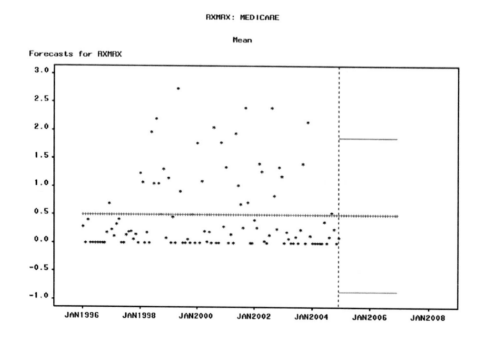

```
OUT=disertation LEAD=0;
ID STARTMEDDATE INTERVAL=MONTH
ACCUMULATE=TOTAL;
FORECAST RXXPX RXPVX RXMDX RXMRX RXQUANTY
DRUG /MODEL=NONE;
BY RXNAME; RUN;
Proc HPF data=disertation out=sasuser.
forecast lead=24;
id startmeddate interval=month;
forecast RXXPX RXPVX RXMRX RXMDX RXQUANTY
DRUG/select=mape holdout=36;
BY RXNAME; Run;
```

Plotting the forecasted series of the antibiotics in one plot is the best way to compare the number of prescriptions, quantity of prescriptions and total payments made between several antibiotics. We plotted all twenty antibiotics in one graph, but looking at Figure 26, we can hardly make comparisons; the reason being the difference in the total number of transactions made for the antibiotics. As a result,

we classified the antibiotics into classes of three based on the number of transactions.

Figure 26 gives the forecasted plot of all the antibiotics for total payments made for all twenty antibiotics.

The total payments made for Keflex are rising starting in January, 2001, while the forecast series for Clarithromycin is decreasing (see Figure 27).

The total payment for Vancomycin is highest on May, 2001; it is an outlier, while Ampicillin, Cipro, Azithromycin and Cephalexin increase through time with the forecast for Azithromycin decreasing (see Figure 28).

The total payment for Tequin is highest in January, 2002, while Dicloxacillin is at its peak around January, 2001 (see Figure 29).

The number of prescriptions of Erythromycin was higher until January, 1999, and then the number of Keflex prescriptions surpassed the number of those for Erythromycin (see Figure 30).

Figure 26. Model forecast for total payments for all antibiotics

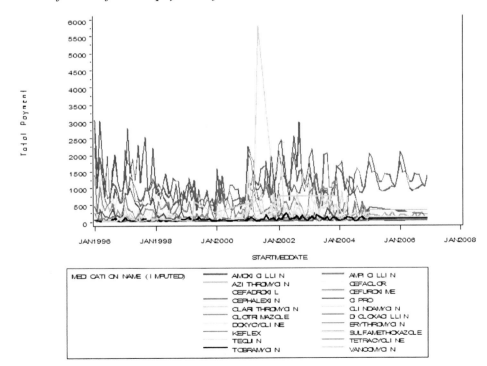

Figure 27. Model forecast for Cefaclor, Cefuroxime, Clarithromycin, Clotrimazole, Erythromycin, Keflex and Tetracycline: total payment

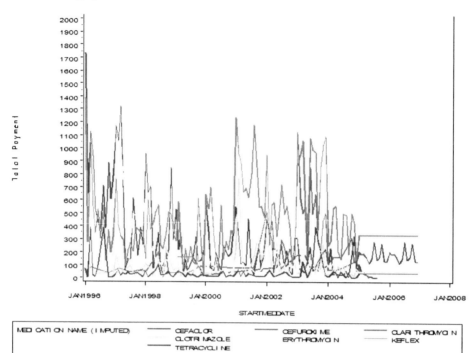

Figure 28. Model forecast for Amoxicillin, Azithromycin, Cephalexin, Cipro, and Vancomycin: total payment

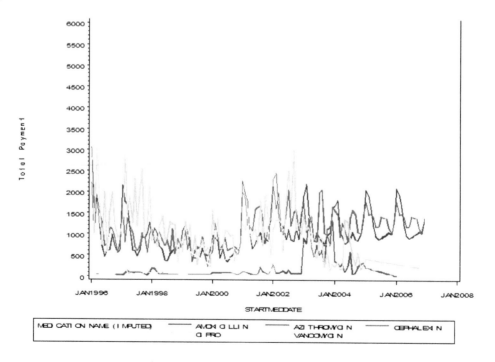

Figure 29. Model forecast for Ampicillin, Cefadroxil, Clindamycin, Dicloxacillin, Doxycycline, Tequin and Tobramycin: total payment

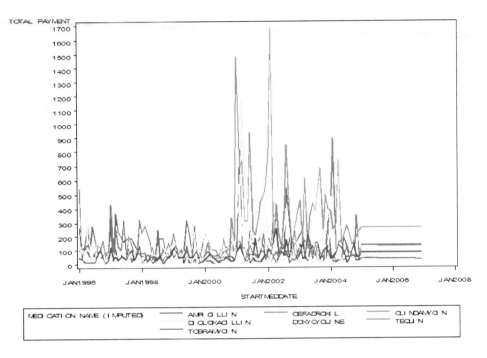

Figure 30. Model forecast for Cefaclor, Cefuroxime, Clarithromycin, Clotrimazole, Erythromycin, Keflex and Tetracycline: number of prescription

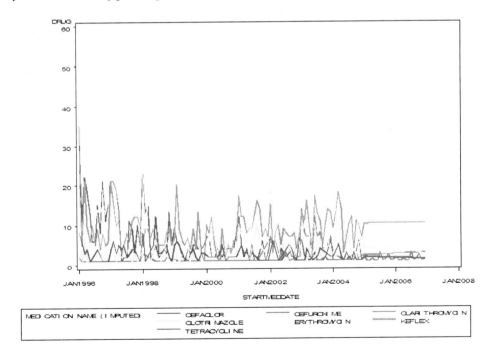

The number of prescriptions of Amoxicillin was greater than the number for Azithromycin, Cephalexin, Cipro, Vancomycin, but all prescriptions were seasonally increasing through time (see Figure 31).

The number of prescriptions for Ampicillin, Cefadroxil, Clindamycin, Dicloxacillin, Doxycycline, Tequin and Tobramycin are close to each other, with Dicloxacillin at its highest value in January, 2001 (see Figure 32).

The quantity of medications prescribed is close for each antibiotic starting January, 1999 with a slightly higher quantity of prescriptions for Keflex around May, 2003 (see Figure 33).

Amoxicillin prescription quantity is higher compared to Cipro, Azithromycin, Cephalexin and Vancomycin, while Cipro and Vancomycin have the smallest quantity of prescriptions (see Figure 34).

Ampicillin prescription quantity is higher from January, 1996 up to May, 1999, but the series of prescription quantity is about the same starting in January, 2000, with a sudden peak for Dicloxacillin, Ampicillin and Clindamycin (see Figure 35).

From an economic stand point, we know that the cost of an item is determined by the market; that means that the supply and demand play a major part. By the same token, the cost of antibiotics depends on the number of prescriptions and the quantity of antibiotics sold. One has to test statistically whether the number of prescriptions and the quantity of prescriptions significantly predict the total payments made for the antibiotics. We regressed the total payment of medication on the quantity of medication and the number of prescriptions. We tested statistically if the quantity of medications and the number of medications affects the total payments made on medication. We picked the antibiotic, Amoxicillin, to demonstrate the effect of predictors (quantity and number of prescriptions) on predicting the total payment.

SAS CODE 7. For regression procedure of total payment of Amoxicillin

Figure 31. Model forecast for Amoxicillin, Azithromycin, Cephalexin, Cipro, and Vancomycin: number of prescriptions

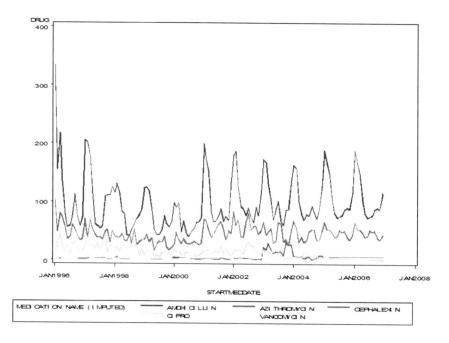

Figure 32. Model forecast for Ampicillin, Cefadroxil, Clindamycin, Dicloxacillin, Doxycycline, Tequin and Tobramycin: number of prescriptions

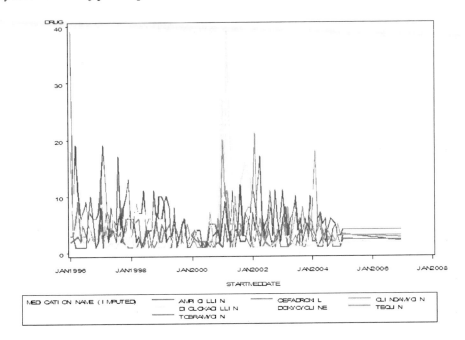

Figure 33. Model forecast for Cefaclor, Cefuroxime, Clarithromycin, Clotrimazole, Erythromycin, Keflex and Tetracycline: quantity

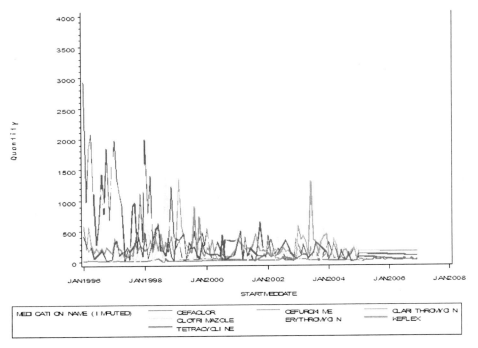

Figure 34. Model forecast for Amoxicillin, Azithromycin, Cephalexin, Cipro, and Vancomycin: quantity

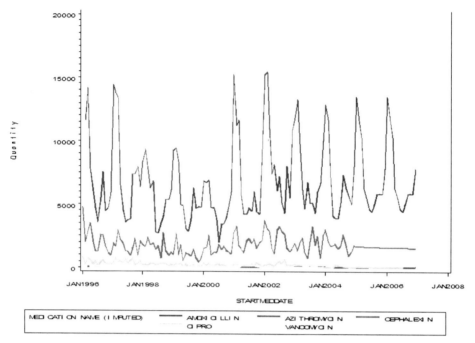

Figure 35. Model forecast for Ampicillin, Cefadroxil, Clindamycin, Dicloxacillin, Doxycycline, Tequin and Tobramycin: quantity

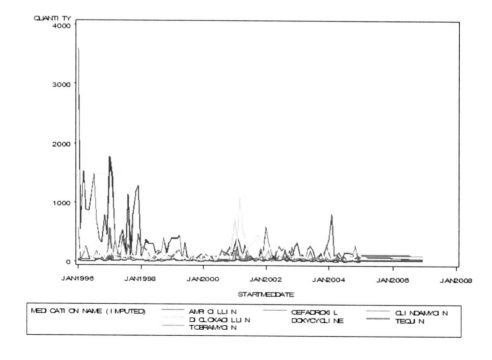

```
DATA AMOXICILLIN;
SET DISER.DISERTATION;
WHERE RXNAME IN ('AMOXICILLIN');
RUN;
PROC HPF DATA=AMOXICILLIN OUT=AMOXICILLIN
LEAD=24;
ID STARTMEDDATE INTERVAL=MONTH
ACCUMULATE=TOTAL;
FORECAST RXXPX/MODEL=NONE;
FORECAST RXQUANTY/MODEL=BESTS
SELECT=MAPE;
FORECAST DRUG/MODEL=WINTERS
TRANSFORM=LOG;
RUN;
PROC AUTOREG DATA=AMOXICILLIN;
MODEL RXXPX=RXQUANTY DRUG;
OUTPUT OUT=TOTAL P=PREDICTED;
LABEL RXQUANTY='QUANTITY';
RUN;
```

SAS CODE 7 was used to create the dataset, Amoxicillin using the Data statement, with no predictive model for total payment, best seasonal model for quantity of medications, and Winter's model with a log transformation for the number of prescriptions (drug).

The parameter estimates for RXQUANTY and DRUG are significant with p-values of 0.0091 and <0.0001 at 5%. The significant parameter estimates the number of prescriptions and the quantity of medications indicates that both can forecast the total payment made for Amoxicillin. About 91% of the time, the variation in total payment is explained by both the quantity of medication and the number of medications. The R-square value close to one indicates that both the predictor variables, quantity and number of prescriptions, predict the total payment. Hence, the model prediction for total payment can include the quantity of medication and the number of prescriptions. We also plotted the model forecast for total payment using the quantity of medication and the number of prescriptions (Table 15).

When we introduced the quantity of prescriptions and the number of prescriptions as predictor variables for total payment for the prescription of Amoxicillin, the R^2 value dramatically increased from -0.094 to 0.9117; this is a great improvement of the predictor variables' influence on the total payment of Amoxicillin. Also, when compared to total payments made for Amoxicillin without the predictor variable (figure 8), Figure 36 gave a better forecast plot with the total payment seasonally increasing or decreasing as we move from January, 1996 up to December, 2006.

Patient Condition Severity

We then used text mining with kernel density estimation to reduce a large number of patient condition codes to make a comparison between the severity of the patient condition on the use of antibiotics. We condensed thousands of patient conditions into an index of 6 levels, and those levels are used to examine the relationship to different target variables of total payment and private

Table 15. Parameter Estimates for Predicting Total Payment

The AUTOREG Procedure			
Dependent Variable		RXXPX	
			TOTAL PAYMENT
Ordinary Least Squares Estimates			
SSE	2513834.41	DFE	105
MSE	23941	Root MSE	154.72970
SBC	1406.49748	AIC	1398.45109

Figure 36. Prediction of total payment using quantity and number of prescriptions for Amoxicillin.

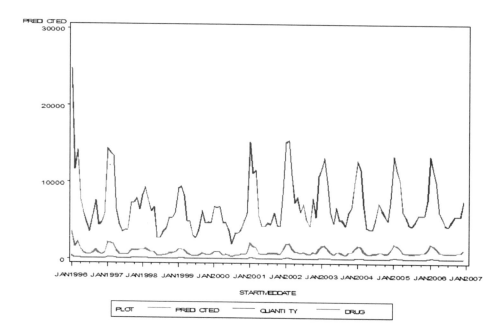

insurance payments. Since there are hundreds of ICD-9 codes, and most patients have more than one ICD-9 code assigned to them, we compress the codes into a total of six clusters. We applied clustering and text mining to group similar patients together so that meaningful analyses can be performed to examine cost. We used text mining to process and analyze the ICD-9 codes and to find similarities between patients. We then group similar patients together.

Clustering was performed using the expectation maximization algorithm. It is a relatively new, iterative clustering technique that works well with nominal data in comparison to the K-means and hierarchical methods that are more commonly used. Six clusters were formed using the ICD9 codes based on the similarity of the text of each ICD-9 code.

SAS CODE 8. To change ICD-9 codes to text and create clusters

```
Proc sort data = sasuser.Antibiotics out=
work.sort_out;
by duid rxicd1x;
Run;

options obs=max;
Data work.sort_out1;
set work.sort_out;
icd9 = translate(left(trim(rxicd1x)),'_'
,' ');
Run;

proc Transpose data=work.sort_out1
out=work.tran
prefix=icd9_;
var icd9 ;
by duid;
run;

data work.concat(keep= duid icd9) ;
length icd9 $32767 ;
set work.tran ;
array rxconcat {*} icd9_: ;
icd9 = left(trim(icd_1)) ;
do i = 2 to dim(rxconcat) ;
icd9 = left(trim(icd9)) || ' ' ||
```

Table 16. Clusters of the ICD-9 Codes

#	Descriptive terms	Freq	Percentage
1	601,562,786,487,465,596,522,496,892,785,575,996,784	760	0.79249218
2	716	2	0.00208551
3	599,593,382,388,493,595	38	0.03962461
4	473,490,519,401,429,477,592,491,311,686,919,428,492, 486,595,478,590	108	0.11261731
5	780,v68,460,41,v25,272,	19	0.0198123
6	244,518,998,590,493,486	32	0.03336809

```
left(trim(rxconcat[i])) ;
end ;
run ;
Proc sql ;
select max(length(icd9)) into:icd9_LEN
from work.concat ;
quit ;
%put icd9_LEN=&icd9_LEN ;
Data work.concat1 ;
length icd9 $ &icd9_LEN ;
set work.concat ;
Run ;
Proc contents data=work.concat1 ; Run;
SAS CODE 15
```

Using SAS CODE 8, six clusters were formed based on the ICD9 codes using Enterprise Miner 5.2. We created six clusters with the cluster number given in Table 7. We will use these clusters to compare the distribution of antibiotics between the clusters using kernel density estimation. Table 16 is the description of the clusters shown in Table 17.

We used kernel density estimation to examine differences within the six clusters. Figures 24 and 25 show the graphs of total payments and private insurance payments respectively by cluster id for the antibiotic, Cipro. Note that cluster 2 has a high probability of total charges and reimbursements compared to the other clusters where the amount is very low. These graphs demonstrate a natural ordering in the clusters that is defined within the text mining tool.

The clusters formed based on the severity of the patient condition were compared using Kernel density estimation to examine private insurance payments for the antibiotic, Cipro (Figure 37). For instance, for patients in cluster 3 taking Cipro, they have a higher probability of paying between 40-80 dollars. As the total payment exceeds 280 dollars, the severity of the disease does not play a role on the size of payment made.

The clusters formed based on the severity of the patient condition were compared using Kernel density estimation to examine private insurance payments for each antibiotic (Figure 38). For instance, for patients in cluster 3 taking Cipro, they have a higher probability of paying between 30-60 dollars, but patients in cluster 6 have a higher probability of paying between 115-180 dollars.

CURRENT AND FUTURE CHALLENGES FACING THE ORGANIZATION

The aim of this project was to develop time series models to investigate prescribing practices and patient usage of medications with respect to the severity of the patient condition. We have analyzed factors that contribute to the cost of medications such as total payments and private insurance payments. The amount of money spent varies between the severities of the patient condition;

Table 17. Text clusters defined by expectation maximization

Cluster Number	ICD-9 Codes	ICD-9 Risk Factors	Frequency	Label
1	601 562 786 487 465 596 522 496 892 785 575 996 784	Prostatitis Diverticula of Intestine Respiratory & Chest symptom Influenza Upper respiratory infection acute Bladder disorder Pulp disease & peripheral tissues Chronic airway obstruction Open wound of foot Symptoms involving cardiovascular system Disorder of gallbladder Anastomosis, graft (bypass), implant Symptoms of head and neck	760	Routine problems
2	716	Other and unspecified arthropathies	2	Arthritis
3	599 593 382 388 493 595	Other disorders of urethra and urinary tract Other disorders of kidney and ureter Suppurative and unspecified otitis media Other disorders of ear Asthma Cystitis	38	Urinary tract infection, asthma
4	473 490 519 401 429 477 592 491 311 686 919 428 492 486 595 478 590	Chronic sinusitis Bronchitis, not specifies as acute or chronic Other diseases of respiratory system Essential hypertension Complications of heart disease Allergic rhinitis, hay fever spasmodic rhinorrhea Calculus of kidney and ureter Chronic bronchitis Depressive disorder Local infections of skin and subcutaneous tissue Superficial injury Heart failure Chronic obstructive pulmonary disease Pneumonia, organism unspecified Cystitis, other disease of urinary system Other disease of upper respiratory tract Infections of kidney	108	Severe complications of respiratory system
5	780 v68 460 041 v25 272	Alteration of consciousness, hallucinations Persons encountering health service Acute nasopharyngitis (common cold) Bacterial infection Contraceptive management, sterilization Disorders of lipoid metabolism	19	Mild risk factors
6	244 518 998 590 493 486	Acquired hypothyroidism, like post-surgical Diseases of lung, pulmonary collapse Postoperative shock, hemorrhage Infections of kidney Asthma Pneumonia	32	Moderate risk factor

that means that patients who are more severely ill spend more money for medications compared to patients who are less ill. Our goal was to develop time series models so that we can compare between several antibiotics. To reach this result, time series models and data mining tools such as

Figure 37. Distributions of total payments for CIPRO

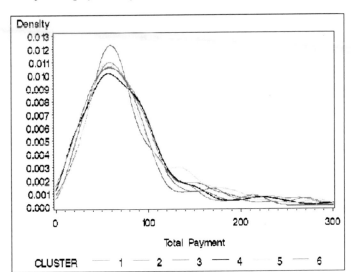

Figure 38. Distributions of private insurance payments for CIPRO

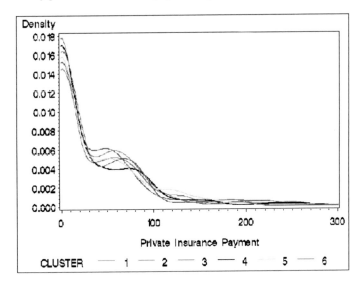

text mining were used to investigate the prescription of medications.

The main analysis idea was to show that the increase in the cost of medication is affected by the increase in private insurance payment, and Medicare and Medicaid payments made. There was also a tremendous change in the number of prescriptions in one antibiotic compared to others.

We also investigated a sudden change, which we call an outlier or event in time series theory. We found out that an outlier or an event does change the predicted payments made for the antibiotics. We studied the effect of the inflation rate in the cost of medications, and found out that the price prediction goes down, meaning that antibiotics get cheaper over time. In other words, we believe that pharmaceutical companies are not gouging people for the price of drugs. Since most of the antibiotics we studied are already available in generic form, or did not change to generic form during the time period under study, we could not take the switch in type into consideration. However, such a switch would involve a step function.

We also found out that the trends in the prescription of antibiotics were increasing over the years 1996-2004. There is a difference in the number of prescriptions of one antibiotic over another, with Amoxicillin mostly prescribed and Vancomycin least prescribed. We also investigated how much patients are spending on the sum and average for antibiotics and found out the spending was increasing over the years, but increasing less than the inflation rate. We examined the average Medicare and Medicaid payments for the antibiotic, Cephalexin, and we found out that the predicted Medicaid payment is three times as large as the Medicare payment. In terms of expenditure, the government's expense for Medicaid was increasing from the model forecast. Text mining was used to reduce a large number of patient condition codes into an index of 6 levels, and to use those levels to examine the relationship between total payment and private insurance payments for different cluster levels.

The results of this study can be used by health care institutions and pharmaceutical companies to predict and forecast the distribution, cost, number of prescriptions, quantity of prescription dose, private insurance payment, Medicare payment and Medicaid payment. The trend of prescription can be used to study what the effect really is on the decrease or increase in the prescriptions of medications

Forecasting has become vital technology for business and research in many fields. Forecasting was mainly used in the financial industry, on which the forecasters have developed time series models through a period of time. In this study, we have taken forecasting path to the health care

industry. The main challenges we faced on this study are the scarcity of data for some antibiotics; as a consequence, no forecasting was done.

REFERENCES

Antibiotics. (n.d.). Retrieved 2007, from http://www.emedicinehealth.com/antibiotics/article_em.htm

Cerrito, P., Badia, A., & Cerrito, J. (2005). *Data mining medication prescriptions for a representative national sample.* Paper presented at: PharmaSug 2005, Phoenix, AZ.

Chan, E., Zhan, C., & Homer, C. J. (2002). *Health care use and costs for children with attention-deficit/hyperactivity disorder: national estimates from the medical expenditure panel survey.* Academy for Health Services Research and Health Policy.

Cohen, J. W., Monheit, A. C., Beauregard, K. M., Cohen, S. B., Lefkowitz, D. C., & Potter, D. E. (1996). The Medical Expenditure Panel Survey: a national health information resource. *Inquiry, 33*(4), 373–389.

Cohen, S. B. (2002). The Medical Expenditure Panel Survey: an overview. [Research Support, U.S. Gov't, P.H.S.]. *Effective Clinical Practice: ECP, 5*(3Suppl), E1.

Cohen, S. B., & Buchmueller, T. (2006). Trends in medical care costs, coverage, use, and access: research findings from the Medical Expenditure Panel Survey. *Medical Care, 44*(5Suppl), 1–3.

Guevara, J. P., Mandell, D. S., Rostain, A. L., Zhao, H., Hadley, T. R., & Guevara, J. P. (2003). National estimates of health services expenditures for children with behavioral disorders: an analysis of the medical expenditure panel survey. [Research Support, Non-U.S. Gov't]. *Pediatrics, 112*(6), 440. doi:10.1542/peds.112.6.e440

Halpern, M. T., Yabroff, K. R., Halpern, M. T., & Yabroff, K. R. (2008). Prevalence of outpatient cancer treatment in the United States: estimates from the Medical Panel Expenditures Survey (MEPS). *Cancer Investigation, 26*(6), 647–651. doi:10.1080/07357900801905519

Law, A. W., Reed, S. D., Sundy, J. S., Schulman, K. A., Law, A. W., & Reed, S. D. (2003). *Direct costs of allergic rhinitis in the United States.* Estimates from the 1996 Medical Expenditure Panel Survey. Research Support, U.S. Gov't, P.H.S.]. *The Journal of Allergy and Clinical Immunology, 111*(2), 296–300. doi:10.1067/mai.2003.68

McGarry, K., Schoeni, R. F., McGarry, K., & Schoeni, R. F. (2005). *Widow(er) poverty and out-of-pocket medical expenditures near the end of life. Research Support, N.I.H.* Extramural.

Miller, J. D., Foster, T., Boulanger, L., Chace, M., Russell, M. W., & Marton, J. P. (2005, September). Direct costs of COPD in the U.S.: an analysis of Medical Expenditure Panel Survey. *COPD, 2*(3), 311–318. doi:10.1080/15412550500218221

Mol, P. G. M., & Wieringa, J. E., NannanPanday, P. V., et al. (2005). Improving compliance with hospital antibiotic guidelines: a time-series intervention analysis. *The Journal of Antimicrobial Chemotherapy, 55*, 550–557. doi:10.1093/jac/dki037

Research Support. (n.d.). U.S. Gov't, P.H.S. *Archives of Pediatrics & Adolescent Medicine, 156*(5), 504-511.

Research Support. (n.d.). U.S. Gov't, P.H.S. *Journals of Gerontology Series B-Psychological Sciences & Social Sciences, 60*(3), S160-168.

Tesfamicael, M. (2005). Calculation of health disparity indices using data mining and the SAS Bridge to ESRI. MWSUG conference, Cincinnati, OH

ADDITIONAL READING

Aldrin, M., & Damsleth, E. (1989). Forecasting Non-seasonal Time Series with Missing Observations. *Journal of Forecasting, 8*, 97–116. doi:10.1002/for.3980080204

Cerrito, P. (2005). *Comparing the SAS Forecasting system with PROC HPF and Enterprise Miner.* Paper presented at: SUGI 30, Philadelphia, PA.

Chan, N. H. (2002). *Time Series Applications to Finance.* New York: John Wiley & Sons, Inc.

Chatfield, C. (1980). *The Analysis of Time Series: An Introduction* (2nd ed.). London: Chapman and Hall.

Chatfield, C., & Yar, M. (1988). Holt-Winters Forecasting: Some Practical Issues. *The Statistician, 37*, 129–140. doi:10.2307/2348687

Migliaro, A., & Jain, C. L. (1984). Understanding business forecasting. Great Neck, New York: Graceway publishing company.

Tesfemicael, M. (2007). *Forecasting prescription of medications and cost analysis using time series analysis* (PhD Dissertation). University of Louisville.

Chapter 16
Cost Models with Prominent Outliers

Chakib Battioui
University of Louisville, USA

ABSTRACT

Government reimbursement programs, such as Medicare and Medicaid, generally pay hospitals less than the cost of caring for the people enrolled in these programs. For many patient conditions, Medicare and Medicaid pay hospitals a fixed amount based upon average cost for a procedure or treatment with local conditions taken into consideration. In addition, while the hospital provides the services, it has little control over the cost of delivery of that service, which is determined more by physician orders. The physician is under no real obligation to control those costs as the physician bills separately for services that are independent of orders charged. However, some patients who are severely ill will cost considerably more than average. This has caused providers to lose money. In this study, we investigate the reimbursement policies and the assumptions that have been made to create these reimbursement policies.

BACKGROUND

According to the US Census Bureau statistics for the year 2004, about 45.8 million people in the United States are without health insurance coverage, which represents 15.7% of the total population. (DeNavas-Walt and Lee, 2004) These uninsured and underinsured individuals have access to many health care facilities even when they are unable to afford the health services costs. The Emergency

Medical Treatment and Labor Act (EMTALA) guarantees that for any individual who comes to the emergency department of a hospital with a request for treatment, the hospital must provide for an appropriate medical screening examination. (EMTALA, 2003) The health care provider does not have any guarantee of any reimbursement from uninsured or underinsured patients.

Government reimbursement programs, such as Medicare and Medicaid, generally pay hospitals less than the cost of caring for the people enrolled in these programs. For many patient conditions, Medicare

DOI: 10.4018/978-1-61520-723-7.ch016

Copyright © 2010, IGI Global. Copying or distributing in print or electronic forms without written permission of IGI Global is prohibited.

and Medicaid pay hospitals a fixed amount based upon average cost for a procedure or treatment with local conditions taken into consideration. In addition, while the hospital provides the services, it has little control over the cost of the delivery of that service, which is determined more by physician orders. The physician is under no real obligation to control those costs as the physician bills separately for services that are independent of orders charged. However, some patients who are severely ill will cost considerably more than average.

Private insurance pays even less than Medicare and Medicaid because they always negotiate discounts with hospitals. A study titled "DRG, costs and reimbursement following Roux-en-Y gastric bypass: an economic appraisal (Angus, et.al. 2004)" (shows that there is a large difference in hospital reimbursement between public and private insurance when DRG codes are used. The study compared the reimbursement rates between a privately-insured group (74 patients) and a publicly-insured group (59 patients) using DRG 228. The two groups were similar in terms of age, sex and BMI. Results show that the hospital received large reimbursements from public insurance compared to private ones ($11,773 public vs $4,435 private).

This situation has caused many health care providers to lose money; some of them have cut their budgets, and others have closed their emergency departments because the reimbursements no longer match costs. In addition, if hospitals were paid the same amount for each admission regardless of its clinical characteristics, they would be encouraged to treat patients who are less ill, and to avoid the cases that require more resources. This policy is observed by looking at the trends in Medicare and total hospital length of stay between 1994 and 2004. The length of stay for Medicare inpatients fell 25% from 7.3 days in 1994 to 5.5 days in 2004 while the length of stay for all hospital discharges fell 11% from 5.0 days in 1994 to 4.5 days in 2004. (MedPac Data

Book, 2005) Figure 1 was developed from the congressional report of the Medicare Payment Advisory Commission's website (www.MedPac.gov) for June 2006. MedPAC is an independent federal body established by the Balanced Budget Act of 1997 to advise the U.S. Congress on issues affecting the Medicare program.

Diagnosis-Related Group (DRG)

The Diagnosis Related Group (DRG) is a classification system developed for Medicare as part of the prospective payment system; it is used as the basis to reimburse hospitals for inpatient services. DRGs are assigned by a software program based on diagnoses, procedures, age, sex, and the presence or absence of complications or comorbidities. A substantial complication or comorbidity is defined as a condition, which, because of its presence with a specific principal diagnosis, would cause an increase in the length of stay by at least one day in at least 75% of the patients. The DRGs are organized into 25 Major Diagnostic Categories (MDC). The diagnoses in each MDC correspond to a single organ system or etiology and, in general, are associated with a particular medical specialty.

Under DRGs, a hospital is paid at a predetermined amount regardless of the costs involved, for each Medicare discharge. Only one DRG is assigned to a patient for a particular hospital admission. One payment is made per patient and that payment is based upon the DRG assignment. For example, if DRG 209 (major joint and limb reattachment procedures of lower extremity) reimburses the hospital $9600 and the hospital incurs $12,000 in costs, then the hospital has lost $2400 on that patient.

The Inpatient Prospective Payment System (IPPS)

Under the Inpatient Prospective Payment System (IPPS), each patient's case is categorized into a

Figure 1.

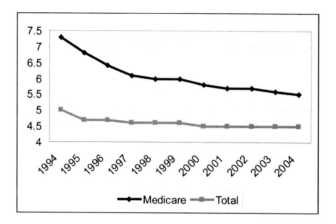

diagnosis related group (DRG). Each DRG has a payment weight assigned to it based on the average resources used to treat cases in that DRG. For example, DRG 205 (Disorders of liver except malign, cirr, alc heap w cc) has a weight of 1.2026, while DRG 206 (Disorders of liver except malign, cirr, alc heap w/o cc) has a weight of 0.7289. Therefore, the reimbursement rate would be higher for the DRG 205 as it has a higher weight.

The base payment rate is divided into a labor-related and non-labor share. The labor-related share is adjusted by the wage index applicable to the area where the hospital is located. This base payment rate is multiplied by the DRG relative weight. The operating payment formula is given below:

[(Labor base rate x Wage index) + Non-labor base rate] x DRG weight.

If the hospital treats a high-percentage of low-income patients, it receives a percentage add-on payment applied to the DRG-adjusted base payment rate. This add-on, known as the disproportionate share hospital (DSH) adjustment, provides for a percentage increase in Medicare payment for hospitals that qualify and serve a disproportionate share of low-income patients. For qualifying hospitals, the amount of this ad-

justment may vary based on the outcome of the statutory calculation.

Also, if the hospital is an approved teaching hospital, it receives a percentage add-on known as the indirect medical education (IME) adjustment, which varies depending on the facility. Finally, for particular cases that are unusually costly, known as outlier cases, the DRG payment is increased. This additional payment is designed to protect the hospital from large financial losses due to unusually expensive cases. Any outlier payment due is added to the DRF-adjusted base payment rate, plus any DSH or IME adjustments.

In healthcare, there are cases with extremely high costs compared with others classified in the same diagnosis-related group. These cases are considered outliers. The Centers for Medicare and Medicaid Services (CMS) explain on their website how hospitals can qualify for outlier payments in addition to the basic prospective payments for cases incurring extraordinarily high costs: "The actual determination of whether a case qualifies for outlier payments takes into account both operating and capital costs and DRG payments. That is, the combined operating and capital costs of a case must exceed the fixed loss outlier threshold to qualify for an outlier payment. The operating and capital costs are computed separately by multiplying the total covered charges by the operating and capital cost-to-charge ratios. The estimated operating and capital costs are compared with the fixed-loss threshold after dividing that threshold into an operating portion and a capital portion. The thresholds are also adjusted by the area wage index before being compared to the operating and capital costs of the case. Finally, the outlier payment is based on a marginal cost factor equal to 80% of the combined operating and capital costs in excess of the fixed-loss threshold.

An example from the CMS website simulates the outlier payment for a case at a generic hospital in the San Francisco, California CBSA, which is a large urban area. (The Center for Health Affairs, 2004) The patient was discharged on or after October 1, 2005, and the hospital incurred Medicare approved charges of $125,000. The DRG assigned to the case was 498 with a relative weight of 2.7791. The hospital is 100% Federal for capital payment purposes. The first step was to determine federal payment with IME and DSH. The formulas for calculating the Federal Rate for Operating and capital Costs were given respectively by:

Federal Rate for Operating Costs = DRG Relative Weight x [(Labor Related Large Urban Standardized Amount x San Francisco Wage Index) + Non labor Related National Large Urban Standardized Amount] x (1 + IME + DSH)

and

Federal Rate for Capital Costs = DRG Relative Weight x Federal Capital Rate x Large Urban Add-On x Geographic Cost Adjustment Factor x (1 + IME + DSH)

The calculations of the formulas were respectively:

$$2.7791 \times [(\$3,297.84 \times 1.4974) + \$1,433.63] \times (1 + 0.0744 + 0.1413) = 21,527.51$$

and

$$2.7791 \times \$420.65 \times 1.03 \times 1.3185 \times (1 + 0.0243 + 0.0631) = \$1,726.36$$

The second step was to determine the operating and capital costs. The operating and capital costs are computed separately by multiplying the total covered charges by the operating and capital cost-to-charge ratios. The cost-to-charge ratio used to adjust covered charges are computed annually by the intermediary for each hospital based on the latest available settled cost report for that hospital, and charge data for the same time period as that covered by the cost report. The cost-to-charge ratio is the ratio between what a day in the hospital costs and what the hospital charges. The operating and capital costs were calculated by using the following.

Operating Costs = (Billed Charges x Operating Cost to Charge Ratio)

($125,000 x .45)=$56,250

and

Capital Costs = (Billed Charges x Capital Cost to Charge Ratio)

($125,000 x .06)= $7,500

In order to qualify for outlier payments, a case must have costs above a fixed-loss cost threshold amount. The threshold amount is defined as a dollar amount by which the costs of a case must exceed payments in order to qualify for outliers. For Federal fiscal year (FY) 2006, the existing fixed-loss outlier threshold was $23,600. The operating and capital Outlier Thresholds were determined by using the following two formulas:

Operating Outlier Threshold = {[Fixed Loss Threshold x ((Labor related portion x San Francisco CBSA Wage Index) + Non labor related portion)] x Operating CCR to Total} + Federal Payment with IME and DSH

and

Capital Outlier Threshold = (Fixed Loss Threshold x Geographic Adj.

Factor x Large Urban Add-On x Capital CCR to Total CCR) + Federal

Payment with IME and DSH

The applications of these two formulas in the example were respectively:

{\$23,600 x [(0.697 x 1.4974) + 0.303] x 0.8824} + \$21,527.51= \$49,571.80

and

(\$23,600 x 1.3185 x 1.03 x 0.1176) + \$1,726.36 = \$5,495.45

Finally, the outlier payment is based on a marginal cost factor equal to 80% of the combined operating and capital costs in excess of the fixed-loss threshold. The operating and capital outlier payment factors were determined by:

Outlier Payment Factor= (Costs - Outlier Threshold) x Marginal Cost

This was applied in the example by:

Operating = (\$56,250 - \$49,571.80) x 0.80 = \$5,342.56

Capital = (\$7,500 - \$5,495.45) x 0.80 = \$1,603.64

In order for a case to qualify for an outlier payment, the combined operating and capital costs must exceed the combined threshold. This threshold value must be between 5 to 6% of total inpatient payments. In recent years, CMS has set the outlier threshold at a level projected to pay 5.1% of total payments for inpatient care. Since these DRG payments are based on average cost, then the threshold value is located about two standard deviations to the right of the mean.

No work has done about analyzing the hospital outlier payments and building new reimbursement models. Very few papers were found about estimating the hospital cost. Mr. S. Greg Potts from the "Arkansas Foundation For Medical Care" has used the Decision Tree model as a tool to estimate the cost of Arkansas Medicaid patients with Diabetes Mellitus. The results of Mr. Potts' paper titled "Data Mining to Determine Characteristics of High-Cost Diabetics in a Medicaid Population" show that one group of recipients with Diabetes accrued average total costs more than three times other recipients with the same diagnosis. (Potts, 2004) This work was missing the problem of taking outlier patients into consideration while looking at the high cost.

SETTING THE STAGE

Under the inpatient Prospective Payment System (PPS), hospitals receive a predetermined amount for treating Medicare patients, determined from the patients' diagnoses. The Payment is based on the diagnosis-related group (DRG) to which a patient is assigned at the time of discharge. The payment is then based upon an average cost with local conditions taken into consideration. However, some patients who are severely ill will cost considerably more than average. The question becomes whether hospitals can afford to care for such patients, or whether they are forced to cost-shift to stay in business. Simulations about the total charges from different distributions were examined to investigate the payment structure.

Simulation is the process of designing a model of a real or imagined system and conducting experiments with that model. The purpose of simulation experiments is to understand the behavior of the system, or to evaluate strategies for the operation of the system. Assumptions are made about this system, and mathematical algorithms and relationships are derived to describe these assumptions. (CMS, n.d.) Simulation is very useful to estimate a complex, real world problem. It is used to develop statistical distribution information about a system by generating sample values for each input variable for the purpose of understanding the behavior of the system.

We have generated three simulations with normal, exponential and gamma distributions in order to consider the difference between the reimbursement payments to the hospital when different distributions about total charges are assumed. In our example below, we assumed that the average total charge amount is $12,000, and the standard deviation is $3,000. We want to discuss the results of using a threshold value for outlier reimbursements. If we assume that the payments are based upon an average cost and the threshold value is located about two standard deviations to the right of the mean assuming a normal distribution, then we can compute how much money the hospitals are losing or making when the distribution of the total charges is exponential or gamma.

Figures 2, 3 and 4 give the normal, exponential and gamma distributions respectively with a dashed line at the value of $18,000 (two standard deviations from the mean). The yellow area is the area after $18,000 and under the distribution curve. It represents the amount that hospitals should receive from the outlier payment if the distribution of the total charge is normal with mean of $12,000 versus what it should receive if the distributions are exponential or gamma.

As shown in figure 2, the total charge is normally distributed. The dashed line is located two standard deviations from the mean. This makes the shaded area represent only about 2.5% of the distribution of total charge. The sum overall total charge for the shaded area is about $396,809.95.

The total charge in figure 3 has an exponential distribution with mean 12,000. The shaded area is clearly higher than 2.5% and the hospital should receive from the outlier payments an amount higher than $396,809.95. This amount is estimated to be $1,724,260.3.

As shown in figure 4, the total charge is assumed a gamma distribution with mean 12,000. Note again that the dashed line is located at 18,000 and the shaded area is again higher than 2.5%. In this case, the hospital should receive again an amount that is greater than $396,809.95. This amount is about $948,722.32.

Figure 2. Normal distribution of the total charges Simulated shown an outlier payments

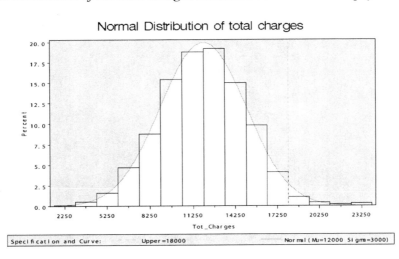

Clearly, the shaded area in figures 3 and 4 is much bigger than the yellow area in figure 2. The conclusion is that if we assume that the distribution of total charges is normal, then by making the outlier payments to be about 5%, the hospital will almost break even. On the other hand, if the true distribution of total charges is exponential or gamma, then hospitals will lose lots of money if the payments are assumed to be normally distributed, and the outlier threshold is about two standard deviations from the mean.

Figure 3. Exponential distribution of the total charges Simulated shown an outlier payments

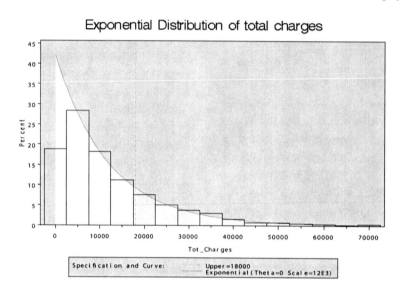

Figure 4. Gamma distribution of the total charges Simulated shown as outlier payments

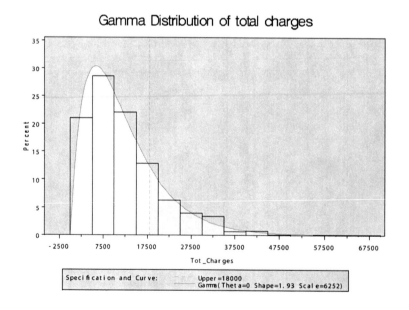

CASE DESCRIPTION

Introduction to MEPS Analysis

We will examine the relationship between the total charges billed by a hospital compared to the payments received for patient care using general and generalized linear models. We will show the effect of outliers into our linear models by using real data. We will compare models with and without outliers.

In addition, we will show how we can use text mining to reduce a large number of patient condition codes into an index of 4 levels, and to use those levels to examine the relationship to the hospital reimbursements by applying linear models. We will compare models with and without the use of the clustering variable.

The data used were obtained from the Medical Expenditure Panel Survey (MEPS). (Sculty, 2003) It gives detailed information on outpatient visits covering calendar year 2002. The data contain 20,535 outpatient event records related to 5894 patients. It contains 86 variables. Out of those variables, we will use only seven: dupersid, evntidx, optc02x, opxp02x, opicd1x, opicd2x, opicd3x, and opicd4x. The variable dupersid identifies each person represented on the data; it is a combination of the dwelling unit and an individual id. Evntidx uniquely identifies each outpatient event. The variables, optc02x and opxp02x, are concerned respectively with total charges and reimbursements. The last four variables are about the 3-digit ICD-9-CM condition code. The first twenty observations of the dataset are given in figure 5.

Summary Statistics and Data Preprocessing

The first analysis step performed was to find the summary statistics about the total charges and reimbursement variables. The output is given in tables 1 and 2.

Notice from tables 1 and 2 that the mean of total charges ($1049.32) is two times higher than the mean of the reimbursements ($480.35). Also, the sum of the overall total charges ($21,498,517.8) is two times higher than the sum of the overall reimbursements ($9,841,519.26). We performed

Figure 5. The first 20 observation of the dataset

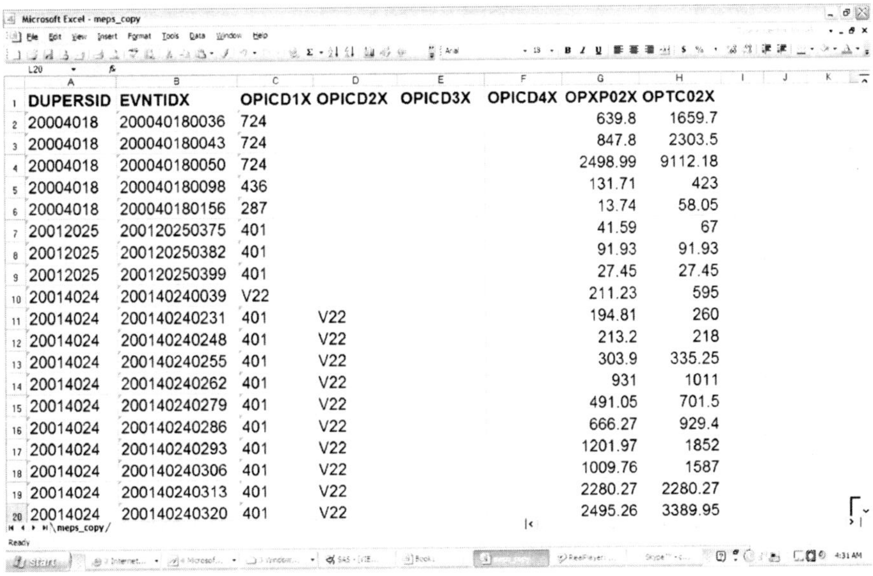

	DUPERSID	EVNTIDX	OPICD1X	OPICD2X	OPICD3X	OPICD4X	OPXP02X	OPTC02X
2	20004018	200040180036	724				639.8	1659.7
3	20004018	200040180043	724				847.8	2303.5
4	20004018	200040180050	724				2498.99	9112.18
5	20004018	200040180098	436				131.71	423
6	20004018	200040180156	287				13.74	58.05
7	20012025	200120250375	401				41.59	67
8	20012025	200120250382	401				91.93	91.93
9	20012025	200120250399	401				27.45	27.45
10	20014024	200140240039	V22				211.23	595
11	20014024	200140240231	401	V22			194.81	260
12	20014024	200140240248	401	V22			213.2	218
13	20014024	200140240255	401	V22			303.9	335.25
14	20014024	200140240262	401	V22			931	1011
15	20014024	200140240279	401	V22			491.05	701.5
16	20014024	200140240286	401	V22			666.27	929.4
17	20014024	200140240293	401	V22			1201.97	1852
18	20014024	200140240306	401	V22			1009.76	1587
19	20014024	200140240313	401	V22			2280.27	2280.27
20	20014024	200140240320	401	V22			2495.26	3389.95

simple data pre-processing by removing all observations with total charges equal to zero because those cases are not meaningful in our analysis. This step only resulted in removing 1001 cases including the 47 missing values.

The four icd-9 codes listed for each outpatient visit were concatenated in order to use the resulting output (icd9 variable) as a classification variable in the linear models. The code used to group the four icd-9 codes is given in table 3.

The frequency distribution of the icd9 variable shows a total of 3164 missing records on the new variable with 1175 icd-9 classes. This large number of classes on our categorical variable was the reason to choose the listwise deletion of the missing values over the other methods. The total

Table 1. Summary statistics for the reimbursements

```
The UNIVARIATE Procedure
Variable: OPXP02X (OPXP02X)
Moments
N 20488 Sum Weights 20488
Mean 480.355294 Sum Observations 9841519.26
Std Deviation 1162.78507 Variance 1352069.11
Skewness 7.0791948 Kurtosis 76.6009151
Uncorrected SS 3.24273E10 Corrected SS 2.76998E10
Coeff Variation 242.067712 Std Error Mean 8.12362118
Basic Statistical Measures
Location Variability
Mean 480.3553 Std Deviation 1163
Median 117.1800 Variance 1352069
Mode 0.0000 Range 24884
Interquartile Range 325.24500
Missing Values
-----Percent Of-----
Missing Missing
Value Count All Obs Obs
. 47 0.23 100.00
```

Table 2. Summary statistics for the total charges

```
The UNIVARIATE Procedure
Variable: OPTC02X (OPTC02X)
Moments
N 20488 Sum Weights 20488
Mean 1049.32242 Sum Observations 21498517.8
Std Deviation 2319.61305 Variance 5380604.72
Skewness 5.45606259 Kurtosis 46.3642818
Uncorrected SS 1.32791E11 Corrected SS 1.10232E11
Coeff Variation 221.058181 Std Error Mean 16.2056241
Basic Statistical Measures
Location Variability
Mean 1049.322 Std Deviation 2320
Median 244.000 Variance 5380605
Mode 0.000 Range 45304
Interquartile Range 741.95500
Missing Values
-----Percent Of-----
Missing Missing
Value Count All Obs Obs
. 47 0.23 100.00
```

Table 3. The code used to concatenate the four icd-9 variables

```
data sasuser.meps;
set sasuser.h67f_TCnot0;
icd9=catx(" ",opicd1x,opicd2x,opicd3x,opicd4x);
run;
```

Table 4. The code used to select records with zero reimbursement

```
data sasuser.meps2;
set sasuser.meps;
if icd9=missing then delete;
if opxp02x = 0 then delete;
run;
```

Table 5. Summary statistics for the reimbursements

```
The UNIVARIATE Procedure
 Variable: OPXP02X (OPXP02X)
 Moments
 N 15729 Sum Weights 15729
 Mean 520.670233 Sum Observations 8189622.09
 Std Deviation 1188.79625 Variance 1413236.52
 Skewness 6.69323812 Kurtosis 67.4259469
 Uncorrected SS 2.64915E10 Corrected SS 2.22274E10
 Coeff Variation 228.320379 Std Error Mean 9.47887659
 Basic Statistical Measures
 Location Variability
 Mean 520.6702 Std Deviation 1189
 Median 143.0000 Variance 1413237
 Mode 8.4300 Range 24882
 Interquartile Range 379.18000
```

number of records with reimbursement equal to zero is 641, which represents the number of patient events with no reimbursement payment. The sum of the overall total charges for these cases is $232,997.80. We removed all these observations from our dataset since the reimbursement variable is used as the dependent variable in the linear models. The code used to remove those cases and the missing records on the icd9 variable is given in table 4.

The summary statistics of the total charges and reimbursement variables for the new dataset is given in tables 5 and 6 respectively.

The Assumptions of the General Linear Model

After preprocessing, our decision was to examine the relationship between the total charges billed by a hospital compared to the payments received for patient care by applying the general linear model. Our dependent variable is the reimbursement variable, while the explanatory variables are total charges and icd9 codes to define patient severity.

However, we need to investigate the assumptions of the model prior to any analysis. Any violation to the assumptions may lead to inaccurate results. We will consider the following assumptions: Normality, Homoscedasticity and Linearity.

Table 6. Summary statistics for the total charges

```
The UNIVARIATE Procedure
Variable: OPTC02X (OPTC02X)
Moments
N 15729 Sum Weights 15729
Mean 1132.24304 Sum Observations 17809050.8
Std Deviation 2402.56128 Variance 5772300.7
Skewness 5.35376125 Kurtosis 45.2061831
Uncorrected SS 1.10951E11 Corrected SS 9.07867E10
Coeff Variation 212.194837 Std Error Mean 19.156842
Basic Statistical Measures
Location Variability
Mean 1132.243 Std Deviation 2403
Median 277.000 Variance 5772301
Mode 50.000 Range 45299
Interquartile Range 841.63000
```

Also, we will investigate in detail the influence of any outliers if they exist on our model. Based on the result of the tests of assumptions, we will use PROC GenMod over PROC GLM to analyze our data and predict the reimbursement values.

Test for Normality

The first step in the data analysis was to examine the reimbursement and total charge variables in order to extract information that can be used to build an accurate linear model. Tables 5 and 6 show that the skewness and kurtosis of the two variables are very high, which indicates that their distributions are not normal. Kernel Density was used on the data to further investigate both the distribution of the total charges and the reimbursements for hospital outpatient services. Kernel Density estimation is a data visualization technique to estimate actual population distributions. It provides a very useful means of investigating an entire population. It is commonly used to test the data sample to make sure it is sufficiently large and to determine whether it follows a normal distribution. The distributions of total charges (optc02x) and reimbursements (opxp02x) are given in Figure 6. The SAS code used to run the kernel density is given in table 7.

Clearly, the two variables have skewed distributions to the right, and both distributions are not

normal. On the other hand, we cannot determine the difference between the two distributions.

A normal, quantile plot, which is called a "qqplot" was also produced to examine the normality of the residuals. It plots the quantiles of the residual variable against the quantiles of the normal distribution. The code and Graph are given in table 8 and figure 7 respectively.

Clearly, the graph is sensitive to non-normality near the two tails, and the residuals are not normally distributed.

Transformation of Variables

A log transformation was used to change the distribution of total charges and reimbursements to normal and to help understand the difference between the two variables. Using the kernel density, we plot the two variables again. The resulting graph is given in Figure 8.

The distribution of the transformed variables is close to normal this time. Also, there is a shift of cost between the payments and reimbursements for hospital outpatient services. Notice that if the charge value is very small (dashed line or smaller), then the probability of the reimbursement value is very high. It is clear that there is a shift between amounts charged by the hospital, and the amount the hospital is reimbursed. Also, if the shift between reimbursements and charges

Figure 6. Distribution of total charges and reimbursements

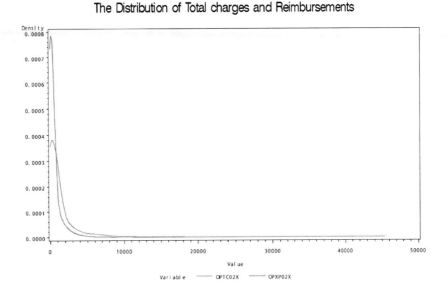

Table 7. Kernel Density Code

```
prockde data =sasuser.meps2 method=SROT gridl=120 gridu=120 bwm=10 out=outchak;
univar optc02x/out=meps1;
univar opxp02x/out=meps2;
run;
quit;
data meps3;
length VAR $ 32 VALUE 8 DENSITY 8 COUNT 8;
set meps1
meps2;
keep VAR VALUE DENSITY COUNT;
run;
quit;
procsort data=meps3 out=chak2;
by var;
run;
quit;
procgplot data=chak2;
symbol1 c=blue i=join w=2 v=none;
symbol2 c=red i=join w=2 v=none;
plot density*value=var/overlay ;
title 'The Distribution of Total charges and Reimbursements';
run;
quit;
```

is linear after a logarithmic transformation, the relationship between the untransformed variables cannot be linear.

Test for Heteroscedasticity & Linearity

The variance of the residuals has to be homogeneous; otherwise, the variance of the residuals is non-constant, and then it is said to be "heterosce-

Figure 7. QQPLOT of residuals

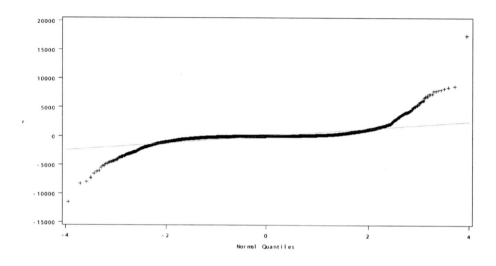

Table 8. Code for creating QQPLOT

```
procglm data=sasuser.meps2;
class icd9;
 model opxp02x=optc02x icd9
 output out=meps_normality (keep= pid oxp02x optc02x icd9 r fv) residual=r predicted=fv;
run;
quit;

procunivariate data=meps_normality normal;
 var r;
 qqplot r / normal(mu=est sigma=est);
run;
```

Figure 8. Distribution of Normal logarithm of Total Charges and reimbursements

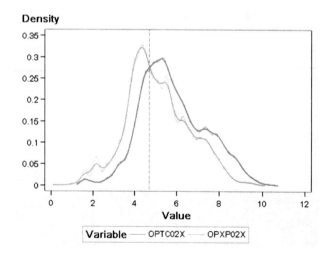

dastic." A graphical method is used to test for homoscedasticity by plotting the residuals versus fitted or predicted values. Results are given in figure 9. The code used to produce the graph is given in table 9.

From the graph in figure 9, we can see that most of the observations are concentrated on the left end, which is a strong indication of heteroscedasticity. This is due to non-strong linearity in the relationship between the reimbursements and total charges variables. The plot of reimbursements (opxp02x) versus total charges (optc02x) is given in Figure 10.

We investigated the distribution of residuals after the log transformation. The plot in figure 11 shows residuals versus predicted values. Certainly, this is not a perfect distribution of residuals, but it is much better than the distribution with the untransformed variables. Also, we checked for

multicollinearity within our predictors. Multicollinearity occurs when the independent variables in the model are correlated among themselves. This can lead to large variance for the estimated coefficients and affect our interpretation of these coefficients. Results show that we do not have this problem within our dataset.

Outlier Diagnostics

An outlier is an observation with a large residual; that is an observation substantially different from the rest of the data. It is very important to examine outliers in our data in order to evaluate their influences in our analysis. The first step to observe outliers is to use graphical methods. Figure 10 shows the existence of many outliers in our data; many observations are at a considerable distance from the general pattern concentrated between

Figure 9. Residuals vs predicted values

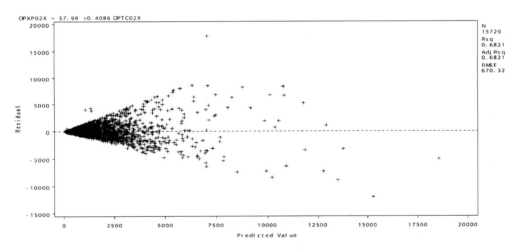

Table 9. Code the Homoscedasticity test

```
/* Tests for Heteroscedasticity */
procreg data=sasuser.meps2;
 model opxp02x=optc02x;
 plot r.*p.;
run;
quit;
```

0 and $10,000. Note that the extreme outliers on total charges and reimbursements are about $45,000 and $25,000 respectively.

Our examination of outliers using studentized residuals indicates that there are 697 outliers in our data. They represent more than 3.7% of the total data. They are all observations located more than 2 standard deviations from the mean. Those cases have high discrepancy; they represent outliers on the reimbursement variable. Table 10 shows the

Figure 10. Plot of Reimbursements versus Total Charges

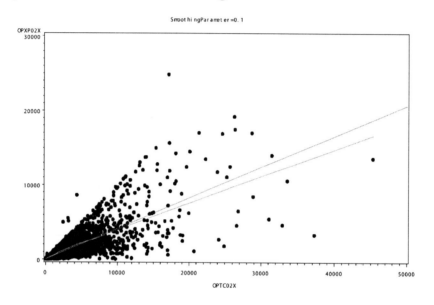

Figure 11. Residuals versus Predicted values after Transformation

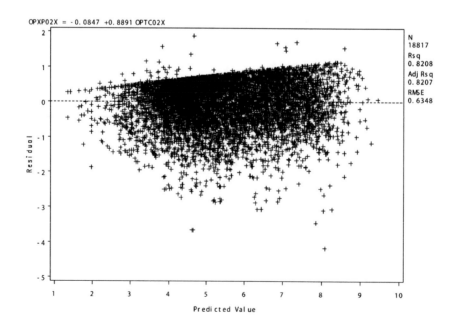

Table 10. The code to check for discrepancy

```
/**test for outliers**/
procglm data=sasuser.meps_final;
 model opxp02x=optc02x ;
 output out=meps_outliers(keep=evntidx opxp02x optc02x r lev cd dffit)
 rstudent=r h=lev cookd=cd dffits=dffit;
run;quit;
/*check the studentized residuals**/
procunivariate data=meps_outliers plots plotsize=30;
 var r;
run;
procsort data=meps_outliers;
 by r;
run;
procprint data=meps_outliers (obs=10);
run;
procprint data=meps_outliers (firstobs=18808 obs=18817);
var evntidx opxp02x optc02x r lev cd dffit;
run;
data meps_outl;
 set meps_outliers;
 if abs(r)<= 2 then delete;run;
```

Table 11. The 10 largest residuals

Obs	EVNTIDX	OPXP02X	OPTC02X	r	lev	cd	dffit
15720	456100150221	13799.4	13958.86	12.0563	.001875759	0.13534	0.52265
15721	226890120041	13760	13828	12.0774	.001838971	0.13314	0.51839
15722	206420330208	17048.05	21354.71	12.4160	.004568069	0.35030	0.84109
15723	453390260545	19208.73	26287.5	12.6517	.007033614	0.56123	1.06481
15724	261530240113	15672.75	17245.86	12.8664	.002923561	0.24019	0.69671
15725	490300270143	15672.75	17245.86	12.8664	.002923561	0.24019	0.69671
15726	209420190390	15000	15372	13.0034	.002297060	0.19259	0.62394
15727	259770200110	15000	15372	13.0034	.002297060	0.19259	0.62394
15728	486660110034	15000	15372	13.0034	.002297060	0.19259	0.62394
15729	265540270194	24884.36	17148.74	27.2407	.002889189	1.02670	1.46634

code used to detect those outliers, while tables 11 and 12 list the 10 largest and 10 smallest residuals respectively along with the event ID, reimbursement and total charge.

Our data contain extreme outliers on the reimbursement variable. We would like to examine also the outliers on the total charge variable. A computation of the cut-off value of the leverage indicates that this value is about 0.000381. There are 561 cases with leverage value higher than the cut-off point (0.000381). They represent more than 3.5% of the total data. The 10 largest values are given in table 13 and the code used to list these cases is given in table 14.

There are extreme outliers on the total charges. Some of them are also outliers on the reimbursement variable. This indicates that we have influential outliers in our data. The overall influence can be measured by computing the value, Dffits, which combines information about residuals and leverage

Table 12. The 10 smallest residuals

Obs	EVNTIDX	OPXP02X	OPTC02X	r	lev	cd	dffit
1	206470110455	3322.76	37281.05	-18.1752	0.014457	2.37318	-2.20131
2	434770171489	4651.85	32922	-13.3666	0.011195	1.00011	-1.42226
3	435770190533	1813.4	24903	-12.6663	0.006287	0.50247	-1.00753
4	221690270189	1113.14	20688.19	-11.1047	0.004276	0.26274	-0.72771
5	497710460401	5478.08	31110	-10.9759	0.009962	0.60155	-1.10102
6	472780150343	2696.89	24180.12	-10.8767	0.005915	0.34934	-0.83898
7	467820360261	634.73	17075.28	-9.5906	0.002863	0.13130	-0.51393
8	457480180283	4600.08	26620.18	-9.5138	0.007219	0.32723	-0.81128
9	257990100159	1242.1	17012.8	-8.6375	0.002841	0.10580	-0.46108
10	487930260305	1242.1	17012.8	-8.6375	0.002841	0.10580	-0.46108

Table 13. The 10 largest leverage values

Obs	EVNTIDX	OPXP02X	OPTC02X	lev	r
15720	490780480263	8475.15	28897.87	0.008555	-5.0860
15721	497710460401	5478.08	31110	0.009962	-10.9759
15722	206770140090	14033.3	31483.82	0.010211	1.6638
15723	206770140103	14033.3	31483.82	0.010211	1.6638
15724	417630110423	14033.3	31483.82	0.010211	1.6638
15725	434770171489	4651.85	32922	0.011195	-13.3666
15726	457800270567	10586.76	33588.73	0.011667	-4.8011
15727	492380100219	10586.76	33588.73	0.011667	-4.8011
15728	206470110455	3322.76	37281.05	0.014457	-18.1752
15729	215000170138	13588.57	45304.29	0.021555	-7.5285

Table 14. The code used to list high leverage observations

```
procsort data=meps_outliers;
 by lev;
run;
procprint data=meps_outliers;
 var evntidx opxp02x optc02x lev r;
 where lev > .000381;
run;
```

to give a statistic for detecting observations that actually influence the estimated parameter. The conventional cut-off point for Dffits is 0.0225. There is a total of 799 influential cases in our dataset. They represent only 5% of all the data.

Data Analysis Without Compression of ICD-9 Codes

a) General Linear Model (GLM)

The first model used to estimate the amount of reimbursement is the general linear model. After ignoring all assumptions of the model, we ran Proc GLM using the code in table 15 in order to compare results with other models.

Results of the analysis are shown in tables 16 and 17. The overall F test is significant ($p<0.0001$), indicating that the model as a whole accounts for a significant amount of the variation in the reimbursement variable. The R^2 indicates that the model accounts for 72% of the variation in optc02x and icd9.

The results show that the model over-fits the data because we have 1156 ICD-9 codes, resulting in 1155 degrees of freedom.

b) Generalized Linear Model (GenMod)

The Generalized Linear Model (PROC GenMod) was used to investigate the shift between total charges and reimbursements to the hospital. The GenMod procedure is needed when the distribution of the data is not normal, or may not have an exact distribution, which applies in our case based on the distribution of the reimbursement shown in Figure 10. It seems that the Gamma distribution would be an appropriate choice since our dependent variable is continuous. It appears also from the transformation that the log function would be suitable as a link function.

Table 15. GLM code

```
procglm data=sasuser.meps2;
class icd9;
model opxp02x = optc02x icd9 / solution;
run;
quit;
```

Table 16. General Linear Model

The GLM Procedure					
Dependent Variable: OPXP02X					
Source	**DF**	**Sum of Squares**	**Mean Square**	**F Value**	**Pr > F**
Model	1156	16078751093	13908954	32.96	<.0001
Error	14572	6148632847	421948		
Corrected Total	15728	22227383940			

R-Square	**Coeff Var**	**Root MSE**	**OPXP02X Mean**		
0.723376	124.7576	649.5756	520.6702		

Table 17. Effects of general Linear Model (type I & III)

Source	**DF**	**Type I SS**	**Mean Square**	**F Value**	**Pr > F**
OPTC02X	1	15160836683	15160836683	35930.5	<.0001
icd9	1155	917914410	794731	1.88	<.0001
Source	DF	Type III SS	Mean Square	F Value	Pr > F
OPTC02X	1	11904668808	11904668808	28213.6	<.0001
icd9	1155	917914410	794731	1.88	<.0001

We ran Proc GenMod on the chosen model by having the total charges and the ICD-9 codes as independent variables. The ICD-9 codes were defined as a class variable. The code used is given in table 18.

The results again show that the model over-fits the data because we have approximately 1156 ICD-9 codes, resulting in 1155 degrees of freedom. Tables 19, 20 and 21 are the outputs of the generalized model. Table 19 displays the "Class Level Information", which identifies the levels of the classification variable (icd9) that are used in the model, while Table 20 gives the results of type 3 analysis; both explanatory variables are significant.

Table 21 lists the first 30 classes about the icd-9 variable and information about whether each

class is significant or not. It shows the need of a compression method to reduce the large number of patient condition codes.

Clustering of the ICD-9 Codes

Since there is no statistical model that can handle a large number of categorical variables without having the problem of over fitting the data, many methods are used to reduce these categorical variables before defining the statistical model. Text mining is an appropriate tool that allows doing that.

Since there are many ICD-9 codes that are used in our data, and most patients have more than one ICD-9 code assigned to them as Table 21 shows,

Table 18. GenMod code before clustering

```
procgenmod data=sasuser.meps2;
class icd9;
model opxp02x = optc02x icd9 / link=log dist=gamma type3 ;
run;
quit;
```

Table 19. Information about the ICD-9 classes

Class Level Information		
Class	**Levels**	**Values**
icd9	1156	008 008 496 492 009 011 034 038 453 041 042 042 070 042 493 714 070 042 780 053 057 070 070 208 070 572 586 075 075 300 V47 078 079 079 490 079 519 079 786 477 088 110 110 110 112 135 135 493 492 135 719 724 135 V72 136 139 149 149 246 153 153 250 V77 ...

Table 20. Goodness of Fit

Criteria For Assessing Goodness Of Fit			
Criterion	**DF**	**Value**	**Value/DF**
Deviance	15E3	12607.1089	0.8652
Scaled Deviance	15E3	17533.1288	1.2032
Pearson Chi-Square	15E3	11446.7538	0.7855
Scaled Pearson X2	15E3	15919.3840	1.0925
Log Likelihood		-101717.0584	

Table 21. Significance of the ICD-9 classes

Analysis Of Parameter Estimates							
Parameter	**DF**	**Estimate**	**Standard Error**	**Wald 95% Conf Limits**		**Chi-Square**	**Pr > ChiSq**
Intercept	1	5.5043	0.4897	4.5446	6.4640	126.36	<.0001
OPTC02X	1	0.0005	0.0000	0.0005	0.0005	8671.36	<.0001
icd9 008	1	-0.5158	0.5234	-1.5416	0.5100	0.97	0.3243
icd9 008 496 492	1	-0.7212	0.6924	-2.0783	0.6359	1.08	0.2976
icd9 009	1	0.0813	0.7742	-1.4361	1.5987	0.01	0.9164
icd9 011	1	-0.7887	0.9792	-2.7079	1.1304	0.65	0.4205
icd9 034	1	-1.0917	0.5653	-2.1997	0.0163	3.73	0.0535
icd9 038 453	1	0.7305	0.9792	-1.1886	2.6496	0.56	0.4556
icd9 041	1	-0.7157	0.5056	-1.7067	0.2753	2.00	0.1569
icd9 042	1	-0.9131	0.5161	-1.9246	0.0984	3.13	0.0768
icd9 042 070	1	-0.8881	0.5996	-2.0633	0.2871	2.19	0.1386
icd9 042 493 714	1	-1.2807	0.6924	-2.6378	0.0764	3.42	0.0644
icd9 042 780	1	0.4053	0.9792	-1.5138	2.3245	0.17	0.6789
icd9 053	1	-0.4779	0.6477	-1.7474	0.7916	0.54	0.4606
icd9 057	1	-0.7232	0.9792	-2.6424	1.1959	0.55	0.4602
icd9 070	1	-0.4850	0.5288	-1.5214	0.5515	0.84	0.3591
icd9 070 208	1	-0.6850	0.9792	-2.6041	1.2342	0.49	0.4842
icd9 070 572 586	1	-0.9235	0.5996	-2.0987	0.2517	2.37	0.1235
icd9 075	1	0.1293	0.9792	-1.7898	2.0484	0.02	0.8949
icd9 075 300 V47	1	-1.9228	0.9792	-3.8420	-0.0037	3.86	0.0496
icd9 078	1	-0.2994	0.5741	-1.4245	0.8258	0.27	0.6020
icd9 079	1	-0.7390	0.5474	-1.8118	0.3338	1.82	0.1770
icd9 079 486	0	0.0000	0.0000	0.0000	0.0000	.	.
icd9 079 490	1	-0.8770	0.9792	-2.7962	1.0422	0.80	0.3704
icd9 079 519	1	0.0034	0.9792	-1.9158	1.9225	0.00	0.9973
icd9 079 786 477	1	-1.3646	0.7741	-2.8819	0.1526	3.11	0.0779
icd9 088	1	-0.3371	0.5852	-1.4840	0.8098	0.33	0.5646
icd9 110	1	-0.4750	0.5741	-1.6002	0.6502	0.68	0.4080
icd9 110 110	1	-0.3403	0.9791	-2.2594	1.5788	0.12	0.7282
icd9 112	1	-1.6309	0.7741	-3.1481	-0.1136	4.44	0.0351
icd9 135	1	0.1462	0.5431	-0.9183	1.2108	0.07	0.7877
icd9 135 493 492	1	0.2097	0.5852	-0.9373	1.3566	0.13	0.7201

Table 22. Clusters of the ICD-9 Codes

#	Descriptive terms	Freq	Percentage
1	444,162,753,304,715,711,195,610,883,955	5980	31%
2	272,429,250,727,312,317,v72,354,159,585	4710	24%
3	518,478,575,185,724,780,593,436,733,410	4063	21%
4	716,729,v56,366,279,285,836,553,492,v57	4781	24%

Table 23. Translation of the ICD-9 codes

Cluster ID	ICD-9	Description
1	444	Arterial embolism and thrombosis.
	162	Malignant neoplasm of trachea, bronchus, and lung.
	753	Congenital anomalies of urinary system.
	304	Drug dependence.
	715	Osteoarthrosis and allied disorders.
	711	Arthropathy associated with infections.
	195	Malignant neoplasm of other and ill-defined sites.
	610	Benign mammary dysplasias.
	883	Open wound of finger(s).
	955	Injury to peripheral nerve(s) of shoulder girdle and upper limb.
2	272	Disorders of lipoid metabolism.
	429	Ill-defined descriptions and complications of heart disease.
	250	Diabetes mellitus.
	727	Other disorders of synovium, tendon, and bursa.
	312	Disturbance of conduct, not elsewhere classified.
	317	Mild mental retardation.
	v72	Special investigations and examinations.
	354	Mononeuritis of upper limb and mononeuritis multiplex.
	159	Malignant neoplasm of other and ill-defined sites within the digestive organs and peritoneum.
	585	Chronic kidney disease (CKD).
3	518	Other diseases of lung.
	478	Other diseases of upper respiratory tract.
	575	Other disorders of gallbladder.
	185	Malignant neoplasm of prostate.
	724	Other and unspecified disorders of back.
	780	General symptoms.
	593	Other disorders of kidney and ureter.
	436	Acute, but ill-defined, cerebrovascular disease.
	733	Other disorders of bone and cartilage.
	410	Acute myocardial infarction.
4	716	Other and unspecified arthropathies.
	729	Other disorders of soft tissues.
	v56	Encounter for dialysis and dialysis catheter care.
	366	Cataract.
	279	Disorders involving the immune mechanism.
	285	Other and unspecified anemias.
	836	Dislocation of knee.
	553	Other hernia of abdominal cavity without mention of obstruction or gangrene.
	492	Emphysema.
	v57	Care involving use of rehabilitation procedures.

clustering and text mining were performed to group similar patients together. The ICD-9 codes are analyzed as text strings. Table 22 shows the results of the analysis.

The clustering variable was created (cluster_ID) with four levels. It can be used in the generalized linear model as an independent variable in order to provide an accurate estimation of the reimbursements by avoiding the over fitting problem. The word translation of the icd-9 codes[9] is given in Table 23.

We used kernel density to examine differences within the four clusters. Figures 12 and 13 are showing the graphs of total charges and reimbursements respectively by cluster id. Note that cluster 2 has a high probability of total charges and reimbursements compared to the other clusters when the amount is very low. These graphs demonstrate a natural ordering in the clusters that is defined within the text mining tool.

Data Analysis with Compression of ICD-9 Codes

The generalized linear model was executed by designating again the distribution and link function to be the gamma and log function respectively. This time, we used the new clustering variable as a class variable. The code used is given in table 24.

Results from type I and type III analysis show that the model is significant. Table 25 displays "criteria for Assessing Goodness of Fit" for this

Figure 12. Kernel Density Estimation of Total Charges by Cluster

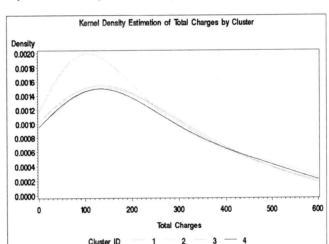

Figure 13. Kernel Density Estimation of Reimbursements by Cluster

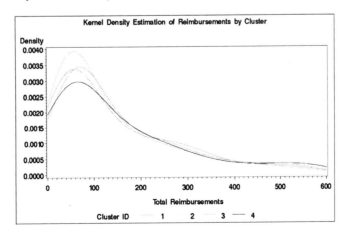

model. It contains statistics that summarize the fit of the model.

In the "Analysis of Parameter Estimates" displayed in table 26, the explanatory variable parameters are significant except for clusters number 1 and 3. Note that the degrees of freedom are high, so the model still over-fits the data. This is due to the fact that our dataset is too large.

We had to choose small samples from our dataset and then run the generalized linear model. Results were almost similar and there is no over-fitting of the data for all these small samples.

Tables 27 and 28 show "criteria for Assessing Goodness of Fit" and "Analysis Of Parameter Estimates" respectively for a model with only 500 observations.

All explanatory variables are significant except for cluster number 1. We removed all the influential outliers, and then ran the same model again. The results show that the scaled deviance and scaled Pearson Chi-square are close to 1, which indicate that this model did not over-fit the data. **Also, every variable is significant this time, including all the four clusters.** This shows

Table 24. GenMod code after Clustering

```
Procgenmod data=sasuser.meps3;
class cluster_id;
model opxp02x = optc02x cluster_id / link=log dist=gamma type3 ;
run;
Quit
```

Table 25. Assessments of GenMod After Clustering

Criteria for Assessing Goodness of Fit			
Criterion	**DF**	**Value**	**Value/DF**
Deviance	16E3	15525.3073	0.9874
Scaled Deviance	16E3	17872.5080	1.1366
Pearson Chi-Square	16E3	13133.9430	0.8353
Scaled Pearson X2	16E3	15119.6042	0.9616
Log Likelihood		-103559.6225	

Table 26. Analysis of Parameter Estimates For GenMod After Clustering

Analysis of Parameter Estimates							
Parameter	**DF**	**Estimate**	**Standard Error**	**Wald 95% Conf Limits**		**Chi-Square**	**Pr > Chi**
Intercept	1	4.9441	0.0140	4.9167	4.9716	124586	<.0001
OPTC02X	1	0.0006	0.0000	0.0006	0.0006	9683.24	<.0001
CLUSTER_ID 1	1	-0.0383	0.0226	-0.0826	0.0059	2.88	0.0898
CLUSTER_ID 2	1	-0.0793	0.0209	-0.1203	-0.0384	14.40	0.0001
CLUSTER_ID 3	1	0.0044	0.0185	-0.0319	0.0407	0.06	0.8118
CLUSTER_ID 4	0	0.0000	0.0000	0.0000	0.0000	.	.
Scale	1	1.1512	0.0116	1.1287	1.1741		

Table 27. criteria For Assessing Goodness of Fit For GenMod After clustering with a sample of 500 obs

Criteria for Assessing Goodness of Fit			
Criterion	**DF**	**Value**	**Value/DF**
Deviance	496	152.0841	0.3682
Scaled Deviance	496	441.7160	1.0695
Pearson Chi-Square	496	87.7086	0.2124
Scaled Pearson X2	496	254.7425	0.6168
Log Likelihood		-2641.7723	

Table 28. Analysis of Parameter Estimates For GenMod After clustering with a sample of 500 obs

Analysis of Parameter Estimates							
Parameter	**DF**	**Estimate**	**Standard Error**	**Wald 95% Confidence Limits**		**Chi-Square**	**ChiSq**
Intercept	1	4.8035	0.0749	4.6566	4.9503	4110.23	<.0001
OPTC02X	1	0.0021	0.0001	0.0019	0.0023	334.89	<.0001
CLUSTER_ID 1	1	-0.1676	0.0965	-0.3568	0.0217	3.01	0.0827
CLUSTER_ID 2	1	-0.4356	0.1221	-0.6748	-0.1964	12.74	0.0004
CLUSTER_ID 3	1	-0.7374	0.0774	-0.8891	-0.5857	90.79	<.0001
CLUSTER_ID 4	0	0.0000	0.0000	0.0000	0.0000	.	.
Scale	1	2.9044	0.1905	2.5541	3.3028		

the effect of the outliers on the data. Tables 29 and 30 display the results

Before clustering, the general and generalized linear models over-fit the data because of the huge number of icd9 codes used as categorical variables. The generalized linear model was used after clustering to predict the reimbursement variable. The problem of over-fitting the data was eliminated by choosing small samples. Results show that cluster 1 was not significant. However, clusters 2, 3 and 4 were significant with the total charges for predicting the reimbursement variable. The removal of the influential outliers was also significant in predicting the reimbursement variable such that all the explanatory variables were significant and the model fits the data very well.

Without the clustering method, we were not able to identify the exact effect in the reimbursement variable. This method proved to be an effective way to reduce a large number of icd-9 codes into an index of 4 levels, and to use those levels to examine the relationship to the hospital reimbursements by applying linear models.

Decision Tree to Analyze a Hospital's Reimbursements

We used some data mining tools, especially Decision Tree Analysis in order to investigate the reimbursement model and to try to extract some patterns from the data so they can be compared to our results from the statistical tools to analyze the reimbursement model. The data used here are the same data used before, so the comparison between statistical and data mining results will be more accurate and effective.

The diagram constructed by Enterprise Miner given in figure 14 was used to compare different

Table 29. Criteria For Assessing Goodness of Fit For GenMod After clustering and removing outliers with a sample of 500 obs

Criteria for Assessing Goodness of Fit			
Criterion	**DF**	**Value**	**Value/DF**
Deviance	413	359.1294	0.7241
Scaled Deviance	413	553.2523	1.1154
Pearson Chi-Square	413	227.8781	0.4594
Scaled Pearson X2	413	351.0547	0.7078
Log Likelihood		-3470.4844	

Table 30. Analysis of Parameter Estimates For GenMod After clustering and removing outliers with a sample of 500 obs

Analysis of Parameter Estimates							
Parameter	**DF**	**Estimate**	**Standard Error**	**Wald 95% Conf Limits**		**Chi-Square**	**Pr > ChiSq**
Intercept	1	5.6889	0.0574	5.5764	5.8015	9818.42	<.0001
OPTC02X	1	0.0006	0.0000	0.0005	0.0007	247.09	<.0001
CLUSTER_ID 1	1	-0.3347	0.1162	-0.5624	-0.1070	8.30	0.0040
CLUSTER_ID 2	1	-0.5716	0.1457	-0.8570	-0.2861	15.40	<.0001
CLUSTER_ID 3	1	-0.8462	0.0869	-1.0166	-0.6759	94.82	<.0001
CLUSTER_ID 4	0	0.0000	0.0000	0.0000	0.0000	.	.
Scale	1	1.5405	0.0888	1.3760	1.7248		

Figure 14. Enterprise Miner screen with the diagram used

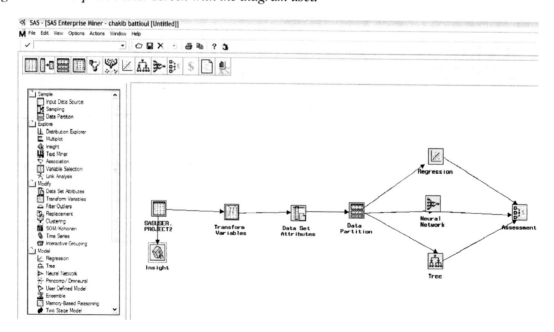

predictive models. The first node to the left of the screen contains the SAS dataset. The data partition node was used to divide the data into two subsets for training and validation. The training subset is used for preliminary model fitting; the validation subset is used to tune model weights during estimation. The assessment node was used to compare between models. The models used were regression, neural network and decision tree.

After running this diagram in order to compare models, the results show that the misclassification rate is high for all models. Since the Decision Tree had the lowest rate; then, we consider this model as the best fit for our data and we will focus our analysis on that model trying to extract some interesting results. Decision Trees produce a set of rules that can be used to generate predictions for a new data set. We ran the Decision Tree on our dataset in order to predict the reimbursement variable.

The first step used was to transform the reimbursement and total charge variables (opxp02x and optc02x respectively) from continuous to nominal in order to obtain meaningful results. The transformation was necessary because the Decision Tree requires the variables to be either interval or nominal. The transformation was based on the creation of five uniform groups. The code used to transform the reimbursement variable is given in table 31.

The new reimbursement variable (Reimblevel) was used as the target variable, while the new total charge variable (chargelevel) was used as an input variable. Cluster_id was also used as an input variable. The rest of the variables were set as rejected. The Data Partition Set node partitions the data into the train and validation sets. All the options are left as default. We ran the Decision Tree on our dataset. Results are given in figures 15 and 16.

Figure 15 shows the assessment plot. The vertical reference line identifies the subtree that optimizes the model assessment measure. This subtree maximizes the assessment value on the training data set. This subtree has the smallest misclassification rate for the validation data (0.36), and the fewest number of leaves (7 leaves). The misclassification rate is still high, but this is the best rate we obtained out of all the predictive models. The tree diagram is given in Figure 16.

The tree diagram displays node (segment) statistics, the names of the variables used to split the data into nodes, and the variable values for several levels of nodes in the tree. In our data, the split variable is the total charges and the cluster id. For each node, there is a separate row for each decision defined in the decision matrix of the target profile. The decision values depend on the type of decision matrix defined. The nodes are colored by the proportion of the reimbursement value.

Table 31. Code used to transform the reimbursements

```
procunivariate data=SASUSER.six ;
var opxp02x; output out=pctlscomp1 pctlpts = 20406080100
pctlpre = _pctl pctlname = pct20 pct40 pct60 pct80 pct100;
run;
procprint data=pctlscomp1;
run;
data sasuser.project;
set sasuser.h67f;
if opxp02x <= 36.78 then ReimbLevel='1';
if 36.78 < opxp02x <= 81 then ReimbLevel ='2';
if 81 < opxp02x <= 180.42 then ReimbLevel ='3';
if 180.42 < opxp02x <= 540.14 then ReimbLevel ='4';
if 540.14 < opxp02x <= 24884.36 then ReimbLevel ='5';
run;
Quit;;
```

Decision tree models involve recursive partitioning of the training data in an attempt to isolate concentrations of cases with identical target values. The first box on the top of the Tree represents the unpartitioned training data. Then

two branches were created. The first branch contains cases with Chargelevel equal to 5, and the second branch contains cases with Chargelevel equal to 1, 2, 3 and 4. In addition, any cases with a missing or unknown Chargelevel are placed in

Figure 15. Assessment plot

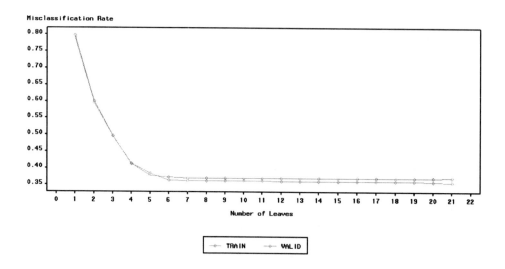

Figure 16. Tree Diagram

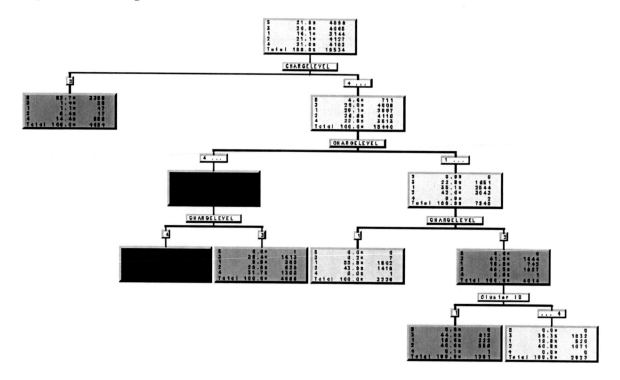

the second branch. Notice that the second branch has more cases than the first. This is indicated not only by the N in node field, but also by the thickness of the line joining the branches to the original, or *root*, node. From the right branch of the initial split, the split continues based on the Chargelevel. When the Chargelevel equals 3, two new branches emerge based on the Cluster id variable. The rules obtained from the tree are given in Table 32. They help predict the reimbursement based on the total charges.

The rules above show the predicted percentage of the reimbursement level for each total charge level. Notice that Cluster_ID 1 is statistically significant in predicting the reimbursement value compared to the rest of the clusters. If the cluster id equals 1 and the total charges equals 2, we will predict 40% of the payments to be in the reimbursement level 2 and 44% on level 3. This result matches the statistical results obtained from linear models.

CURRENT AND FUTURE CHALLENGES FACING THE ORGANIZATION

The aim of this study was to show that Medicare's inpatient reimbursement system is not a fair system for many hospitals. Some patients are severely ill and stay at the hospital more than others, and thus cost a lot more than an average inpatient's cost. Our goal was not to build a new outlier reimbursement system but only to show a gap in the current system. To reach this result, statistical and data mining tools were used to investigate two sets of data.

The main analysis idea was to prove that whenever the hospitals are receiving payments based upon an average cost, they are losing considerable revenue because the distribution of the hospital's cost and charges is usually exponential or gamma, but not a normal distribution as the Centers for Medicare and Medicaid Services assume.

Table 32. English rules of Decision Tree

Rule 1:
IF CHARGELEVEL EQUALS 5
THEN
 NODE : 2
 N : 4094
 5 : 82.7%
 3 : 1.4%
 1 : 1.1%
 2 : 0.4%
 4 : 14.4%

Rule 2:
IF CHARGELEVEL EQUALS 4
THEN
 NODE : 6
 N : 4101
 5 : 17.3%
 3 : 18.2%
 1 : 4.6%
 2 : 6.0%
 4 : 53.9%

Rule 3:
IF CHARGELEVEL EQUALS 3
THEN
 NODE : 7
 N : 4099
 5 : 0.0%
 3 : 39.4%
 1 : 8.9%
 2 : 20.0%
 4 : 31.7%

Rule 4:
IF CHARGELEVEL EQUALS 1
THEN
 NODE : 8
 N : 3226
 5 : 0.0%
 3 : 0.2%
 1 : 55.9%
 2 : 43.9%
 4 : 0.0%

Rule 5:
IF Cluster ID EQUALS 1
AND CHARGELEVEL EQUALS 2
THEN
 NODE : 14
 N : 1391
 5 : 0.0%
 3 : 44.0%
 1 : 16.0%
 2 : 40.0%
 4 : 0.1%

Simulations about normal, exponential and gamma distributions were generated to examine the outlier payments on each distribution whenever the outlier threshold is about two standard deviations from the mean. Results from simulations show that when we assume that the distribution of total charges is normal, and the outlier threshold is about two standard deviations from the mean, then the hospitals will almost break even. On the other hand, if the true distribution of total charges is exponential or gamma, then hospitals will lose a considerable amount if the payments are assumed to be normally distributed, and the outlier threshold is about two standard deviations from the mean.

The results were then applied to actual payment data to investigate the cost mechanism. The analysis was done on the hospital's total charges and also on specific DRG's. Results show that the distribution of the hospital's charges is exponential, or comes from an exponential family. We estimated the hospital's lost amount from the outlier payments.

Text mining was used to reduce a large number of patient condition codes into an index of 4 levels, and to use those levels to examine the relationship to the hospital reimbursements by applying linear models. We compare models with and without the use of a clustering variable to define patient severity, and we compare models with and without outliers.

Results show that the generalized linear model was the best fit to the data because it takes into consideration the fact that the distribution of the total charges is a gamma distribution by applying a log transformation. In addition, results show that the clustering variable was significant for predicting the reimbursement variable, and the removal of the influential outliers was also significant in predicting the reimbursement variable such that all the explanatory variables were significant and the model fits the data very well. Almost the same results were confirmed using Decision Tree analysis. If hospitals were paid the same amount for each admission regardless of its clinical characteristics, they would be encouraged to treat patients who are less ill, and to avoid the cases that require more resources. This situation has caused many health care providers to lose money; some of them have cut their budgets, and others have closed their emergency departments because the reimbursements no longer match the cost.

Clearly, this analysis has many advantages and benefits. The results of this study are very useful by hospitals to negotiate with CMS their outlier payments and show how much money they are losing by the current payment system. In addition, this work is very good proof to show the effect of different predictors on their total charges and then ask Medicare to take these variables into consideration whenever they are making their payments to hospitals. This study is an attempt to improve the healthcare payment system.

REFERENCES

Angus, L. D., Gorecki, P. J., Mourello, R., Ortega, R. E., & Adamski, J.(n.d.). DRG, costs and reimbursement following Roux-en-Y gastric bypass: an economic appraisal . In Potts, S. G. (Ed.), *Data Mining to Determine Characteristics of High-Cost Diabetics in a Medicaid Population.*

Camen DeNavas-Walt, B. D. P.,Lee, C. H. (n.d.). *Income, Poverty, and Health Insurance Coverage in the United States: 2004.* US Census Burea News (Press Kit/ Reports. P60-229).

Commission, M. P. A. (2006, June). MedPac Data Book 2006: Section 7: Acute inpatient services. Retrieved from Center of Medicare and Medicaid, http://www.cms.hhs.gov/AcuteInpatientPPS/downloads/outlier_example.pdf

Medical Expenditure Panel Survey (MEPS). (n.d.). Retrieved from http://www.meps.ahrq.gov/PUFFiles/H67G/H67Gdoc.pdf

Smith, R.D. (n.d.). *Simulation Article. Encyclopedia of Computer Science.* Basingstoke, UK: Nature Publishing Group.

Snyder, D. (2006, May 1). *In U.S Hospitals, Emergency Care in Critical Condition.* Retrieved from http://www.foxnews.com/story/0,2933,193883,00.html

The Emergency Medical Treatment and Labor Act (EMTALA). (n.d.). *The regulations, incorporating all of the revisions as made in 2000 and 2003. The primary regulation: 42 CFR 489.24 (a) 1).* Retrieved from http://www.emtala.com/law/index.html

ADDITIONAL READING

Battioui, C. (2007). *Cost Models with Prominent Outliers.* Louisveille, KY: University of Louisville.

Dallas, E., Johnson, K. S. U., & Manhattan, K. S. (2003). An Introduction to the Analysis of Mixed Models. In SUGI 28, Paper 253-28

Dorr, D. A., Horn, S. D., & Smout, R. J. (2005). Cost analysis of nursing home registered nurse staffing times. *Journal of the American Geriatrics Society, 53*(5), 840–845. doi:10.1111/j.1532-5415.2005.53267.x

Englesbe, M. J., Dimick, J. B., Fan, Z., Baser, O., & Birkmeyer, J. D. (2009). Case mix, quality and high-cost kidney transplant patients. *American Journal of Transplantation, 9*(5), 1108–1114. doi:10.1111/j.1600-6143.2009.02592.x

Raddish, M., Horn, S. D., & Sharkey, P. D. (1999). Continuity of care: is it cost effective? *The American Journal of Managed Care, 5*(6), 727–734.

Schabenberger, O. (n.d.). *Introducing the GLIMMIX Procedure for Generalized Linear Mixed Models.* Cary, NC: SAS Institute Inc

Section 3
Modeling EEG Images for Analysis

Chapter 17
The Relationship between Sleep Apnea and Cognitive Functioning

M. S. S. Khan
University of Louisville, USA

ABSTRACT

The brain is the most complicated and least studied area of Neuro Sceince. In recent times, it has been one of the fastest growing areas of study in the Medical Sciences. This is mostly due to computers and computational techniques that have emerged in the last 10-15 years. Cognitive Neuropsychology aims to understand how the structure and function of the brain relates to psychological processes. It places emphasis on studying the cognitive effects of brain injury or neurological illness with a view to inferring models of normal cognitive functioning. We investigate the relationship between sleep apnea and learning disorders. Sleep apnea is a neural disorder, where individuals find it difficult to sleep because they stop breathing. We want to see if patients with learning disabilities should be treated for sleep apnea.

BACKGROUND

Sleep Apnea

We have a number of different datasets of EEG data of children collected concerning both the reactions to different stimuli and from sleep apnea studies. These data have been completely de-identified and will be used throughout this project. Generally, EEG data are collected using a Geodesic Sensor Net.(Johnson et al., 2001; Tucker, 1993) This is a

system that allows the mapping of brain activity data using a cap containing 128 electrodes. The cap is placed on the subject's head. This system makes it much easier to collect brain activity data from children since previously, collecting these type of data required electrodes to be placed on a person's head one-at-a-time using applicator gel. Most children will not sit still for this type of research. The Geodesic Sensor Net allows all of the electrodes to be placed on a child's head at once and collection of data is much faster than using the old EEG or electro-encephalogram method. Data are recorded at fixed time intervals, usually measured in seconds.

DOI: 10.4018/978-1-61520-723-7.ch017

Copyright © 2010, IGI Global. Copying or distributing in print or electronic forms without written permission of IGI Global is prohibited.

Figure 1. Geodesic sensor net configuration

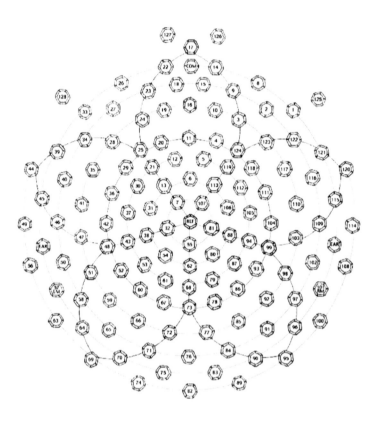

Geodesic Sensor Net
128 Channel V2.0

For example, in the data analyzed for any one child, an entire collection of 250 data points can be recorded in under 20 minutes.

Figure 1 represents the positioning of the electrodes for a 128 channel Geodesic Sensor Net.

The electrodes that appear vertically in the center of the chart, running from top to bottom, divide the other electrodes into left and right sections. For statistical analyses, all electrode readings from the left side of the brain can be averaged to one value as can all values from the right side of the brain. The brain positioning of all electrodes is shown in Table 1.

The EEG data, then, have hundreds, sometimes, thousands of data points recorded in sequence from each of the net sensors. There may be just a handful of subjects in a study, with each subject having these multiple recordings of data. The methods used to model the data must be able to accommodate the type of data collected.

For each electrode, then, we have a sequence X_{i1}, X_{i2}, ..., X_{in} representing the first to the last timed reading (assuming a total of n readings). The value i represents the specific electrode. This sequence is not a random sample since it is clear that $X_{i,t}$ is related to $X_{i,t+1}$. It is also questionable whether we can assume stationarity, meaning that $X_{i,t}$ and $X_{i,t+1}$ have the same probability distribution. For the purposes of this study, we will make such an assumption. Moreover, if i and j are in

Table 1. Electrode/Brain position

Position	Brain Position	Electrodes
FL	Front Left	18 19 20 22 23 24 25 26 27 28 33 34 39 128
FR	Front Right	1 2 3 4 8 9 10 14 15 121 122 123 124 125
CL	Center Left	7 12 13 21 29 30 31 32 35 36 37 38 41 42 43 46 47 48 51
CR	Center Right	5 81 88 94 98 99 103 104 105 106 107 109 110 111 112 113 117 118 119
PL	Parietal Left	54 61 67 53 60 52 59 58 64 63
PR	Parietal Right	78 79 80 87 86 93 92 97 96 100
OL	Occipital Left	65 66 69 70 71 72 74 75
OR	Occipital Right	77 83 84 85 89 90 91 95
TL	Temporal Left	40 44 45 49 50 56 57
TR	Temporal Right	101 102 108 114 115 116 120

the same general location, we must assume that $X_{i,t}$ and $X_{j,t}$ are related in some way.

Because of these relationships and the lack of randomness in the variables, we cannot use standard regression techniques to investigate the data because these techniques make the assumption that the data are both independent and identically distributed, as well as coming from a normal distribution. Such assumptions are clearly false in data collected from EEG monitoring. In the past, attempts have been made to classify, or group the EEG readings to simplify the problem. (Kook, Gupta, Kota, & Molfese, 2007) Another approach, specifically used in hypothesis testing, has been to reduce the sample data to its averages, and to analyze the average.(Mayes, Molfese, Key, & Hunter, 2005) Such an approach greatly reduces the amount of information from the EEG data that is used in the analysis. By using techniques that were specifically designed to work with these types of data, we can greatly expand the amount of knowledge extracted from the data. Therefore, we must work with techniques that do not assume independence in the data points.

The three techniques that will be used in the proposed short course are part of the general topic of data mining. Data mining is a general term that is used to describe a process of data analysis, beginning with required data preprocessing followed by exploration and hypothesis generation and ending with the validation of results and their use in making decisions from the data.

DATA MINING

Data mining techniques are the result of a long process of research and product development. This evolution began when business data were first stored on computers, continued with improvements in data access, and generated technologies that allow users to navigate through their data in real time. Data mining goes beyond retrospective data access and navigation to prospective and proactive information delivery. Data mining is ready for application in the business community because it is supported by three technologies:

- Massive data collection
- Powerful multiprocessor computers
- Data mining algorithms

Commercial databases are growing at unprecedented rates. A recent META Group survey of data warehouse projects found that 19% of respondents are beyond the 50 gigabyte level, while 59% expected to be there by the second quarter of 1996.[1] In some industries, these num-

Table 2. Steps in the evolution of data mining

Evolutionary Step	Business Question	Enabling Technologies	Product Providers	Characteristics
Data Collection (1960s)	"What was my total revenue in the last five years?"	Computers, tapes, disks	IBM, CDC	Retrospective, static data delivery
Data Access (1980s)	"What were unit sales in New England last March?"	Relational databases (RD-BMS), Structured Query Language (SQL), ODBC	Oracle, Sybase, Informix, IBM, Microsoft	Retrospective, dynamic data delivery at record level
Data Warehousing & Decision Support (1990s)	"What were unit sales in New England last March? Drill down to Boston."	On-line analytic processing (OLAP), multidimensional databases, data warehouses	Pilot, Comshare, Arbor, Cognos, Microstrategy	Retrospective, dynamic data delivery at multiple levels
Data Mining (Emerging Today)	"What's likely to happen to Boston unit sales next month? Why?"	Advanced algorithms, multiprocessor computers, massive databases	Pilot, Lockheed, IBM, SGI, numerous startups (nascent industry)	Prospective, proactive information delivery

bers can be much larger. The accompanying need for improved computational engines can now be met in a cost-effective manner with parallel multiprocessor computer technology. Data mining algorithms embody techniques that have existed for at least 10 years, but have only recently been implemented as mature, reliable, understandable tools that consistently outperform older statistical methods.

Dynamic data access is critical for drill-through in data navigation applications, and the ability to store large databases is critical to data mining. The four steps listed in Table 2 were revolutionary because they allowed new business questions to be answered accurately and quickly.

The core components of data mining technology have been under development for decades, in research areas such as statistics, artificial intelligence, and machine learning. Today, the maturity of these techniques, coupled with high-performance relational database engines and broad data integration efforts, make these technologies practical for current data warehouse environments.

Data mining derives its name from the similarities between searching for valuable business information in a large database, for example, finding linked products in gigabytes of store scanner data and mining a mountain for valuable ore. Both processes require either sifting through an immense amount of material, or intelligently probing it to find exactly where the value resides. Given databases of sufficient size and quality, data mining technology can generate new business opportunities by providing these capabilities:

- **Automated prediction of trends and behaviors**. Data mining automates the process of finding predictive information in large databases. Questions that traditionally required extensive hands-on analysis can now be answered directly from the data and quickly. A typical example of a predictive problem is targeted marketing. Data mining uses data on past promotional mailings to identify the targets most likely to maximize return on investment in future mailings. Other predictive problems include forecasting bankruptcy and other forms of default, and identifying segments of a population likely to respond similarly to given events.

- **Automated discovery of previously unknown patterns**. Data mining examines databases and identifies previously hidden patterns. An example of pattern discovery is the analysis of retail sales data to identify seemingly unrelated products that are often purchased together. Other pattern discovery problems include detecting fraudulent credit card transactions and identifying anomalous data that could represent data entry keying errors.

Data mining techniques can yield the benefits of automation on existing software and hardware platforms, and can be implemented on new systems as existing platforms are upgraded and new products developed. When data mining tools are implemented on high performance parallel processing systems, they can analyze massive databases in minutes. Faster processing means that users can automatically experiment with more models to understand complex data. High speed makes it practical for users to analyze huge quantities of data. Larger databases, in turn, yield improved predictions. Databases can be larger in both depth and breadth:

- **More columns.** Analysts must often limit the number of variables they examine when doing hands-on analysis due to time constraints. Yet variables that are discarded because they seem unimportant may carry information about unknown patterns. High performance data mining allows users to explore the full depth of a database, without pre-selecting a subset of variables.
- **More rows.** Larger samples yield lower estimation errors and variance, and allow users to make inferences about small but important segments of a population.

A recent Gartner Group Advanced Technology Research Note listed data mining and artificial intelligence at the top of the five key technology areas that "will clearly have a major impact across a wide range of industries within the next 3 to 5 years."[2] Gartner also listed parallel architectures and data mining as two of the top 10 new technologies in which companies will invest during the next 5 years. According to a recent Gartner HPC Research Note, "With the rapid advance in data capture, transmission and storage, large-systems

users will increasingly need to implement new and innovative ways to mine the after-market value of their vast stores of detail data, employing MPP [massively parallel processing] systems to create new sources of business advantage.

The most commonly used techniques in data mining are:

- **Artificial neural networks:** Non-linear predictive models that learn through training and resemble biological neural networks in structure.
- **Decision trees:** Tree-shaped structures that represent sets of decisions. These decisions generate rules for the classification of a dataset. Specific decision tree methods include Classification and Regression Trees (CART) and Chi Square Automatic Interaction Detection (CHAID).
- **Genetic algorithms:** Optimization techniques that use process such as genetic combination, mutation, and natural selection in a design based on the concepts of evolution.
- **Nearest neighbor method:** A technique that classifies each record in a dataset based on a combination of the classes of the k record(s) most similar to it in a historical dataset (where $k > 1$). Sometimes called the k-nearest neighbor technique.
- **Rule induction:** The extraction of useful if-then rules from data based on statistical significance.

Many of these technologies have been in use for more than a decade in specialized analysis tools that work with relatively small volumes of data. These capabilities are now evolving to integrate directly with industry-standard data warehouse and OLAP platforms.

The primary technique that is used to perform data mining is called modeling. Modeling is simply the act of building a model in one situation where you know the answer and then applying it

Table 3. Data Mining for prospecting

	Customers	Prospects
General information (e.g. demographic data)	Known	Known
Proprietary information (e.g. customer transactions)	Known	Target

to another situation where you do not. This act of model building is something that people have been doing for a long time, certainly before the advent of computers or data mining technology. What happens on computers, however, is not much different than the way people build models. Computers are loaded with lots of information about a variety of situations where an answer is known, and then the data mining software on the computer must run through that data and distill the characteristics of the data that should go into the model. Once the model is built, it can then be used in similar situations. For example, say that you are the director of marketing for a telecommunications company and you would like to acquire some new long distance phone customers. You could just randomly go out and mail coupons to the general population. However, you would not achieve the desired results and, of course, you have the opportunity to do much better than random if you could use your business experience stored in your database to build a model.

As the marketing director, you have access to a lot of information about all of your customers: their age, sex, credit history and long distance calling usage. The good news is that you also have a lot of information about your prospective customers: their age, sex, credit history, etc. Your problem is that you do not know the long distance calling usage of these prospects (since they are most likely now customers of your competition). You'd like to concentrate on those prospects who have large amounts of long distance usage. You can accomplish this by building a model. Table 3 illustrates the data used for building a model for new customers prospecting in a data warehouse.

The goal in prospecting is to make some calculated guesses about the information about prospects based on the model that we build going from Customer General Information to Customer Proprietary Information. For instance, a simple model for a telecommunications company might be:

98% of my customers who make more than $60,000/year spend more than $80/month on long distance.

This model could then be applied to the prospect data to try to tell something about the proprietary information that this telecommunications company does not currently have access to. With this model in hand, new customers can be selectively targeted. Test marketing is an excellent source of data for this kind of modeling. Mining the results of a test market representing a broad but relatively small sample of prospects can provide a foundation for identifying good prospects in the overall market. Table 4 shows another common scenario for building models: predict what is going to happen in the future.

If someone told you that he had a model that could predict customer usage, how would you know if he really had a good model? The first thing you might try would be to ask him to apply his model to your customer base, where you already knew the answer. With data mining, the best way to accomplish this is by setting aside some of your data in a vault to isolate it from the mining process. Once the mining is complete, the results can be tested against the data held in the vault to confirm the model's validity. If the model works, its observations should hold for the vaulted data.

Table 4. Data Mining for predictions

	Yesterday	Today	Tomorrow
Static information and current plans (e.g. demographic data, marketing plans)	Known	Known	Known
Dynamic information (e.g. customer transactions)	Known	Known	Target

To best apply these advanced techniques, they must be fully integrated with a data warehouse as well as flexible interactive business analysis tools. Many data mining tools currently operate outside of the warehouse, requiring extra steps for extracting, importing, and analyzing the data. Furthermore, when new insights require operational implementation, integration with the warehouse simplifies the application of results from data mining. The resulting analytic data warehouse can be applied to improve business processes throughout the organization, in areas such as promotional campaign management, fraud detection, new product rollout, and so on.

The ideal starting point is a data warehouse containing a combination of internal data tracking all customer contact coupled with external market data about competitor activity. Background information on potential customers also provides an excellent basis for prospecting. This warehouse can be implemented in a variety of relational database systems: Sybase, Oracle, Redbrick, and so on, and should be optimized for flexible and fast data access.

An OLAP (On-Line Analytical Processing) server enables a more sophisticated end-user business model to be applied when navigating the data warehouse. The multidimensional structures allow the user to analyze the data as they want to view their business, summarizing by product line, region, and other key perspectives of their business. The Data Mining Server must be integrated with the data warehouse and the OLAP server to embed ROI-focused business analysis directly into this infrastructure. An advanced, process-centric metadata template defines the data mining objectives for specific business issues such as campaign management, prospecting, and promotion optimization. Integration with the data warehouse enables operational decisions to be directly implemented and tracked. As the warehouse grows with new decisions and results, the organization can continually mine the best practices and apply them to future decisions.

This design represents a fundamental shift from conventional decision support systems. Rather than simply delivering data to the end user through query and reporting software, the Advanced Analysis Server applies users' business models directly to the warehouse and returns a proactive analysis of the most relevant information. These results enhance the metadata in the OLAP Server by providing a dynamic metadata layer that represents a distilled view of the data. Reporting, visualization, and other analysis tools can then be applied to plan future actions and confirm the impact of those plans.

Wavelet Analysis

The discrete wavelet transform decomposes a function as a sum of basis functions called wavelets. These basis functions have the property that they can be obtained by dilating and translating two basic types of wavelets known as the *scaling function* or *father wavelet φ,* and the *mother wavelet ψ.* These translations and dilations are defined as follows:

$$\varphi_{j,k}(x) = 2^{j/2}\varphi(2^j x - k)$$
$$\psi_{j,k}(x) = 2^{j/2}\psi(2^j x - k)$$

The index j defines the dilation or *level* while the index k defines the translate. Loosely speaking, sums of the $\Phi_{j,k}(x)$ capture low frequencies and sums of the $\psi_{j,k}(x)$ represent high frequencies in the data. More precisely, for any suitable function $f(x)$ and for any j_0,

$$f(x) = \sum_k c_k^{jo} \phi_{jo,k}(x) + \sum_{j \geq jo} \sum_k d_k^j \varphi_{j,k}(x)$$

where the c_k^j and d_k^j are known as the scaling coefficients and the detail coefficients, respectively. For orthonormal wavelet families, these coefficients can be computed by

$$c_k^j = \int f(x) \phi j, k(x) dx$$
$$d_k^j = \int f(x) \varphi j, k(x) dx .$$

The key to obtaining fast numerical algorithms for computing the detail and scaling coefficients for a given function $f(x)$ is that there are simple recurrence relationships that enable you to compute the coefficients at level j-1 from the values of the scaling coefficients at level j. These formulae are

$$c_k^{j-1} = \sum_i h_{i-2k} c_i^j$$
$$d_k^{j-1} = \sum_i g_{i-2k} c_i^j$$

The coefficients h_k and g_k that appear in these formulae are called *filter coefficients*. The h_k are determined by the father wavelet and they form a low-pass filter; $g_k = (-1)^k h_{1-k}$ that defines a high-pass filter. The preceding sums are formally over the entire (infinite) range of integers. However, for wavelets that are zero except on a finite interval, only finitely many of the filter coefficients are non-zero, and so, in this case, the sums in the recurrence relationships for the detail and scaling coefficients are finite.

Conversely, if you know the detail and scaling coefficients at level j-1, then you can obtain the scaling coefficients at level j using the relationship

$$c_k^j = \sum_i h_{k-2i} c_i^{j-1} + \sum_i g_{k-2i} d_i^{j-1}$$

Suppose that you have data values

$$y_k = f(x_k), k = 0,1,2, ..., N\text{-}1$$

at $N=2^J$ equally spaced points x_k. It turns out that the values $2^{-J/2} y_k$ are good approximations of the scaling coefficients c_k^J. Then, using the recurrence formula, you can find c_k^{J-1} and d_k^{J-1}, $k = 0,1,2, ..., N/2\text{-}1$. The discrete wavelet transform of the y_k at level J-1 consists of the $N/2$ scaling and $N/2$ detail coefficients at level J-1. A technical point that arises is that in applying the recurrence relationships to finite data, a few values of the c_k^J for $k<0$ or $k \geq N$ may be needed. One way to cope with this difficulty is to extend the sequence c_k^J to the left and right using some specified boundary treatment.

Continuing by replacing the scaling coefficients at any level j by the scaling and detail coefficients at level j-1 yields a sequence of N coefficients

$$\{c^0_0, d^0_0, d^1_0, d^1_1, d^2_0, d^2_1, d^2_2, d^2_3, d^3_1, ..., d^3_7, ..., d^{J-1}_0, ..., d^{J-1}_{N/2-1}\}$$

This sequence is the finite discrete wavelet transform of the input data $\{y_k\}$. At any level j_0, the finite dimensional approximation of the function $f(x)$ is

$$f(x) \approx \sum_k c_k^{j0} \varphi_{j0,k}(x) + \sum_{j=j0}^{J-1} \sum_k d_k^j \psi_{j,k}(x)$$

Obstructive sleep apnea syndrome (OSAS) is a respiratory disorder characterized by the repeated cessations of breathing during sleep due to obstruction of the upper airways. Classic features include excessive snoring, nocturnal hypoxemia, and disruption of normal sleep patterns. Excessive daytime sleepiness has been reported in a majority of the individuals with the disorder and has been associated with difficulty in maintaining adequate arousal to complete occupational or domestic activities. Sleepiness during driving is particularly problematic, and individuals with OSAS are at higher risk for motor vehicle accidents.

OSAS and related deficits have been reported across a range of neuropsychological domains, including motor speed, attention, information processing speed, working memory, long-term episodic memory and executive control. The etiologies of such impairments have been explored in number of studies.

Ridge Regression

Data regression analysis is a technique used for the modeling and analysis of numerical data consisting of values of a dependent variable (response variable) and of one or more independent variables (explanatory variables). The dependent variable in the regression equation is modeled as a function of the independent variables, corresponding parameters ("constants"), and an error term. The error term is a random variable. It represents unexplained variation in the dependent variable. The parameters are estimated so as to give a "best fit" of the data. Most commonly, the best fit is evaluated by using the least squares method, but other criteria have also been used. Regression can be divided to sub-topics of linear regression and Non-Linear regression. We discuss linear regression.

In linear regression, the model specification is that the dependent variable, y_i is a linear combination of the *parameters* (but need not be linear in the *independent variables*). For example, in simple linear regression for modeling N data points, there is one independent variable: x_i, and two parameters, β_0 and β_1:

straight line: $y_i = \beta_0 + \beta_1 x_i + \in_i, \ i = 1, \dots, N$

In multiple linear regression, there are several independent variables or functions of independent variables. For example, adding a term in x_i^2 to the preceding regression gives:

parabola: $y_i = \beta_0 + \beta_1 x_i + \beta_2 x_i^2 + \in_i, i = 1, N$

This is still linear regression; although the expression on the right hand side is quadratic in the independent variable x_i but linear in the parameters β_0, β_1 and β_2.

In both cases, ε_i is an error term and the subscript i indexes a particular observation. Given a random sample from the population, we estimate the population parameters and obtain the sample linear regression model: $y_i = \hat{\beta}_0 + \hat{\beta}_1 X_i + e_i$. The term e_i is the residual, $e_i = y_i - \hat{y}_i$. One method of estimation is ordinary least squares. This method obtains parameter estimates that minimize the sum of squared residuals, SSE:

$$SSE = \sum_{i-1}^{N} e_i^2$$

Minimization of this function results in a set of normal equations, a set of simultaneous linear equations in the parameters, which are solved to yield the parameter estimators, $\hat{\beta}_0, \hat{\beta}_1$.

Figure 2. llustration of linear regression on a data set (red points)

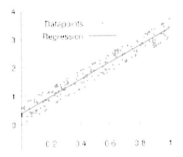

In the case of simple regression, the formulas for the least squares estimates are:

$$\hat{\beta}_1 \frac{\sum(x_i - \bar{x})(y_i - \bar{y})}{\sum(x_i - \bar{x})^2} \quad and \quad \hat{\beta}_0 = \bar{y} - \hat{\beta}_1 \bar{x}$$

where $\bar{x}$ is the mean (average) of the x values and $\bar{y}$ is the mean of the y values. The process of linear least squares (straight line fitting) is used for a derivation of these formulas. Under the assumption that the population error term has a constant variance, the estimate of that variance is given by:

$$\hat{\sigma}_\epsilon = \sqrt{\frac{SSE}{N-2}}$$

This is called the root mean square error (RMSE) of the regression. The standard errors of the parameter estimates are given by

$$\hat{\sigma}_{\beta_0} = \hat{\sigma}_\epsilon \sqrt{\frac{1}{N} \frac{\bar{x}^2}{\sum(x_i - \bar{x})^2}}$$

$$\hat{\sigma}_{\beta_1} = \hat{\sigma}_\epsilon \sqrt{\frac{1}{\sum(x_i - \bar{x})^2}}$$

Under the further assumption that the population error term is normally distributed, the researcher can use these estimated standard errors to create confidence intervals and conduct hypothesis tests about the population parameters.

In the more general multiple regression model, there are p independent variables:

$$y_i = \beta_0 + \beta_1 x_{1i} + \cdots + \beta_p x_{pi} + \epsilon_i,$$

The least square parameter estimates are obtained by p normal equations. The residual can be written as

$$e_i = y_i - \hat{\beta}_0 - \hat{\beta}_1 x_1 - \cdots - \hat{\beta}_p x_p$$

The normal equations are

$$\sum_{i-1}^{N} \sum_{k-1}^{p} X_{ij} X_{ik} \hat{\beta}_k = \sum_{i-1}^{N} X_{ij} y_i, j = 1, p$$

In matrix notation, the normal equations are written as

$$(X^\mathrm{T} X)\hat{\beta} = X^\mathrm{T} y$$

Around the middle of the 20th century, the Russian theoretician, Andre Tikhonov, was working on the solution of *ill-posed problems*. These are mathematical problems for which no unique solution exists because, in effect, there is not enough information specified in the problem. It is necessary to supply extra information (or assumptions), and the mathematical technique Tikhonov developed for this is known as regularization.

Tikhonov's work only became widely known in the West after the publication in 1977 of his book. Meanwhile, two American statisticians, Arthur Hoerl and Robert Kennard, published a paper in 1970 on ridge regression, a method for solving badly conditioned linear regression problems. Bad conditioning means there are numerical difficulties in performing the inverse step necessary to obtain the variance matrix. It is also a symptom of an ill-posed regression problem in Tikhonov's sense, and Hoerl & Kennard's method was in fact a crude form of regularization, known now as zero-order regularization.

In the 1980's, when neural networks became popular, weight decay was one of a number of techniques `invented' to help prune unimportant network connections. However, it was soon recognized that weight decay involves adding the same penalty term to the sum-squared-error as in ridge regression. Weight-decay and ridge regression are equivalent.

Ridge regression is mathematically and computationally convenient. We present Ridge regression from the perspective of bias and variance and how it affects the equations for the optimal weight vector, the variance matrix and the projection matrix. A method to select a good value for the regularization parameter, based on a re-estimation formula, is then presented, followed by a generalization of ridge regression which, if radial basis functions are used, can be justly called local ridge regression. It involves multiple regularization parameters and we describe a method for their optimization.

When the input is x, the trained model predicts the output as f(x) . If we had many training sets (which we never do, but just suppose) and if we knew the true output, y(x), we could calculate the mean-squared-error as:

$$MSE = \left\langle (y(x) - f(x))^2 \right\rangle$$

where the expectation (averaging) indicated by the value of MSE is taken over the training sets. This score, which defines how good the average prediction is, can be broken down into two components, namely

$$MSE = (y(x) - \langle f(x) \rangle)^2 + \left\langle (f(x) - \langle f(x) \rangle)^2 \right\rangle$$

The first part is the *bias* and the second part is the *variance*.

If f(x)=y(x) for all values of x, then the model is unbiased (the bias is zero). However, an unbiased model may still have a large mean-squared-error if it has a large variance. This will be the case if f(x) is highly sensitive to the peculiarities (such as noise and the choice of sample points) of each particular training set, and it is this sensitivity that causes regression problems to be ill-posed in the Tikhonov sense. Often, however, the variance can be significantly reduced by deliberately introducing a small amount of bias so that the net effect is a reduction in mean-squared-error.

Introducing bias is equivalent to restricting the range of functions for which a model can account. Typically, this is achieved by removing degrees of freedom. Examples would be lowering the order of a polynomial or reducing the number of weights in a neural network. Ridge regression does not explicitly remove degrees of freedom, but instead reduces the effective number of parameters. The resulting loss of flexibility makes the model less sensitive.

A convenient, if somewhat arbitrary, method of restricting the flexibility of linear models is to augment the sum-squared-error with a term that penalizes large weights,

$$C = \sum_{i=1}^{P} (\hat{y}_i - f(x_i))^2 + \lambda \sum_{j=1}^{m} w_j^2$$

This is ridge regression (weight decay) and the regularization parameter $\lambda > 0$ controls the balance between fitting the data and avoiding the penalty. A small value for λ means that the data can be fit tightly without causing a large penalty; a large value for λ means that a tight fit has to be sacrificed if it requires large weights. The bias introduced favors solutions involving small weights, and the effect is to smooth the output function since large weights are usually required to produce a highly variable (rough) output function. The optimal weight vector for the above cost function has already been dealt with, as have the variance matrix and the projection matrix. In summary,

$$A = H^{\mathsf{T}} H + \lambda I_m,$$
$$\hat{w} = A^{-1} H^{\mathsf{T}} \hat{y},$$
$$P = I_P - H A^{-1} H^{\mathsf{T}}$$

Some sort of model selection must be used to choose a value for the regularization parameter, λ. The value chosen is the one associated with the lowest prediction error. The popular choices to optimize the error are leave-one-out cross-validation, generalized cross-validation, final prediction error and Bayesian information criterion. There are also bootstrap methods. The most convenient method is generalized cross validation (GCV). It leads to the simplest optimization formula, especially in local optimization.

Since all the model selection criteria depend nonlinearly on λ, we need a method of nonlinear optimization. We could use any of the standard techniques for this, such as the Newton method. Alternatively, we can exploit the fact that when the derivative of the GCV error prediction is set to zero, the resulting equation can be manipulated so that only the estimate for λ appears on the left hand side,

$$\hat{\lambda} = \frac{\hat{y}^{\mathsf{T}} P^2 \hat{y} \, trace(A^{-1} - \lambda A^{-2})}{\hat{w}^{\mathsf{T}} A^{-1} \hat{w} \, trace(P)}$$

This is not a solution; it is a re-estimation formula because the right hand side depends on λ (explicitly as well as implicitly through A^{-1} and P). To use it, an initial value of $\hat{\lambda}$ is chosen and used to calculate a value for the right hand side. This leads to a new estimate and the process can be repeated until convergence.

The selection criteria depend mainly on the projection matrix P, and therefore, we need to deduce its dependence on the individual regularization parameters. The relevant relationship is one of the incremental operations. Adapting the notation somewhat, it is

$$P = P_j - \frac{P_j h_j h_j^{\mathsf{T}} P_j}{\lambda_j + h_j^{\mathsf{T}} P_j h_j},$$

where P_j is the projection matrix after the jth basis function has been removed and h_j is the jth column of the design matrix λ_j. In contrast to the case of standard ridge regression, there is an analytic solution for the optimal value of λ_j based on GCV minimization; no re-estimation is necessary. The trouble is that there are $m - 1$ other parameters

to optimize and each time one λ_j is optimized, it changes the optimal value of each of the others. Optimizing all the parameters together has to be done as a kind of re-estimation, doing one at a time and then repeating until they all converge.

When $\lambda_j = \infty$ the two projection matrices, P and P_j are equal. This means that if the optimal value of λ_j is ∞, then the jth basis function can be removed from the network. In practice, especially if the network is initially very flexible (high variance, low bias), infinite optimal values are very common and local ridge regression can be used as a method of pruning unnecessary hidden units.

The algorithm can get stuck in local minima, like any other nonlinear optimization, depending on the initial settings. For this reason, it is best in practice to give the algorithm a head start by using the results from other methods rather than starting with random parameters. For example, standard ridge regression can be used to find the best global parameter, $\hat{\lambda}$, and the local algorithm can then start from

$$\lambda_j = \lambda, \, 1 \leq j \leq m$$

Alternatively, forward selection can be used to choose a subset, S, of the original m basis functions, in which case, the local algorithm can start from

$$\lambda_j = \begin{cases} 0 \; if \; j \in S \\ \infty \; otherwise \end{cases}$$

SETTING THE STAGE

Time Series Analysis

We can use time series techniques to model any one EEG node, or to examine several in one area of the brain. We can use autoregression techniques to investigate the relationship of one series of EEG responses to another, and to examine patterns in

Figure 3. Graph of left and right side data

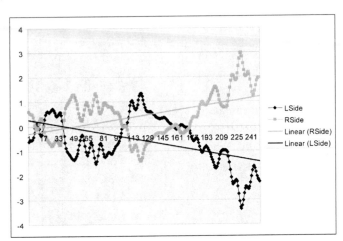

relationship to external stimuli. The predictor and response variable are almost mirror images of each other as shown in Figure 3.

Right side data were chosen because the model that is developed for the predictor series will also be applied to the response series. For the right side data analysis, the default number of lags was kept at 24. The data show significant autocorrelation through lag 14. This plot shows, for example, that at lag 1, the correlation between a right side value and the right side value for the previous time point is significant. The diagnostics of the model indicate that some autocorrelation is present. The Inverse Autocorrelation function stays near zero throughout the entire series (except lag 1 which is normal).

Wavelet Analysis

Our Data are part of an ongoing research at the Department of Pediatrics, University of Louisville. These Data were collected from the children who suffer from Sleep Apnea. They are kept under observation at the onsite facility of the Department. In this process, they wear a EEG scalp meter. There brain function is recorded in the form of medical time series, which is recorded in the Eu-

ropean Data Format (EDF), which is a standard in recording medical time series. To make these data useful for our research, we have to convert these EDF files first into ASCII format, with the help of HypoLab software. Once this is done, we import these converted files into the SAS environment. The data have been de-identified to satisfy HIPAA regulations.

We use wavelets, a mathematical function used to divide a given function into different frequency components and we study each component with a resolution that matches its scale. Data were measured by the scalp Electroencephalography, or EEG. These are brain waves patterns, which carry very important information. We are interested in EEG patterns that are related to learning disabilities, using data mining techniques to uncover information. Since high frequencies occur in discrete intervals, we model brain function using discrete wavelet analysis to decode information. In SAS /IML, we can model the EEG using wavelet analysis to see if a particular wave is associated with a level of cognitive functioning.

We compare the wavelet decomposition of various EEG data. These decompositions are then smoothed at various decomposition levels. Since this is an ongoing work, we are still in the process in implementing these techniques on more of the dataset and weighing our options in the use of Data mining Algorithms.

The discrete wavelet transform decomposes a function as a sum of basis functions called wavelets. These basis functions have the property that they can be obtained by dilating and translating two basic types of wavelets known as the *scaling function* or *father wavelet φ*, and the *mother wavelet ψ*. These translations and dilations are defined as follows:

$$\varphi_{j,k}(x) = 2^{j/2}\varphi(2^j x - k)$$
$$\psi_{j,k}(x) = 2^{j/2}\psi(2^j x - k)$$

The index j defines the dilation or *level* while the index k defines the translate. Loosely speaking, sums of the $\Phi_{j,k}(x)$ capture low frequencies and sums of the $\psi_{j,k}(x)$ represent high frequencies in the data. More precisely, for any suitable function $f(x)$ and for any j_0,

$$f(x) = \sum_k c_k^{j_0}\phi_{j_0,k}(x) + \sum_{j \geq j_0}\sum_k d_k^j\varphi_{j,k}(x)$$

where the c_k^j and d_k^j are known as the scaling coefficients and the detail coefficients, respectively. For orthonormal wavelet families, these coefficients can be computed by

$$c_k^j = \int f(x)\phi_{j,k}(x)dx$$
$$d_k^j = \int f(x)\varphi_{j,k}(x)dx$$

The key to obtaining fast numerical algorithms for computing the detail and scaling coefficients for a given function $f(x)$ is that there are simple recurrence relationships that enable you to compute the coefficients at level j-1 from the values of the scaling coefficients at level j. These formulae are

$$c_k^{j-1} = \sum_i h_{i-2k}c_i^j$$
$$d_k^{j-1} = \sum_i g_{i-2k}c_i^j$$

The coefficients h_k and g_k that appear in these formulae are called *filter coefficients*. The h_k are determined by the father wavelet and they form a low-pass filter; $g_k = (-1)^k h_{1-k}$ that defines a high-pass filter. The preceding sums are formally over the entire (infinite) range of integers. However, for wavelets that are zero except on a finite interval, only finitely many of the filter coefficients are non-zero, and so, in this case, the sums in the recurrence relationships for the detail and scaling coefficients are finite.

Conversely, if you know the detail and scaling coefficients at level j-1, then you can obtain the scaling coefficients at level j using the relationship

$$c_k^j = \sum_i h_{k-2i}c_i^j + \sum_i g_{k-2i}d_i^{j-1}$$

Suppose that you have data values

$$y_k = f(x_k), k = 0,1,2, ..., N\text{-}1$$

at $N=2^J$ equally spaced points x_k. It turns out that the values $2^{-J/2}y_k$ are good approximations of the scaling coefficients c_k^J. Then, using the recurrence formula, you can find c_k^{J-1} and d_k^{J-1}, $k = 0,1,2, ..., N/2\text{-}1$. The discrete wavelet transform of the y_k at level J-1 consists of the $N/2$ scaling and $N/2$ detail coefficients at level J-1. A technical point that arises is that in applying the recurrence relationships to finite data, a few values of the c_k^J for $k<0$ or $k \geq N$ may be needed. One way to cope with this difficulty is to extend the sequence c_k^J to the left and right using some specified boundary treatment.

Continuing by replacing the scaling coefficients at any level j by the scaling and detail coefficients at level j-1 yields a sequence of N coefficients

$$\{c^0{}_0, d^0{}_0, d^1{}_0, d^1{}_1, d^2{}_0, d^2{}_1, d^2{}_2, d^2{}_3, d^3{}_1, ..., d^3{}_7, ..., d^{J-1}{}_0,$$
$$..., d^{J-1}{}_{N/2-1}\}$$

This sequence is the finite discrete wavelet transform of the input data $\{y_k\}$. At any level j_0, the finite dimensional approximation of the function $f(x)$ is

$$f(x) \approx \sum_k c_k^{j0} \varphi_{j0,k}(x) + \sum_{j=j0}^{J-1} \sum_k d_k^j \psi_{j,k}(x)$$

Obstructive sleep apnea syndrome (OSAS) is a respiratory disorder characterized by the repeated cessations of breathing during sleep due to obstruction of the upper airways. Classic features include excessive snoring, nocturnal hypoxemia, and disruption of normal sleep patterns. Excessive daytime sleepiness has been reported in a majority of the individuals with the disorder and has been associated with difficulty in maintaining adequate arousal to complete occupational or domestic activities. Sleepiness during driving is particularly problematic, and individuals with OSAS are at higher risk for motor vehicle accidents.

OSAS and related deficits have been reported across a range of neuropsychological domains, including motor speed, attention, information processing speed, working memory, long-term episodic memory and executive control. The etiologies of such impairments have been explored in number of studies.

Ridge Regression

Below, it shows four different fits (the red curves) to a training set of $p=50$ patterns randomly sampled from the sine wave

$$y=\sin(12x)$$

between $x=0$ and $x=1$ with Gaussian noise of standard deviation $\sigma=0.1$ added. The training set input-output pairs are shown by blue circles and

the true target by the dashed curves. The model used is a radial basis function network with $m = 50$ Gaussian functions of width $r = 0.05$, whose positions coincide with the training set input points. Each fit uses standard ridge regression, but with four different values of the regularization parameter λ.

The first fit (Figure 4, top left) is for $\lambda = 1 \times 10^{-10}$ and is too rough; high weights have not been penalized enough. The last fit (bottom right) is for $\lambda = 1 \times 10^5$ and is too smooth; high weights have been penalized too much. The other two fits are for $\lambda = 1 \times 10^{-5}$ (top right) and $\lambda = 1$ (bottom left), which are just about right; there is not much to choose between them.

The variation of the effective number of parameters, γ, as a function of λ is shown in the figure below. Clearly γ decreases monotonically as λ increases and the RBF network loses flexibility. The other figure shows the root-mean-squared-error (RMSE) as a function of λ. RMSE was calculated using an array of 250 noiseless samples of the target between $x=0$ and $x=1$. Figure 5 sug-

Figure 4. Our different RBF fits (solid curves) to data (crosses) sampled from a sine wave (dashed curve)

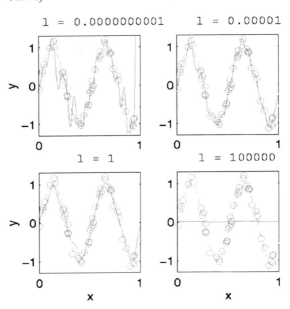

Figure 5. RMSE as functions of λ. The optimal value is shown with a star

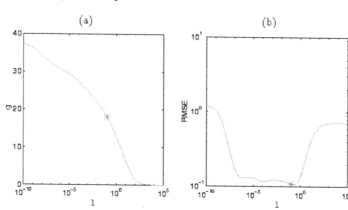

Figure 6. GCV as functions of λ with the optimal value shown with a star

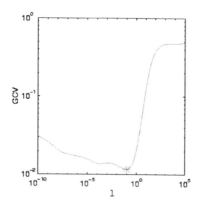

gests λ≈0.1 as the best value (minimum RMSE) for the regularisation parameter.

In real applications where the target is, of course, unknown, we do not, unfortunately, have access to RMSE. Then we must use one of the model selection criteria to find parameters such as λ. The solid red in Figure 6 shows the variation of GCV over a range of λ values. The re-estimation formula based on GCV gives $\hat{\lambda} = 0.10$ starting from the initial value of $\hat{\lambda} = 0.01$. Note, however, that had we started the re-estimation at $\hat{\lambda} = 10^{-5}$, then the local minima at $\hat{\lambda} = 2.1 \times 10^{-4}$ would have been the final resting place. The values of γ and RMSE at the optimum, $\hat{\lambda} = 0.1$, are marked with stars in the figures above.

The values $\hat{\lambda}_j = 0.1$ were used to initialize a local ridge regression algorithm, which continually sweeps through the regularization parameters optimizing each in turn until the GCV error prediction converges. This algorithm reduced the error prediction from an initial value of $\hat{\sigma}^2 = 0.016$ at the optimal global parameter value to $\hat{\sigma}^2 = 0.009$. At the same time, 18 regularization parameters ended up with an optimal value of ∞, enabling the 18 corresponding hidden units to be pruned from the network.

CASE DESCRIPTION

Time Series Analysis

The use of SAS/ETS has been well established, and now there exists a point-and-click interface in SAS to develop time series models. Data were aggregated into left lobe and right lobe data. Data averaged for the left side of the brain will represent the dependent or response variable (y) and data averaged for the right side of the brain will represent the independent or predictor variable (x). Because there is only one response and one predictor variable, it is tempting to use linear regression to forecast one set of data based on the other. However, using linear regression would result in a less precise model. Because time also

Figure 7. A patient with period oscillations

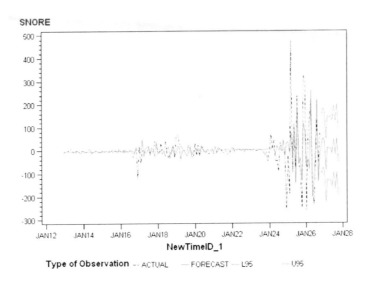

Figure 8. A patient with no oscillations

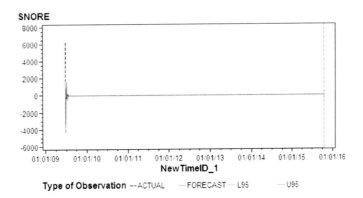

represents a predictor variable, the data will likely exhibit autocorrelation. Autocorrelation indicates that the most recent measurements are dependent on, or predictable from, past observations. This is often the case in time series data, since the observations in the data are usually not independent from one another.

Diagnosis is based on lab test and patient history.

The Data for these time series model in figures 7 and 8 are taken from the Sleep Center of Department of Pediatrics at University of Louisville, Kentucky.

These time series models were generated based on stepwise autoregressive. Also, we assume that the model has 95% confidence interval and the degree of time is linear.

We can see from the figure 7 that snoring in this particular patient is at a regular interval. At certain times, it is very low but it has become very strong. Snoring happens due to the fact of obstructive sleep. Similarly in figure 8, this patient has no obstructive sleep issues and hence not much of snoring is recorded for this patient.

Wavelet Analysis

The data were measured by the scalp Electroencephalography, or EEG. These are brain waves patterns, which carry very important information recorded on electronic impulses. The data were originally stored in EDF format (European Database Format), which is commonly used for brain wave patterns, and which must be translated into SAS. We are interested in EEG patterns that are related to learning disabilities, using data mining techniques to uncover information. Since high frequencies occur in discrete intervals, we model brain function using discrete wavelets analysis to decode the information. In SAS /IML, we can model the EEG using wavelet analysis to see if a particular wave is associated with a level of cognitive functioning. Due to the size of the original data set, we used a 1% sample to get the given plot in Figure 9.

The discrete wavelet transform decomposes a function as a sum of basis functions called wavelets. These basis functions have the property that they can be obtained by dilating and translating two basic types of wavelets known as the *scaling function* or *father wavelet* φ and the *mother wavelet* ψ. These translates and dilations are defined as follows:

$$\varphi_{j,k}(x) = 2^{j/2}\varphi(2^j x - k)$$
$$\psi_{j,k}(x) = 2^{j/2}\psi(2^j x - k)$$

So, we can now approximate our original EEG data using the final linear combination of the above functions

$$f(x) \approx \sum_k c_k^{j0}\varphi_{j0,k}(x) + \sum_{j=j0}^{J-1}\sum_k d_k^j\psi_{j,k}(x)$$

The $f(x)$ function defined above is the most central idea in using the wavelet analysis for data of this nature. It essentially captures the high and low frequencies of the EEG.

.We ran the following SAS/ IML code to produce the figure 10a, 10b, 11a, 11b. These figures were from two different data sets.

```
%wavginit;
proc iml;
%wavinit;
use sasuser.iml610NCB;
read all var{F1} into absorbance;
optn = &waveSpec; /* optn=j(1,4,.); */
```

Figure 9. Line plot of 1% of the original data

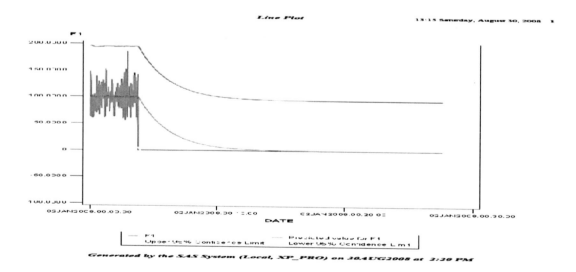

416

```
optn[&family] = &daubechies; /* optn[3] =
1; */
optn[&member] = 3; /* optn[4] = 3; */
optn[&boundary] = &polynomial; /* optn[1]
= 3; */
optn[&degree] = &linear; /* optn[2] = 1;
*/
call wavft(decomp,absorbance,optn);
call wavprint(decomp,&summary);
call wavprint(decomp,&detailCoeffs,1,4);
call wavget(tLevel,decomp,&topLevel);
call wavget(noiseCoeffs,decomp,&detailCoe
ffs,tLevel-1);
```

```
noiseScale=mad(noiseCoeffs,"nmad");
print "Noise scale = " noiseScale;
call coefficientPlot(decomp,,,,, "Wavelet
Comparison");
%wavhelp(coefficientPlot);
call coefficientPlot(decomp,, 7,,
'uniform',"Wavelet Comparison");
call coefficientPlot(decomp,&SureShrin
k,6,,, "Wavelet Comparison");
```

Above in the Figures 10a and 11a, we compute the wavelet decomposition. Coefficients of these decompositions for the family of Daubechies

Figure 10.

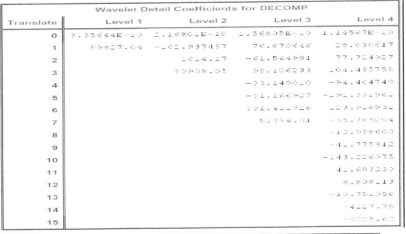

Wavelet Detail Coefficients for DECOMP				
Translate	Level 1	Level 2	Level 3	Level 4
0	3.35644E-10	2.16801E-10	1.56805E-10	1.14567E-10
1	99827.04	-162.937437	76.670646	28.030617
2		1614.17	-61.564981	77.724927
3		80909.03	98.106233	104.485759
4			-33.149010	-94.464749
5			-51.166927	-191.331961
6			881.411726	123.916951
7			51754.01	-35.765204
8				-12.938600
9				-41.775812
10				-143.226073
11				41.693230
12				8.808113
13				-10.751056
14				-4127.79
15				-8223.62

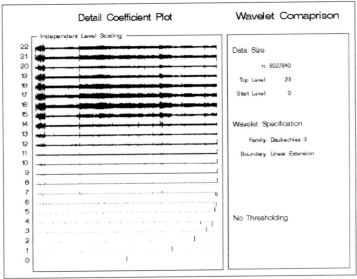

Figure 11.

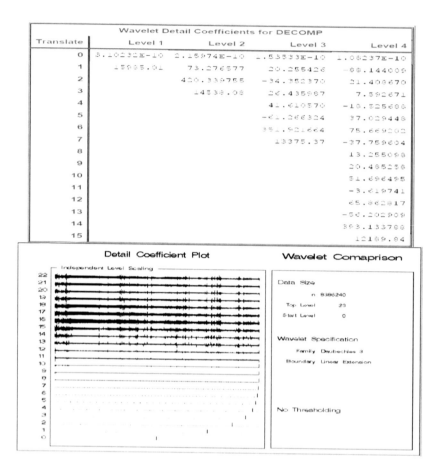

wavelet for D2-D16 (Multiple of 2) are given. The wavelet coefficients are derived by reversing the order of the scaling function coefficients and then reversing the sign of every second one. Mathematically, this looks like $bk = (-1)kaN - 1 - k$, where k is the coefficient index, b is a coefficient of the wavelet sequence and a is a coefficient of the scaling sequence. N is the wavelet index.

In Figures 10b and 11b, the detail coefficients at each level are scaled independently. The oscillations present in the data are captured in the detailed coefficients at levels 12, 13, and 14. There are two data sets, one with children with learning disorders and another group without, but both have sleep apnea. As a control, we have been blinded as to which group is which. At first glance, we notice that 10b has a lot more thick bands of signals when compared to 11b. Thus, it suggests that 10b has lot more information and more hidden patterns, which could be of a similar nature to the signal in 11b.

Since this is an ongoing study, we are using other Data mining algorithms to study further into these isolated oscillations to detect patterns. These include time series analysis and ridge regression.

CURRENT AND FUGURE CHALLENGES FACING THE ORGANIZATION

The use of all of these models remains under-developed when researching problems with sleep apnea and cognitive functioning. This study represents the beginning; much more effort will be required before these techniques are used routinely. This is also the beginning of an ongoing study to examine the relationship between sleep apnea and learning disabilities.

REFERENCES

Johnson, M. H., deHaan, M., Oliver, A., Smith, W., Hatzakis, H., & Tucker, L. (2001). Recording and analyzing high-density event related potentials with infants using the Geodesic Sensor Net. *Developmental Neuropsychology, 19*(3), 295–323. doi:10.1207/S15326942DN1903_4

Kook, H., Gupta, L., Kota, S., & Molfese, D. (2007). *A dynamic multi-channel decision-fusion strategy to classify differential brain activity.* Paper presented at the 29th Annual International Conference of the IEEE EMBS, Lyon, France.

Mayes, L. C., Molfese, D. L., Key, A. P., & Hunter, N. C. (2005). Event-related potentials in cocaine-exposed children during a Stroop task. *Neurotoxicology and Teratology, 27*, 797–813. doi:10.1016/j.ntt.2005.05.011

Tucker, D. (1993). Spatial sampling of head electrical fields: the geodesic sensor net. *Electroencephalography and Clinical Neurophysiology, 87*(3), 154–163. doi:10.1016/0013-4694(93)90121-B

ADDITIONAL READING

Cazelles, B., Chavez, M., Magny, G. C., Guegan, J. F., Hales, S., & Cazelles, B. (2007). Time-dependent spectral analysis of epidemiological time-series with wavelets. *Journal of the Royal Society, Interface, 4*(15), 625–636. doi:10.1098/rsif.2007.0212

Demongeot, J. (2007). A brief history about analytic tools in medical imaging: splines, wavelets, singularities and partial differential equations. In *Conference Proceedings: Annual International Conference of the IEEE Engineering in Medicine & . Biology and Society, 2007*, 3474–3480.

Katz, S. L. (2009). Assessment of sleep-disordered breathing in pediatric neuromuscular diseases. *Pediatrics, 123*(Suppl 4), 222–225. doi:10.1542/peds.2008-2952E

Poza, J., Caminal, P., Vallverdu, M., Hornero, R., Romero, S., Barbanoj, M. J., et al. (2007). Study of the EEG changes during the combined ingestion of alcohol and H1-antihistamines by using the wavelet transform. *Conference Proceedings: Annual International Conference of the IEEE Engineering in Medicine & Biology Society, 2007*, 23-26.

Ramachandran, S. K., & Josephs, L. A. (2009). A meta-analysis of clinical screening tests for obstructive sleep apnea. *Anesthesiology, 110*(4), 928–939. doi:10.1097/ALN.0b013e31819c47b6

Shidahara, M., Ikoma, Y., Kershaw, J., Kimura, Y., Naganawa, M., & Watabe, H. (2007). PET kinetic analysis: wavelet denoising of dynamic PET data with application to parametric imaging. *Annals of Nuclear Medicine, 21*(7), 379–386. doi:10.1007/s12149-007-0044-9

Tonelli de Oliveira, A. C., Martinez, D., Vasconcelos, L. F., Cadaval Goncalves, S., do Carmo Lenz, M., & Costa Fuchs, S. (2009). Diagnosis of obstructive sleep apnea syndrome and its outcomes with home portable monitoring. *Chest, 135*(2), 330–336. doi:10.1378/chest.08-1859

Compilation of References

Ait-Khaled, N., Enarson, D., Bissell, K., & Billo, N. (2007). Access to inhaled corticosteroids is key to improving quality of care for asthma in developing countries. *Allergy, 62*(3), 230–236. doi:10.1111/j.1398-9995.2007.01326.x

Akita, R. M. (2002). Silver Bullet Solutions Inc., San Diego, CA. "User Based Data Fusion Approaches". Information Fusion. In *Proceedings of the Fifth International Conference*. (Volume: 2, pp 1457- 1462).

Alberg, A. J. (2003). Epidemiology of Lung Cancer. *Chest, 123*, 21–49. doi:10.1378/chest.123.1_suppl.21S

American Diabetes Association. (2008, March). Economic Costs of Diabetes in the U.S. in 2007. *DIABETES CARE, 31*(3).Retrieved Dec.10th, 2008, from http://care.diabetesjournals.org/misc/econcosts.pdf

American Diabetes Association. (n.d.). *Diabetes and Cardiovascular (Heart) Disease*.Retrieved Feb.5th, 2009, fromhttp://www.diabetes.org/diabetes-statistics/heart-disease.jsp

Aneziokoro, C. O., Cannon, J. P., Pachucki, C. T., & Lentino, J. R.. The effectiveness and safety of oral linezolid for the primary and secondary treatment of osteomyelitis. *Journal of Chemotherapy (Florence, Italy), 17*(6), 643–650.

Angus, L. D., Gorecki, P. J., Mourello, R., Ortega, R. E., & Adamski, J.(n.d.). DRG, costs and reimbursement following Roux-en-Y gastric bypass: an economic appraisal . In Potts, S. G. (Ed.), *Data Mining to Determine Characteristics of High-Cost Diabetics in a Medicaid Population*.

Anonymous. (2006, June). *The GLIMMIX Procedure*. Retrieved Nov.10th, 2008, from http://support.sas.com/rnd/app/papers/glimmix.pdf

Anonymous. (n.d.). *Cluster Analysis*. Retrieved Feb.20th, 2009, from http://www.statsoft.com/textbook/stcluan.html

Anonymous-1985 recommendations. (1985). Diphtheria, tetanus, and pertussis: guidelines for vaccine prophylaxis and other preventive measures. Recommendation of the Immunication Practices Advisory Committee. Centers for Disease Control, Department of Health and Human Services. *Annals of Internal Medicine, 103*(6), 896-905.

Anonymous-asthma. (2007). Trends in asthma morbidity and mortality. Retrieved September, 2008, from http://www.lungusa.org/site/c.dvLUK9O0E/b.22884/k.7CE3/Asthma_Research__Studies.htm

Anonymous-attorney. (2008). *Gardasil Lawyers*. Retrieved 2008, from http://www.brownandcrouppen.com/gardasil-attorney.asp

Anonymous-Mayoasthma. (2008). Asthma. Retrieved September, 2008, from http://www.mayoclinic.com/health/asthma/DS00021/DSECTION=treatments-and-drugs

Anonymous-Medstat. (2007). *Thomson Healthcare*. Retrieved from http://home.thomsonhealthcare.com/

Anonymous-MEPS. (2007). *Medical Expenditure Panel Survey* [Electronic Version]. Retrieved December, 2007, from http://www.meps.ahrq.gov/mepsweb/.

Copyright © 2010, IGI Global, distributing in print or electronic forms without written permission of IGI Global is prohibited.

Anonymous-MMWR. (2004, September 3). Suspension of rotavirus vaccine after reports of intussusception-United States, 1999. *MMWR*, 786–789.

Anonymous-MMWR. (2008). Syncope after vaccination-United States, January 2005-2007. *MMWR*, *57*(17), 457–460.

Anonymous-MMWRpertussis. (2002). Pertussis-United States, 1997-2000. *MMWR*, *51*(4), 73–76.

Anonymous-NICE. (2008). *Drug Eluting Stents for the Treatment of coronary artery disease*. London: National Institute for Health and Clinical Excellence.

Anonymous-NIHasthma. (2008). What is Asthma? Retrieved September, 2008, from http://www.nhlbi.nih.gov/health/dci/Diseases/Asthma/Asthma_WhatIs.html

Anonymous-NIS. (2007). *Overview of the National Inpatient Sample*. Retrieved December, 2007, from http://www.hcup-us.ahrq.gov/nisoverview.jsp.

Anonymous-NIS. (2008). *Introduction to the HCUP Nationwide Inpatient Sample (NIS)*. Retrieved 2005, from http://www.hcup-us.ahrq.gov/db/nation/nis/NIS_Introduction_2005.jsp

Anonymous-VAERS. (2008). Vaccine Adverse Event Reporting System. Retrieved September, 2008, from http://vaers.hhs.gov/

Anonymous-asthma. (2007). *Trends in asthma morbidity and mortality*. Retrieved September, 2008, from http://www.lungusa.org/site/c.dvLUK9O0E/b.22884/k.7CE3/Asthma_Research__Studies.htm

Antibiotics. (n.d.). Retrieved 2007, from http://www.emedicinehealth.com/antibiotics/article_em.htm

Austin, P. C., Alter, D. A., & Tu, J. V. (2003). The use of fixed- and random-effects models for classifying hospitals as mortality outliers: a monte carlos assessment. *Medical Decision Making*, *23*, 526–539. doi:10.1177/0272989X03258443

Barker, N. (2005). *A Practical Introduction to the Bootstrap Using the SAS System*. In Proceedings of SAS Conference, Oxford Pharmaceutical Science.

Barlow, W. E., White, E., Ballard-Barbash, R., Vacek, P. M., Titus-Ernstoff, L., & Carney, P. A. (2006). Prospective breast cancer risk prediction model for women undergoing screening mammography. *Journal of the National Cancer Institute*, *98*(17), 1204–1214.

Barlow, W. E., White, E., Ballard-Barbash, R., Vacek, P. M., Titus-Ernstoff, L., & Carney, P. A. (2006). Prospective breast cancer risk prediction model for women undergoing screening mammography. *Journal of the National Cancer Institute*, *98*(17), 1204–1214.

Barnes Jewish Hospital. (n.d.). Retrieved 2007, from http://www.bjc.org

Barrentt, B., & Wi. C.-E. A. (2002, March 11). Retrieved from http://www.here.research.med.va.gov/FAQ_AL.htm.

Barrentt, P. (2002, March 11). *W. i. C.-E. A.* Retrieved from http://www.here.research.med.va.gov/FAQ_AL.htm

Berry, M. J. A., & Linoff, G. (1999). *Mastering Data Mining: The Art and Science of Customer Relationship Management*. New York: John Wiley & Sons, Inc.

Berzuini, C., & Larizza, C. (1996). A unified approach for modeling longitudinal and failure time data, with application in medical monitoring. *IEEE Transactions on Pattern Analysis and Machine Intelligence*, *16*(2), 109–123. doi:10.1109/34.481537

Bines, J. E. (2005). Rotavirus vaccines and intussusception risk. *Current Opinion in Gastroenterology*, *21*(1), 20–25.

Binh An Diep, P. H. F. C., Graber, C. J., Szumowski, J. D., Miller, L. G., Han, L. L., Chen, J. H., et al. (n.d.). *Emergence of Multidrug-Resistant, Community-Associated, Methicillin-Resistant Staphylococcus aureus Clone USA300 in Men Who Have Sex with Men (Annals of Internal Medicine website)*. Retrieved February 19, 2008, from: http://www.annals.org/cgi/content/full/0000605-200802190-00204v1

Blanchard, E. (2001). *Irritable bowel syndrome: psychosocial assessment and treatment*. Washington, DC: American Psychological Association. doi:10.1037/10393-000

Blanchard, E., Lackner, J., Carosella, A., Jaccard, J., Krassner, S., & Kuhn, E. (2008). The role of stress in symptom exacerbation among IBS patients. *Journal of Psychosomatic Research, 64*, 119–128. doi:10.1016/j.jpsychores.2007.10.010

Blue Cross Blue Shield of Texas. (n.d.). *W. I. t. R. A. C.* Retrieved from http://www.bcbstx.com/provider/bluechoice_solutions_tool_raci.htm.

Brophy, J., & Erickson, L. (2004). An economic analysis of drug eluting coronary stents: a Quebec perspective. *AETMIS, 4*(4), 38.

Brophy, J., & Erickson, L. (2005). *Cost Effectiveness of Drug Eluting Coronary Stents A Quebec Perspective.* Cambridge, UK: Cambridge University Press.

Brown, R. (2001). Behavioral issues in asthma management. *Pediatric Pulmonology, 21*(Supplement), 26–30. doi:10.1002/ppul.2003

Brown, R. (2001). Behavioral issues in asthma management. *Pediatric Pulmonology, 21*(Supplement), 26–30. doi:10.1002/ppul.2003

Bruin, J. S. d., Cocx, T. K., Kosters, W. A., Laros, J. F., & Kok, J. N. (2006). *Data mining approaches to criminal career analysis.* Paper presented at the Proceedings of the Sixth International Conference on Data Mining, Hong Kong.

Brus, T., Swinnen, G., Vanhoof, K., & Wets, G. (2004). Building an association rules framework to improve produce assortment decisions. *Data Mining and Knowledge Discovery, 8*, 7–23. doi:10.1023/B:DAMI.0000005256.79013.69

Camen DeNavas-Walt, B. D. P., Lee, C. H. (n.d.). *Income, Poverty, and Health Insurance Coverage in the United States:2004.* US Census Burea News (Press Kit/ Reports. P60-229).

Center for Studying Health System Change. (2004). Retrieved 2007, from http://www.hschange.com/CONTENT/799/

Centers for Disease Control and Prevention. (2007). *National Diabetes Fact Sheet, 2007.* Retrieved Nov.3rd, 2008, from http://www.cdc.gov/diabetes/pubs/pdf/ndfs_2007.pdf

Centers for Disease Control. (1996). Retrieved from http://www.cdc.gov/nchs/products/pubs/pubd/series/sr13/150-141/sr13_150.htm

Centers for Disease Control. (2003). Retrieved 2007, from http://www.cdc.gov/nchs/products/pubs/pubd/ad/300-291/ad293.htm

Centers for Disease Control. (n.d.). Retrieved 2007, from http://www.cdc.gov/nchs/about/major/ahcd/ahcd1.htm

Cerrito, J. C. & Pharm (Personal Communication, October, 2005).

Cerrito, P. (2007) *Exploratory Data Analysis: An Introduction to Data Analysis Using SAS.* Retrieved from Lulu.com

Cerrito, P. (2008). *Student Papers in Introductory Statistics for Mathematics Majors.* Retrieved from Lulu.com

Cerrito, P. (2010). *Clinical Data Mining for Physician Decision Making and Investigating Health Outcomes.* Hershey, PA: IGI Global Publishing.

Cerrito, P. B. (2009). *Data Mining Healthcare and Clinical Databases.* Cary, NC: SAS Press.

Cerrito, P. B. (2009). *Text Mining Techniques for Healthcare Provider Quality Determination: Methods for Rank Comparisons.* Hershey, PA: IGI Global Publishing.

Cerrito, P. B., & Cerrito, J. C. (2006). *Data and text mining the electronic medical record to improve care and to lower costs.* Paper presented at the SUGI31, San Francisco.

Cerrito, P. C., & Cerrito, J. (2008). C. *Survival Data Mining: Treatment of Chronic Illness.* in *SAS Global Forum*, SAS Institute Inc. Retrieved 2009, from http://sasglobalforum.org

Cerrito, P., & Cerrito, J. C. (2006). Data and Text Mining the Electronic Medical Record to Improve Care and to Lower Costs [Electronic Version]. In *SUGI 31 Proceedings, 31.* Retrieved January, 2007, from http://www2.sas.com/proceedings/sugi31/077-31.pdf.

Cerrito, P., Badia, A., & Cerrito, J. (2005). *Data mining medication prescriptions for a representative national sample.* Paper presented at: PharmaSug 2005, Phoenix, AZ.

Chan, E., Zhan, C., & Homer, C. J. (2002). *Health care use and costs for children with attention-deficit/hyperactivity disorder: national estimates from the medical expenditure panel survey.* Academy for Health Services Research and Health Policy.

CHi-Ming, C., Hsu-Sung, K., Shu-Hui, C., Hong-Jen, C., Der-Ming, L., Tabar, L., et al. (2005). Computer-aided disease prediction system: development of application software with SAS component language. *Journal of Evaluation in Clinical Practice, 11*(2), 139–159. doi:10.1111/j.1365-2753.2005.00514.x

Chipps, B., & Spahn, J. (2006). What are the determinates of asthma control? *The Journal of Asthma, 43*(8), 567–572. doi:10.1080/02770900600619782

Circulation, American Heart Association. (2006) *Heart disease and Strok Statistics.* Retrieved from http://circ.ahajournals.org/cgi/reprint/113/6/e85.pdf.

Circulation, J. A. H. A. (n.d.). *Heart Association Statistics Committee and Stroke Statistics Subcommittee.* Retrieved from http://circ.ahajournals.org/cgi/reprint/113/6/e85.pdf.

Claus, E. B. (2001). Risk models used to counsel women for breast and ovarian cancer: a guide for clinicians. *Familial Cancer, 1,* 197–206. doi:10.1023/A:1021135807900

Cleveland Clinic. (n.d.). Retrieved from: http://www.clevelandclinic.org/health/health-info/docs/2700/2702.asp?index=9495

Cluett, J. (2006) *"What is arthroscopic surgery?"* Retrieved from http://orthopedics.about.com/cs/arthroscopy/a/arthroscopy.htm

Cohen, B. (2008). *Drug-Eluting Stent overview.* Retrieved from http://www.ptca.org/stent.html

Cohen, D. J., Bakhai, A., Shi, C., Githiora, L., Lavelle, T., & Berezin, R. H. (2004). *Cost-Effectiveness of Sirolimus-Eluting Stents for Treatment of Complex Coronary Stenoses.* Boston: Harvard Clinical Research Institute.

Cohen, J. W., Monheit, A. C., Beauregard, K. M., Cohen, S. B., Lefkowitz, D. C., & Potter, D. E. (1996). The Medical Expenditure Panel Survey: a national health information resource. *Inquiry, 33*(4), 373–389.

Cohen, S. B. (2002). The Medical Expenditure Panel Survey: an overview. [Research Support, U.S. Gov't, P.H.S.]. *Effective Clinical Practice: ECP, 5*(3Suppl), E1.

Cohen, S. B., & Buchmueller, T. (2006). Trends in medical care costs, coverage, use, and access: research findings from the Medical Expenditure Panel Survey. *Medical Care, 44*(5Suppl), 1–3.

Commission, M. P. A. (2006, June). MedPac Data Book 2006: Section 7: Acute inpatient services. Retrieved from Center of Medicare and Medicaid, http://www.cms.hhs.gov/AcuteInpatientPPS/downloads/outlier_example.pdf

Conboy-Ellis, K. (2006). Asthma pathogenesis and management. *The Nurse Practitioner, 31,* 24–44. doi:10.1097/00006205-200611000-00006

Cox, J. L. A. (2005). Some limitations of a proposed linear model for antimicrobial risk management. *Risk Analysis, 25*(6), 1327–1332. doi:10.1111/j.1539-6924.2005.00703.x

Creed, F. (1999). The relationship between psychosocial parameters and outcome in irritable bowel syndrome. *The American Journal of Medicine, 107,* 74S–80S. doi:10.1016/S0002-9343(99)00083-2

Creed, F., Guthrie, E., Ratcliffe, J., Fernandes, L., Rigby, C., & Tomenson, B. (2005). Does psychological treatment help only those patients with severe irritable bowel syndrome who also have a concurrent psychiatric disorder? *The Australian and New Zealand Journal of Psychiatry, 39,* 807–815.

Cugnet, P. (1997). *Confidence Interval Estimation for Distribution Systems Power Consumption By using the Bootstrap Method.* Virginia Tech University.

David, J., Bakhai, C., Shi, A., Githiora, C., Lavelle, L., & Berezin, T. (2004). Cost-Effectiveness of Sirolimus-Eluting Stents for Treatment of Complex Coronary Stenoses. *ACC Current Journal Review, 13*(11), 55–56. doi:10.1016/j.accreview.2004.10.053

Demetriou, N., Tsami-Pandi, A., & Parashis, A. (1995). Compliance with suportive periodontal treatment in private Periodonatal Practice. A 14 year retrospective study. *Journal of Periodontology, 66*(2), 145–149.

Drossman, D., Camilleri, M., Mayer, E., & Whitehead, W. (2002). AGA technical review on irritable bowel syndrome. *Gastroenterology, 123*, 2108–2131. doi:10.1053/gast.2002.37095

Earle, C. C., & Earle, C. C. (2004). Outcomes research in lung cancer. [Review]. *Journal of the National Cancer Institute. Monographs, 33*, 56–77. doi:10.1093/jncimonographs/lgh001

Eleuteri, A., Tagliaferri, R., Milano, L., Sansone, G., Agostino, D. D., Placido, S. D., et al. (2003). *Survival analysis and neural networks.* Paper presented at the 2003 Conference on Neural Networks, Portland, Oregon.

Faculty Practice Plan boosts emergency room operations.(1999). Retrieved 2007, from http://record.wustl.edu/archive/1999/09-09-99/articles/practice.html

Fajadet, J. P. M., Hayashi, E. B., et al. (2002, March 18) *American College of Cardiology 51st Annual Scientific Session* (Presentation # 0032-1). Retrieved from http://www.stjohns.com/doctorclark/AnswerPage.aspx?drclark_id=22

Fausett, L. (n.d.). *Fundamentals of Neural Networks: Architectures, Algorithms, and Applications.* Englewood Cliffs, NJ: Prentice Hall.

FDA. (2003, April). *Food and Drug administration news, Media Inquiries: 301-827-6242, Consumer Inquiries: 888-INFO-FDA.* Retrieved from http://www.fda.gov/bbs/topics/NEWS/2003/NEW00896.html

Fisher, B., Anderson, S., & Bryant, J. (2002). Twenty-Year Follow-Up of a Randomized Trial Comparing Total Mastectomy, Lumpectomy, and Lumpectomy plus Irradiation for the Treatment of Invasive Breast Cancer. *The New England Journal of Medicine, 347*(16), 1233–1241. doi:10.1056/NEJMoa022152

Fisher, B., Anderson, S., & Redmond, C. K. (1995). Reanalysis and Results after 12 years of Follow up in a Randomized Clinical Trial Comparing Total Mastectomy with Lumpectomy with or without Irradiation in the Treatment of Breast Cancer. *The New England Journal of Medicine, 333*(22), 1456–1461. doi:10.1056/NEJM199511303332203

Foster, D. P., & Stine, R. A. (2004). Variable selection in data mining: building a predictive model for bankruptcy. *Journal of the American Statistical Association, 99*(466), 303–313. doi:10.1198/016214504000000287

Foster, D. P., & Stine, R. A. (2004). Variable selection in data miing: building a predictive model for bankruptcy. *Journal of the American Statistical Association, 99*(466), 303–313. doi:10.1198/016214504000000287

Freedman, A. N., Seminara, D., Mitchell, H., Hartge, P., Colditz, G. A., & Ballard-Barbash, R. (2005). Cancer risk prediction models: a workshop on developmnet, evaluation, and application. *Journal of the National Cancer Institute, 97*(10), 715–723.

Freedman, L. S., & Pee, D. (1989). Return to a note on screening regression equations. The American Statistician, 43, 279–282. doi:10.2307/2685389doi:10.2307/2685389

Freedman, N. (2005). Cancer risk prediction models: a workshop on development, evaluation, and application. *Journal of the National Cancer Institute, 97*, 715–723.

Friedman, J., Hastie, T. & Tibshirani, R. (n.d.). *The Elements of Statistical Learning: Data Mining, Inference and Prediction.* New York: Springer Verlag.

Gail, M. H. (1989). Projecting individualized probabilities of developing breast cancer for white females who are being examined annually. *Journal of the National Cancer Institute, 81*, 1879–1886. doi:10.1093/jnci/81.24.1879

Gardner, P., Pickering, L., Orenstein, W., Gershon, A., & Nichol, K. (2002). Infectious diseases society of

America. Guidelines for quality standards for immunization. *Clinical Infectious Diseases*, 35(5), 503–511. doi:10.1086/341965

Gaylor, D. W. (2005). Risk/benefit assessments of human diseases: optimum dose for intervention. *Risk Analysis*, 25(1), 161–168. doi:10.1111/j.0272-4332.2005.00575.x

Gillette, B. (2005, September). *Manage Health Care Executive, E. G. c. W. I. o. H. S. o. C. a. Q.* Retrieved from http://www.managedhealthcareexecytive.com/mhe/article.

Gillette, B. (2005, September). *Manage Health Care Executive.* Retrieved from http://www.managedhealthcareexecytive.com/mhe/article

Giudiei, P., & Passerone, G. (2002). Data mining of association structures to model consumer behaviour. *Computational Statistics & Data Analysis*, 38, 533–541. doi:10.1016/S0167-9473(01)00077-9

Giudier, P., & Passerone, G. (2002). Data mining of association structures to model consumer behavior. *Computational Statistics & Data Analysis*, 38(4), 533–541. doi:10.1016/S0167-9473(01)00077-9

Government Accounting Office. (2002). Retrieved 2007, from www.gao.gov/new.items/d03460.pdf, www.gao.gov/new.items/d03769t.pdf

Guevara, J. P., Mandell, D. S., Rostain, A. L., Zhao, H., Hadley, T. R., & Guevara, J. P. (2003). National estimates of health services expenditures for children with behavioral disorders: an analysis of the medical expenditure panel survey. [Research Support, Non-U.S. Gov't]. *Pediatrics*, 112(6), 440. doi:10.1542/peds.112.6.e440

Hakim, S., Venegas, J. G., & Burton, J. D. (1976). The physics of the cranial cavity, hydrocephalus and normal pressure hydrocephalus: mechanical interpretation and mathematical model. Surgical Neurology, 5(3), 187–210. PubMed

Hall, D. L., & McMullen, S. A. H. (2004). *Mathematical Techniques in Multisensor Data Fusion.* Norwood, MA: Artech House, Inc.

Halpern, M. T., Yabroff, K. R., Halpern, M. T., & Yabroff, K. R. (2008). Prevalence of outpatient cancer treatment in the United States: estimates from the Medical Panel Expenditures Survey (MEPS). *Cancer Investigation*, 26(6), 647–651. doi:10.1080/07357900801905519

Hand, D. J., & Bolton, R. J. (2004). Pattern discovery and detection: a unified statistical methodology. *Journal of Applied Statistics*, 8, 885–924. doi:10.1080/0266476042000270518

Hand, D. J., & Bolton, R. J. (2004). Pattern discovery and detection: a unified statistical methodology. *Journal of Applied Statistics*, 8, 885–924. doi:10.1080/0266476042000270518

Hernandez, M. A., & Stolfo, S. J. (1998). Real-world data is dirty: data cleansing and the merge/purge problem. *Data Mining and Knowledge Discovery*, 2, 9–17. doi:10.1023/A:1009761603038

Hillilä, M., Hämäläinen, J., Heikkinen, M., & Färäkkilä, M. (2008). Gastrointestinal complaints among subjects with depressive symptoms in the general population. *Alimentary Pharmacology & Therapeutics*, 28, 648–654. doi:10.1111/j.1365-2036.2008.03771.x

Hopenhayn-Rich, C. (2001). Lung cancer in the commonwealth: A closer look at the data. *Lung Cancer Policy Brief 2001, 1*(2).

Hosking, J. R., Pednault, E. P., & Sudan, M. (1997). Statistical perspective on data mining. *Future Generation Computer Systems*, 13(2-3), 117–134. doi:10.1016/S0167-739X(97)00016-2

Howell. (2002). *Bootstrapping Medians.* Burlington, VT: University of Vermont.

Huang, J.-Q., Sridhar, S., & Hunt, R. H. (2002). Role of helicobacter pylori infection and non-steroidal anti-inflammatory drugs in peptic-ulcer disease: a meta-analysis. *Lancet, 359*(9300), 14,19.

ICD9.chrisendres website (n.d.). *Free online searchable ICD-9-CM.* Retrieved 2009, from www.ICD9.chrisendres.com

Iezzoni, L. I., Ash, A. S., Shwartz, M., Daley, J., Hughes, J. S., & Mackleman, Y. D. (1995). Predicting who dies depends on how severity is measured: implications for evaluating patient outcomes. *Annals of Internal Medicine, 123*(10), 763–770.

Igor Singer, M. (n.d.). *FRACP, FACP, FACC, FACA, Executive Medical Director, Cardiovascular Services, Methodist Medical Center.* Retrieved from http://week.com/health_med/health_med.asp?id=4495

Inadomi, J., Fennerty, M., & Bjorkman, D. (2003). Systematic review: the economic impact of irritable bowel syndrome. *Alimentary Pharmacology & Therapeutics, 18,* 671–682. doi:10.1046/j.1365-2036.2003.t01-1-01736.x

Institute, N. C. (2006). *The nation's investment in cancer research. A plan and budget proposal for the year 2006.* Retrieved from http://plan.cancer.gov/

Jackson, J., O'Malley, P., Tomkins, G., Balden, E., Santoro, J., & Kroenke, K. (2000). Treatment of functional gastrointestinal disorders with anti-depressants: a meta-analysis. *The American Journal of Medicine, 108,* 65–72. doi:10.1016/S0002-9343(99)00299-5

Jacobsen, R., Møller, H., & Mouritsen, A. (1999). Natural variation in the human sex ratio. Human Reproduction (Oxford, England), 14, 3120–3125. PubMeddoi:10.1093/humrep/14.12.3120doi:10.1093/humrep/14.12.3120

Jiang, T., & Tuxhilin, A. (2006). *Improving personalization solutions through optimal segmentation of customer bases.* Paper presented at the Proceedings of the Sixth International Conference on Data Mining, Hong Kong.

John, T. T., & Chen, P. (2006). Lognormal selection with applications to lifetime data. *IEEE Transactions on Reliability, 55*(1), 135–148. doi:10.1109/TR.2005.858098

Johnson, M. H., deHaan, M., Oliver, A., Smith, W., Hatzakis, H., & Tucker, L. (2001). Recording and analyzing high-density event related potentials with infants using the Geodesic Sensor Net. *Developmental Neuropsychology, 19*(3), 295–323. doi:10.1207/S15326942DN1903_4

Joint Commission on Healthcare Quality. (2004). Retrieved 2007, from www.jcrinc.com/generic.asp?durki=9649

Kannel, W. B. (1976). A general cardiovascular risk profile: the Framingham Study. *The American Journal of Cardiology, 38,* 46–51. doi:10.1016/0002-9149(76)90061-8

Kantardzic, M. (2003). *Data Mining: Concepts, Models, Methods, and Algorithms.* Hoboken, NJ: IEEE.

Keim, D. A., Mansmann, F., Schneidewind, J., & Ziegler, H. (2006). Challenges in visual data analysis. *Information Visualization, 2006,* 9–16.

Keucher, T. R., & Mealey, J. (1979). Long-term results after ventriculoatrial and ventriculoperitoneal shunting for infantile hydrocephalus. Journal of Neurosurgery, 50(2), 179–186. PubMeddoi:10.3171/jns.1979.50.2.0179doi:10.3171/jns.1979.50.2.0179

Kim, X., Back, Y., Rhee, D. W., & Kim, S.-H. (2005). *Analysis of breast cancer using data mining & statistical techniques.* Paper presented at the Proceedings of the Sixth International Conference on Software Engineering, Artificial Intelligence, Networking, and Parallel/Distributed Computing, Las Vegas, NV.

Kook, H., Gupta, L., Kota, S., & Molfese, D. (2007). *A dynamic multi-channel decision-fusion strategy to classify differential brain activity.* Paper presented at the 29th Annual International Conference of the IEEE EMBS, Lyon, France.

Krzysztof, J., Cios, G., & Moore, W. (2002). Uniqueness of Medical Data Mining. *Artificial Intelligence in Medicine, 26*(1), 1–24. doi:10.1016/S0933-3657(02)00049-0

Lavengood, K. A., & Kiser, P. (2007) Information Professionals in the Text Mine. *ONLINE, 31*(3) Retrieved Mar. 3rd, 2009, from http://www.infotoday.com/online/may07/Lavengood_Kiser.shtml

Law, A. W., Reed, S. D., Sundy, J. S., Schulman, K. A., Law, A. W., & Reed, S. D. (2003). *Direct costs of allergic rhinitis in the United States.* Estimates from the 1996 Medical Expenditure Panel Survey. Research Support,

U.S. Gov't, P.H.S.]. *The Journal of Allergy and Clinical Immunology, 111*(2), 296–300. doi:10.1067/mai.2003.68

Lee, S. (1995). *Predicting atmospheric ozone using neural networks as compared to some statistical methods.* Paper presented at the Northcon 95. I EEE Technical Applications Conference and Workshops Northcon95, Portland, Oregon.

Levy, R., Cain, K., Jarrett, M., & Heitkemper, M. (1997). The relationship between daily life stress and gastrointestinal symptoms in women with irritable bowel syndrome. *Journal of Behavioral Medicine, 20*, 177–193. doi:10.1023/A:1025582728271

Linoff, G. S. (2004). *Survival Data Mining for Customer Insight. 2007.* Retrieved from www.intelligententerprise. com/showArticle.jhtml?articleID=26100528

Loebstein, R., Katzir, I., Vasterman-Landes, J., Halkin, H., & Lomnicky, Y. (2008). Database assessment of the effectiveness of brand versus generic rosiglitazone in patients with type 2 diabetes mellitus. *Medical Science Monitor, 14*(6), 323–326.

Loren, K. (n.d.). *Heart Disease: Number One Killer.* Retrieved from http://www.heart-disease-bypass-surgery. com/data/footnotes/f5.htm

Louis Anthony Cox, J. (2005). Some limitations of a proposed linear model for antimicrobial risk management. *Risk Analysis, 25*(6), 1327–1332. doi:10.1111/j.1539-6924.2005.00703.x

Mannila, H. (1996). *Data mining: machine learning, statistics and databases.* Paper presented at the Eighth International Conference on Scientific and Statistical Database Systems, 1996. Proceedings, Stockholm.

Mauldin, P. D., Salgado, C. D., Durkalski, V. L., & Bosso, J. A. (2008). (n.d.). Nosocomial infections due to methicillin-resistant Staphylococcus aureus and vancomycin-resistant enterococcus: relationships with antibiotic use and cost drivers. *The Annals of Pharmacotherapy, 42*(3), 317–326. doi:10.1345/aph.1K501

Mayes, L. C., Molfese, D. L., Key, A. P., & Hunter, N. C. (2005). Event-related potentials in cocaine-exposed children during a Stroop task. *Neurotoxicology and Teratology, 27*, 797–813. doi:10.1016/j.ntt.2005.05.011

Mc, L. T. C., & Allaster, D. L. (n.d.). *B. U. o. S. E. S. t. F. a. T. S.*Fort Lee, VA . *Us Army Logistics Management Collage.*

McGarry, K., Schoeni, R. F., McGarry, K., & Schoeni, R. F. (2005). *Widow(er) poverty and out-of-pocket medical expenditures near the end of life. Research Support, N.I.H.* Extramural.

McKerrow, P. J., & Volk, S. J. (1996, November). "A Systems Approach to Data Fusion". In *Proceedings of ADFS-96, IEEE* (pp 217-222).

McLaughlin, J. F., Loeser, J. D., & Roberts, T. S. (1997). Acquired hydrocephalus associated with superior vena cava syndrome in infants. Child's Nervous System, 13, 59–63. PubMeddoi:10.1007/s003810050042doi:10.1007/s003810050042

Medfriendly, Inc. (n.d.). *Functional Independence Scores.* Retrieved 2004, from http://www.medfriendly.com/functionalindependencemeasure.html

MedlinePlus. (n.d.). *MedlinePlus.* Retrieved 2009, from: www.medlineplus.gov

Medscape.com. (2006, July 10). *Methicillin-Resistant Staphylococcus aureus Skin Infections Among Tattoo Recipients — Ohio, Kentucky, and Vermont, 2004–2005.* Retrieved from http://www.medscape.com/viewarticle/537433

Medstatmarketscan.com. (n.d.). *Marketscan Research Database, Thomson MedStat; Ph.D. Dissertation Support Program.* Retrieved from http://www.medstatmarketscan.com/

Meier, U., Zeilinger, F. S., & Kintzel, D. (1999). Diagnostic in Normal Pressure Hydrocephalus: A Mathematical Model for Determination of the ICP-Dependent Resistance and Compliance. Acta Neurochirurgica, 141, 941–948. PubMeddoi:10.1007/s007010050400doi:10.1007/s007010050400

Menon, R., Tong, L. H., Sathiyakeerthi, S., Brombacher, A., & Leong, C. (2004). The needs and benefits of applying textual data mining within the product development process. *Quality and Reliability Engineering International*, *20*, 1–15. doi:10.1002/qre.536

Menon, R., Tong, L. H., Sathiyakeerthi, S., Brombacher, A., & Leong, C. (2004). The needs and benefits of applying textual data mining within the product development process. *Quality and Reliability Engineering International*, *20*, 1–15. doi:10.1002/qre.536

Merberg, A., & Miller, S. (2006). *The Sampling Distribution of the Median. Efron, B., & Tibshirani, R. J. (1998). An Introduction to the Bootstrap.* Boca Raton, FL: CRC Press LLC.

Middleton, D. B., Zimmerman, R. K., & Mitchell, K. B. (2007). Vaccine schedules and procedures, 2007. *The Journal of Family Practice*, *56*(2), 42–60.

Miller, D. P. (n.d.). Bootstrap 101: Obtain Robust Confidence Intervals for Any Statistic. In *Proceedings of SUGI 29, Ovation Research Group* (pp.193-229).

Miller, J. D., Foster, T., Boulanger, L., Chace, M., Russell, M. W., & Marton, J. P. (2005, September). Direct costs of COPD in the U.S.: an analysis of Medical Expenditure Panel Survey. *COPD*, *2*(3), 311–318. doi:10.1080/15412550500218221

Miyamoto, T., Kumagai, T., Jones, J. A., Van Dyke, T. E., & Nunn, M. E. (2006). Compliance as a Prognostic Indicator: Retrospective Study of 505 Patients Treated and Maintained for 15 Years. *Journal of Periodontology*, *77*(2), 223–232. doi:10.1902/jop.2006.040349

Moches, T. A. (2005). *Text data mining applied to clustering with cost effective tools.* Paper presented at the IEEE International Conference on Systems, Mand, and Cybernetics, Waikoloa, HI.

Moffat, M. (2003). History of Physical Therapy Practice in the United States, The. *Journal of Physical Therapy Education.* Retrieved from FindArticles.com

Mol, P. G. M., & Wieringa, J. E., NannanPanday, P. V., et al. (2005). Improving compliance with hospital antibiotic guidelines: a time-series intervention analysis. *The Journal of Antimicrobial Chemotherapy*, *55*, 550–557. doi:10.1093/jac/dki037

Moses, J. W., & Leon, M. B. (n.d.). Lenox Hill Hospital and the Cardiovascular Research Foundation, U.S. SIRIUS Study:1,058 Patients, Retrieved from http://www.investor.jnj.com/releaseDetail.cfm?ReleaseID=90711&year=2002

Nagashima, T., Tamaki, N., Matsumoto, S., & Seguchi, Y. (1986). Biomechanics and a theoretical model of hydrocephalus: application of the finite element method. In J. D. Miller (Ed.), Intracranial Pressure VI (pp. 441–446). New York: Springer.

National HeartLung and Blood Institute. (n.d.). *D. a. C. I., Angioplasty.* Retrieved from http://www.nhlbi.nih.gov/health/dci/Diseases/Angioplasty/Angioplasty_WhatIs

National Institute of Diabetes and Digestive and Kidney Diseases. (2008). *National Diabetes Statistics, 2007.* Retrieved November 3rd, 2008, from http://diabetes.niddk.nih.gov/dm/pubs/statistics/

Newsome, L. T., Kutcher, M. A., Gandhi, S. K., Prielipp, R. C., & Royster, R. L. (2008). *A Protocol for the Perioperative Management of Patients With Intracoronary Drug-Eluting Stents.* Winston-Salem, NC: Wake Forest University School of Medicine.

NIS. (n.d.). *The National Inpatient Sample.* Retrieved 2009, from http://www.ahrq.gov.n.d

Nursing Center. com. (2004). Retrieved 2007, from http://www.nursingcenter.com/prodev/ce_article.asp?tid=512689

O'Reilly, K. B. (2008). *Time to get tough? States increasingly offer ways to opt out of vaccine mandates.* Retrieved September, 8, 2008, from http://www.ama-assn.org/amednews/2008/09/08/prsa0908.htm

O'Ryan, M., Lucero, Y., Pena, A., & Valenzuela, M. T. (2003). Two year review of intestinal intussusception in six large public hospitals of Santiago, Chili. *The Pediatric Infectious Disease Journal*, *22*, 717–721.

Obedian, E., & Fischer, D. B., Haffty, & B. G. (2000). Second malignancies After Treatment of Early-Stage Breast Cancer: Lumpectomy and Radiation Therapy Verus Mastectomy. *Journal of Clinical Oncology*, *18*(12), 2406–2412.

Parkin, D. (2005). Max Global Cancer Statistics, 2002. *CA: a Cancer Journal for Clinicians*, *55*, 74–108. doi:10.3322/canjclin.55.2.74

Pazzani, M. J. (2000). Knowledge discovery from data? *IEEE Intelligent Systems*, (March/April): 10–13. doi:10.1109/5254.850821

Pear, R. (2007, August 19). Medicare Says It Won't Cover Hospital Errors. *New York Times*.

Peduzzi, P., Concato, J., Kemper, E., Holford, T. R., & Feinstein, A. R. (1996). A Simulation Study of the Number of Events per Variable in Logistic Regression Analysis. Journal of Clinical Epidemiology, 49(12), 1373–1379. PubMeddoi:10.1016/S0895-4356(96)00236-3doi:10.1016/S0895-4356(96)00236-3

Pfizer (2007, March). *Zyvox.* (distributed by Pfizer). Retrieved 2009, from http://www.pfizer.com/files/products/uspi_zyvox.pdf

Pinna, G., Maestri, R., Capomolla, S., Febo, O., Mortara, A., & Riccardi, P. (2000). Determinant role of short-term heart rate variability in the prediction of mortality in patients with chronic heart failure. *IEEE Computers in Cardiology*, *27*, 735–738.

Poisal, J. A., Truffer, C., & Smith, S. (2007). Health Spending Projections Through 2016: Modest Changes Obscure Part D's Impact. Health Affairs, 26(2), 242–253. doi:10.1377/hlthaff.26.2.w242doi:10.1377/hlthaff.26.2.w242

Popescul, A., Lawrence, S., Ungar, L. H., & Pennock, D. M. (2003). *Statistical relational learning for document mining.* Paper presented at the Proceedings of the Third IEEE International Conference on Data Mining, Melbourne, FL.

Poses, R. M., McClish, D. K., Smith, W. R., Huber, E. C., Clomo, F. L., & Schmitt, B. P. (2000). Results of report cards for patients with congestive heart failure depend on the method used to adjust for severity. *Annals of Internal Medicine*, *133*, 10–20.

Potts, W. (2000). *Survival Data Mining. 2007,*Retrieved from http://www.data-miners.com/resources/Will%20Survival.pdf

Quality, A. H. R. a. (2000). *Healthcare Cost and Utilization Project (HCUP)* Retrieved September 14, 2008, from www.hcup-us.ahrq.gov/nisoverview.jsp

Refaat, M. (2007). *Data Preparation for Data Mining Using SAS.* San Francisco: Morgan Kaufmann Publications.

Research Support. (n.d.). U.S. Gov't, P.H.S. *Archives of Pediatrics & Adolescent Medicine, 156*(5), 504-511.

Reuters, T. (2008). *Health Care, Medical Episode Grouper - Government.* Retrieved from http://research.thomsonhealthcare.com/Products/view/?id=227

Ried, R., Kierk, N. D., Ambrosini, G., Berry, G., & Musk, A. (2006). The risk of lung cancer with increasing time since ceasing exposure to asbestos and quitting smoking. *Occupational and Environmental Medicine*, *63*(8), 509–512. doi:10.1136/oem.2005.025379

Robertson, S., & Maddux, J. (1986). Compliance in Pediatric Orthodontic Treatment: Current Research and Issues. *Children's Health Care*, *15*(1), 40–48. doi:10.1207/s15326888chc1501_7

Rotavirus, A.-M. (2008, April 18). Rotavirus vaccination coverage and adherence to the advisory committee on immunization practices (ACIP)-recommended vaccination schedule-United States, February 2006-May 2007. *MMWR*, 398–401.

Royal Military Academy. (n.d.). *Introduction to Data Fusion.* Retrieved from http://www.sic.rma.ac.be/Research/Fusion/Intro/content.html

Roy-Byrne, P., Davidson, K., Kessler, R., Asmundson, G., Goodwin, R., & Kubzansky, L. (2008). Anxiety disorders and co morbid medical illness. *General Hospital Psychiatry*, *30*, 208–225. doi:10.1016/j.genhosppsych.2007.12.006

Sabate, J. (1999). Nut consumption, vegetarian diets, ischemic heart disease risk, and all-cause mortality: evidence from epidemiologic studies. *The American Journal of Clinical Nutrition*, *70*(Suppl), 500–503.

Sahai, H., & Ageel, M. I. (2000). *The Analysis of variance: Fixed, Random and mixed models*, library of Boston: Birkhausser

Sahoo, P. (2002). *Probability and Mathematical Statistics.* Louisville, KY: Department of Mathematics, University of Louisville.

Sargan, J. D. (2001). Model building and data mining. *Econometric Reviews, 20*(2), 159–170. doi:10.1081/ETC-100103820

SAS 9.1.3 (n.d.). High-Performance Forecasting, User's Guide, Third Edition. Retrieved 2007, from http://support.sas.com/documentation/onlinedoc/91pdf/sasdoc_913/hp_ug_9209.pdf

SAS Institute. (1999). *SAS/STAT User's Guide.* Cary, NC: SAS Publishing.

SAS. (n.d.). *Introduction to Time Series Forecasting Using SAS/ETS Software Course Notes, C. b. S. I. I.* Cary, NC . *SAS Publishing.*

SAS.com. (n.d.). *SAS 9.1.3 Help and Documentation.* Retrieved 2009, from http://www.sas.com

SAS® (2004). *Text Miner Manual.* Cary, NC: SAS Institute.

Schwartz, M. (2007). *Wanted: Emergency Care Just For Kids.* Retrieved from http://www.lpfch.org/fundraising/news/spring03/emergency.html

Seker, H., Odetayo, M., Petrovic, D., Naguib, R., Bartoli, C., Alasio, L., et al. (2002). *An artificial neural network based feature evaluation index for the assessment of clinical factors in breast cancer survival analysis.* Paper presented at the IEEE Canadian Conference on Electrical & Computer Engineering, Winnipeg, Manitoba.

Sengupta, D., & Jammalamadaka, S. R. (2003). *Linear Models: An Integrated Approach.* Washington, DC: World Scientific Publishing Co.

Senneville, E., Legour, L., Valette, M., Yazdanpanah, Y., Beltrand, E., & Caillaux, M. (2006). Effectiveness and tolerability of prolonged linezolid treatment for chronic osteomyelitis: a retrospective study. *Clinical Therapeutics, 28*(8), 1155–1163. doi:10.1016/j.clinthera.2006.08.001

Shah, S. S., Hall, M., Slonim, A. D., Hornig, G. W., Berry, J. G., & Sharma, V. (2008). A multicenter study of factors influencing cerebrospinal fluid shunt survival in infants and children. Neurosurgery, 2008, 1095–1103. doi:10.1227/01.neu.0000325871.60129.23doi:10.1227/01.neu.0000325871.60129.23

Shaw, B., & Marshall, A. H. (2006). Modeling the health care costs of geriatric inpatients. *IEEE Transactions on Information Technology in Biomedicine, 10*(3), 526–532. doi:10.1109/TITB.2005.863821

Siegrist, M., Keller, C., & Kiers, H. A. (2005). A new look at the psychometric paradigm of perception of hazards. *Risk Analysis, 25*(1), 211–222. doi:10.1111/j.0272-4332.2005.00580.x

Silverman, B. W. (1986). Density Estimation for Statistics and Data Analysis (Monographs on Statistics and Applied Probability. Boca Raton, FL: Chapman & Hall/CRC.

Simonsen, L., Viboud, C., Elixhauser, A., Taylor, R., & Kapikian, A. (2005). More on Rotashield and intussusception: the role of age at the time of vaccination. *The Journal of Infectious Diseases, 192*(Supple 1), 36–43. doi:10.1086/431512

Smith, P. J. (2008). Controversial HPV vaccine causing one death per month: FDA report. *LifeSiteNews.* Retrieved from http://www.lifesitenews.com/ldn/2008/jul/08070316.html

Smith, R.D. (n.d.). *Simulation Article. Encyclopedia of Computer Science.* Basingstoke, UK: Nature Publishing Group.

Snyder, D. (2006, May 1). *In U.S Hospitals, Emergency Care in Critical Condition.* Retrieved from http://www.foxnews.com/story/0,2933,193883,00.html

Sokol, L., Garcia, B., West, M., Rodriguez, J., & Johnson, K. (2001). *Precursory steps to mining HCFA health care claims.* Paper presented at the 34th Hawaii International Conference on System Sciences, Hawaii.

Soll, A. H., & Gastroenterology, C. A. C. o. (1996). Medical treatment of peptic ulcer disease: practice guidelines. *Journal of the American Medical Association, 275*(8), 622–629. doi:10.1001/jama.275.8.622

Sollid, L. (2007). *The Evolution Of Emergency Room Medecine: Today's patients often need a high level of medical care,* Calgary Health Region's hospital Emergency Departments. Retrieved from http://www.calgaryhealthregion.ca/newslink/er_pack052103/evol_er052103.html

Sousa, J. E., Costa, M. A., & Sousa, A. G. (2003). Two-year angio-graphic and intravascular ultrasound follow-up after implantation of sirolimus-eluting stents in human coronary arteries. *Circulation, 107,* 381–383. doi:10.1161/01.CIR.0000051720.59095.6D

StatSoft. (1984-2004)., *Inc.* Retrieved 2009, from www.statsoft.com

StatSoft. (2007). Electronic Statistics Textbook. Tulsa, OK: StatSoft.

Tan, P. -N., Steinbach, M., & Kumar, Vi. (2006). *Introduction to Data Mining.* . Boston: Pearson Education

Tebbins, R. J. D., Pallansch, M. A., Kew, O. M., Caceres, V. M., Jafari, H., & Cochi, S. L. (2006). Risks of Paralytic disease due to wild or vaccine-derived poliovirus after eradication. *Risk Analysis, 26*(6), 1471–1505. doi:10.1111/j.1539-6924.2006.00827.x

Tesfamicael, M. (2005). Calculation of health disparity indices using data mining and the SAS Bridge to ESRI. MWSUG conference, Cincinnati, OH

Texas Heart Institute. H. I. C. (n.d.). *Coronary Artery Bypass, at St. Lukes'Episcopal Hospital.* Retrieved from http://texasheart.org/HIC/Topics/Proced/cab.cfm

The Diabetes Control and Complications Trial/Epidemiology of Diabetes Interventions and Complications (DCCT/EDIC) Study Research Group. (2005,December). Intensive Diabetes Treatment and Cardiovascular Disease in Patients with Type 1 Diabetes. *The New England Journal of Medicine, 353,* 2643-2653. Retrieved Dec.12th, 2008, from http://content.nejm.org/cgi/content/full/353/25/2643

The Glimmix Procedure. (2005, November). Retrieved 2007, from http://support.sas.com/rnd/app/papers/glimmix.pdf

The Statistics Homepage. (1984-2005). *Statsoft,Inc.* Retrieved from http://www.statsoft.com/textbook/stathome.html=

The Emergency Medical Treatment and Labor Act (EMTALA). (n.d.). *The regulations, incorporating all of the revisions as made in 2000 and2003. The primary regulation: 42 CFR 489.24 (a) 1).* Retrieved from http://www.emtala.com/law/index.html

Thomas, J. W. (1998). Research evidence on the validity of adjusted mortality rate as a measure of hospital quality of care. *Medical Care Research and Review, 55*(4), 371–404. doi:10.1177/107755879805500401

Thomas, J. W. (2006). Should Episode-Based Economic Profiles Be Risk Adjusted to Account for Differences in Patients' Health Risks? *Health Services Research, 41*(2), 581–598. doi:10.1111/j.1475-6773.2005.00499.x

Thompson Cancer Survival Center. (2008). *Lung Cancer Diagnosis and Staging.* Retrieved from Thompson Cancer Survival Center web site http://www.thompsoncancer.com/tcsc-lungcancer-diagnosis.cfm

Thompson, K. M., & Tebbins, R. J. D. (2006). Retrospective cost-effectiveness analyses for polio vaccination in the United States. *Risk Analysis, 26*(6), 1423–1449. doi:10.1111/j.1539-6924.2006.00831.x

Thomson Medstat. (2002). *MarketScan® Research Databases User Guide and Database Dictionary.* Ann Arbor, MI: Michigan University Press.

Tosh, P. K., Boyce, T., & Poland, G. A. (2008). Flu Myths: Dispelling the Myths Associated With Live Attenuated Influenza Vaccine. *Mayo Clinic Proceedings, 83*(1), 77–84. doi:10.4065/83.1.77

Travis, W. D. (1995). Lung cancer. *Cancer, 75*(Suppl. 1), 191–202. doi:10.1002/1097-0142(19950101)75:1+<191::AID-CNCR2820751307>3.0.CO;2-Y

Tsanakas, A., & Desli, E. (2005). Measurement and pricing of risk in insurance markets. *Risk Analysis, 23*(6), 1653–1668. doi:10.1111/j.1539-6924.2005.00684.x

Tucker, D. (1993). Spatial sampling of head electrical fields: the geodesic sensor net. *Electroencephalog-*

raphy and Clinical Neurophysiology, 87(3), 154–163. doi:10.1016/0013-4694(93)90121-B

United States Renal Data System. (2007). *USRDS 2007 Annual Data Report.* Retrieved Dec.10th, 2008, from http://www.usrds.org/atlas_2007.htm

University of Iowa Health Science Relations. (2005, December). *Glucose Control Cuts Risk Of Heart Disease In Type 1 Diabetes.* Retrieved from http://www.news-releases.uiowa.edu/2005/december/122205glucose_control.html

Upton, G., & Cook, I. (2004). *Dictionary of Statistics.* Oxford, UK: Oxford University Press.

Urban Institute. (2002). Retrieved 2007, from http://www.urban.org/publications/1000728.html

USFDA. (n.d.). *US. Food and Drug Administration website,*www.fda.org;*used to concert NDC Numbers.* Retrieved 2009, from http://www.fda.gov/cder/ndc/database/Default.htm

Verbeke, G. (1997). *Linear Mixed Models in Practice: A SAS-Oriented Approach.* New York: Springer Verlag.

W. I. t. R. A. C. (n.d.). *Blue Cross Blue Shield of Texas.* Retrieved from http://www.bcbstx.com/provider/bluechoice_solutions_tool_raci.htm.

Wang, K., & Zhou, X. (2005). Mining customer value: from association rules to direct marketing. *Data Mining and Knowledge Discovery*, 11, 57–79. doi:10.1007/s10618-005-1355-x

Wang, Y., Dunham, M. H., Waddle, J. A., & McGee, M. (2006). *Classifier Fusion for Poorly-Differentiated Tumor Classification using Both Messenger RNA and MicroRNA Expression Profiles.* Accepted by the 2006 Computational Systems Bioinformatics Conference (CSB 2006). Stanford, California.

Weis, S. M., Indurkhya, N., Zhang, T., & Damerau, F. J. (2005). *Text Mining: Predictive Methods for Analyzing Unstructured Information.* New York: Springer.

Whitehead, W. (1994). Assessing the effects of stress on physical symptoms. *Health Psychology*, 13, 99–102. doi:10.1037/0278-6133.13.2.99

Wickedly, D. D., Mendenhall, W. III, & Scheaffer, R. L. (2002). *Mathematical Statistics with Applications.* Sixth Edition. Casella, G., & Berger, R. (2002). *Statistical Inference.* Second Edition. Albrecht, G., &Hoogstraten, J. (n.d.). *Satisfacion as a determinant of Compliance.* (1998). *Community Dentistry and Oral Epidemiology*, 26(2), 139–146.

Wilcox, R. R. (2005). Introduction to Robust Estimation and Hypothesis Testing. Second Edition.

Wingo, P. A. (2003). Long-Term Trends in Cancer Mortality in the United States, 1930–1998. *Cancer*, 97(11Suppl), 3133–3275. doi:10.1002/cncr.11380

Wong, K., Byoung-ju, C., Bui-Kyeong, H., Soo-Kyung, K., & Doheon, L. (2003). A taxonomy of dirty data. *Data Mining and Knowledge Discovery*, 7, 81–99. doi:10.1023/A:1021564703268

Wong, R. C.-W., & Fu, A. W.-C. (2005). Data mining for inventory item selection with cross-selling considerations. *Data Mining and Knowledge Discovery*, 11, 81–112. doi:10.1007/s10618-005-1359-6

Wong, R. C.-W., & Fu, A. W.-C. (2005). Data mining for inventory item selection with cross-selling considerations. *Data Mining and Knowledge Discovery*, 11, 81–112. doi:10.1007/s10618-005-1359-6

Medical Expenditure Panel Survey (MEPS). (n.d.). Retrieved from http://www.meps.ahrq.gov/PUFFiles/H67G/H67Gdoc.pdf

Vancomycin (n.d.). *vancomycin Description.* Retrieved 2009, from http://www.drugs.com/pro/vancomycin.html

Xiangchun, K. X., Back, Y., Rhee, D. W., & Kim, S.-H. (2005). *Analysis of breast cancer using data mining & statistical techniques.* Paper presented at the Proceedings of the Sixth International Conference on Software Engineering, Artificial Intelligence, Networking, and Parallel/Distributed Computing, Las Vegas, NV.

Xie, H., Chaussalet, T. J., & Millard, P. H. (2006). A model-based approach to the analysis of patterns of length of stay in institutional long-term care. *IEEE Transac-*

tions on Information Technology in Biomedicine, *10*(3), 512–518. doi:10.1109/TITB.2005.863820

Yock, C. A., Boothroyd, D. B., Owens, D. K., Garber, A. M., & Hlatky, M. A. (2003, October 1). Cost-effectiveness of Bypass Surgery versus Stenting in Patients with Multivessele Coronary Artery Disease. *The American Journal of Medicine*, *115*, 382–389. doi:10.1016/S0002-9343(03)00296-1

Yuhua Li, D. M., Bandar, Z. A., O'Shea, J. D., & Crockett, K. (2006). Sentence similarity based on semantic nets and corpur statistics. *IEEE Transactions on Knowledge and Data Engineering*, *18*(6), 1138–1148.

Zhu, X., Wu, X., & Chen, Q. (2006). Bridging local and global data cleansing: identifying class noise in large, distributed data datasets. *Data Mining and Knowledge Discovery*, *12*(2-3), 275. doi:10.1007/s10618-005-0012-8

About the Contributors

Patricia Cerrito (PhD) has made considerable strides in the development of data mining techniques to investigate large, complex medical data. In particular, she has developed a method to automate the reduction of the number of levels in a nominal data field to a manageable number that can then be used in other data mining techniques. Another innovation of the PI is to combine text analysis with association rules to examine nominal data. The PI has over 30 years of experience in working with SAS software, and over 10 years of experience in data mining healthcare databases. In just the last two years, she has supervised 7 PhD students who completed dissertation research in investigating health outcomes. Dr. Cerrito has a particular research interest in the use of a patient severity index to define provider quality rankings for reimbursements.

* * *

M. S. S. Khan received his B.S degree in Mathematics from the University of Leicester, Leicester, England in 1999. He then moved across the Atlantic to pursue his Graduate studies. He received his first M.A in Mathematics from the University of Missouri in 2002 and he earned his second M.A in Mathematical Sciences from the University of Montana, Missoula in 2005. He is working on his PhD in Computer Science and Computer Engineering in the Speed School of Engineering from the University of Louisville. His research interests span several fields, including Statistical Modeling, Wavelets, Network Tomography, Data Mining, Algorithm Development, Ring Theory and Mathematical Biology

Jennifer Ferrell Pleiman received her MS in Public Health from the University of Louisville. She is currently working on her PhD at UofL. She presently works in healthcare insurance where she uses datamining techniques to solve internal business problems. In addition to presenting at regional and national conferences, Jennifer has published her research in journals. Jennifer's independent research has primarily focused on health outcomes and quality of life. Since 2003, Jennifer uses SAS to conduct her research. She hopes to continue her research to help make changes to improve patient's quality of life.

Mussie A. Tesfamicael, PhD, is a Statistical Analyst at Kendle International, Inc. Actively involved in biostatistical analysis and SAS programming. Dr. Tesfamicael received his Ph.D. in Applied and Industrial mathematics from University of Louisville in 2007. He also holds masters in Mathematics and Biostatistics from the University of Louisville and Southern Illinois University at Carbondale respectively. Dr. Tesfamicael has research interest on Time Series, Health outcome Datamining and Biostatistical Research.

Copyright © 2010, IGI Global, distributing in print or electronic forms without written permission of IGI Global is prohibited.

Joseph Twagilimana was born in Rwanda and studied Mathematics and engineering sciences at the National University of Rwanda. He resettled in USA in 1998 following the tragedy that happened in Rwanda in 1994. He completed his studies at the University of Louisville, where he graduated with a Master degree in Arts and sciences in August 2002, and a PhD in applied and industrial Mathematics, in the application area of Data Mining and Data Analyst, in May 2006. He is married and has three children. He now works at WellPoint, Inc., a heath care insurance company, as a Data Mining Analyst.

Xiao Wang is currently pursuing her Ph.D. degree in Industrial and Applied Mathematics at the University of Louisville. Xiao earned her master's degree in Applied Mathematics in 2008, another master's degree in Economics in 2006 and a bachelor's degree in Finance in 2002. Xiao's research focuses on healthcare outcomes and cost using SAS Enterprise Miner. She has finished 4 projects with a concentration on the costs of patients with diabetes in the Medicare population. Her current project is to investigate the impact of Medicare, Part D on diabetic medications. Xiao has also used SAS Enterprise Guide, SAS Enterprise Miner and is familiar with Base SAS and SAS SQL. So far, she has published several papers and posters. Xiao has twice been awarded "SAS Student Ambassador".

Damien Wilburn received a B.S. in Biology and Mathematics from the University of Louisville in 2009. He graduated *summa cum laude*, and completed senior theses in both biology and mathematics that yielded two publications. This work was presented at regional conferences, and as posters at the national meetings of the Association of Biomolecular Resource Facilities and International Society for Pharmacoeconomics and Outcomes Research. Currently, he is a pre-doctoral student in Biochemistry and Molecular Biology at the University of Louisville studying the evolution and regulation of pheromone signaling.

Hamed Zahedi grew up in Iran and has a degree in Applied Mathematics from the University of Esfahan, Esfahan, Iran. He has a PhD degree in Applied Mathematics from the University of Louisville, where his dissertation work was focused on analytics in the healthcare industry. He won an award to present his work at M2006, F2007, SESUG 2007 and PharmaSUG 2008 and he is a 2007 SAS Student Ambassador. His work has also been presented at the SAS Global Forum 2007, Data Mining conferences (M2007 and M2008) and INFORMS Annual meeting 2007. He is currently working on analytics, data mining and predictive modeling in healthcare at the Humana Insurance Company.

Index

Copyright © 2010, IGI Global, distributing in print or electronic forms without written permission of IGI Global is prohibited.

Z